FOOD, NUTRITION *and the* NITRIC OXIDE PATHWAY

HOW TO ORDER THIS BOOK

BY PHONE: 866-401-4337 or 717-290-1660, 9AM–5PM Eastern Time

BY FAX: 717-509-6100

BY MAIL: Order Department

DEStech Publications, Inc.

439 North Duke Street

Lancaster, PA 17602, U.S.A.

BY CREDIT CARD: American Express, VISA, MasterCard, Discover

BY WWW SITE: http://www.destechpub.com

FOOD, NUTRITION *and* *the* NITRIC OXIDE PATHWAY

Biochemistry and Bioactivity

Edited by NATHAN S. BRYAN, Ph.D.
The University of Texas Health Science Center

Foreword by Louis J. Ignarro
1998 Nobel Laureate in Physiology or Medicine

DES*tech* Publications, Inc.

Food, Nutrition and the Nitric Oxide Pathway

DEStech Publications, Inc.
439 North Duke Street
Lancaster, Pennsylvania 17602 U.S.A.

Printed in the United States of America

10 9 8 7 6 5 4 3 2 1

Main entry under title:
Food, Nutrition and the Nitric Oxide Pathway: Biochemistry and Bioactivity

A DEStech Publications book
Bibliography: p.
Includes index p. 217

ISBN: 978-1-932078-84-8

To Drs. Mark P. Richards and Robert G. Brannan for their efforts in bringing the biomedical science of nitrite and nitrate to nutritionists, food professionals and laypersons. It is through their efforts this book was made possible.

Contents

Foreword

THE field of nitric oxide continues to evolve, and recent research confirms NO is one of the most important molecules produced by the human body. Over 100,000 papers have appeared on the topic of nitric oxide. We have learned a great deal since the endothelium-derived relaxing factor was identified as nitric oxide. Nitric oxide or NO was for many years stigmatized as a toxic air pollutant in automobile exhaust. You can imagine the impact when it was discovered that such a gaseous molecule is produced in the human body. Even more remarkable is the fact that such a gas is produced *in vivo* to serve as a signal for cell-to-cell communication and the transduction of nerve impulses. NO is a molecule that regulates blood pressure, causes penile erection, and controls the action of almost every cell in our body. The immune system uses nitric oxide in fighting viral, bacterial and parasitic infections, as well as tumors. NO transmits messages between nerve cells and is associated with learning, memory, sleeping, feeling pain, and depression. It is a key mediator in inflammation. Early studies on NO stemmed from work with nitroglycerin and other nitrovasodilators as we attempted to understand how these medicines, used for hundreds of years, actually worked. It was discovered that nitroglycerin makes NO, which accounts for its therapeutic efficacy for angina through dilating constricted and diseased blood vessels in the heart.

The discovery of the L-arginine: NO pathway was transformational for science and medicine. NO is formed from the semi-essential amino acid precursor L-arginine by the enzyme NO synthase. From this discovery a well-described pathway became known whereby NO was generated within the human body. In most studies, acute and chronic administration of L-arginine has been shown to improve endothelial function and increase NO output in numerous animal models. However due to the "arginine paradox" it is still unclear how supplemental L-arginine can enhance NO production when the baseline plasma concentration is about 25- to 30-fold higher than the Michaelis-Menten constant Km of the isolated, purified NOS enzyme. Since L-arginine is considered a semi-essential amino acid, it must come partly from the diet since endogenous production from the urea cycle is not sufficient to maintain steady-state levels necessary for all metabolic functions. Therefore, L-arginine supplementation has been used for years to attempt to restore NO production, particularly in individuals who are NO deficient, with mixed results.

Despite previous work, there is still much to be learned about the production and regulation of NO within the body. The limitations in our understanding arise from the fact that its production is very complex and once produced, the NO gas is degraded in less than one second as it diffuses to reach its cellular target or it is quickly inactivated by reaction with oxygen, oxygen radicals, or proteins.

Among the complexities associated with NO is its relationship to dietary intake. For example, diets rich in fruits and vegetables have been postulated to enhance NO production availability due to their high antioxidant capacity. However, there may be more to the story than simple dietary antioxidants affecting NO homeostasis, and this is where the present volume makes an important contribution. It explores the fertile concept that nitric oxide activity can be modulated by certain foods independent of L-arginine. It shows how research over the past several years has revealed a heretofore unknown activity in certain foods of nitrogen oxides that can then be metabolized to NO in the body when consumed. An essential metabolic pathway in plants is nitrogen fixation facilitated by bacteria in the soil. Nitrogen fixation is the process by which nitrogen is taken from its relatively inert molecular form (N_2) in the atmosphere and converted into nitrogen compounds (such as ammonia, nitrate, nitrite, nitric oxide and nitrogen dioxide). This is an essential process for life because fixed nitrogen is required to make nucleotides, which are needed to make DNA and also to make amino acids, necessary for producing proteins. As part of their metabolism, plants are enriched with nitrogen oxides as intermediates in this pathway. Consuming plant-based foods then provides the body with a rich pool of nitrogen oxides, such as nitrite and nitrate, from which we now know nitric oxide can be produced. Interestingly, the connections between NO and nitrite and nitrate have been known for many years, but were largely confined to the belief that both of the latter simply existed as inert breakdown products of NO. We now understand the reversibility of this process, specifically under conditions where NO is insufficiently produced.

The body of work cotnained in this volume, linking NO to food and nutrition, may have revolutionary implications in terms of developing strategies to combat heart disease and many other contemporary diseases associated with a NO deficiency. Proving that a natural and inexpensive regimen of foods rich in nitric oxide activity does restore NO homeostasis can have profound effects on public health. As is suggested by the important research in this book, dietary guidelines for nitrite and nitrate must be re-evaluated in terms of their protective nature and considered as essential nutrients. This is a relatively new area of nitric oxide research and one that is very exciting. The L-arginine pathway to make NO may turn out to be only part of the story. The symbiosis between humans and the bacteria that reside in and on our body may be just as important in terms of utilizing nitrate and nitrite to make NO under conditions where the oxidation of L-arginine is dysfunctional. After all a simple one-electron reduction is energetically and kinetically much easier than a five electron oxidation.

The research presented in this text provides an important expansion of NO work by linking food and nutrition to NO chemistry and biochemistry. Dr. Nathan S. Bryan, the editor, is one of the leading pioneers in this field and is to be congratulated for the present effort in communicating new knowledge and assembling the world's experts in their respective fields, who in these pages present and explain a biological pathway critical to human health.

LOUIS J. IGNARRO
1998 Nobel Laureate in Physiology or Medicine

Preface

THE discovery of the nitric oxide (NO) pathway in the 1980s represented a critical advance in cardiovascular medicine. Continuous generation of NO is essential for the integrity of the cardiovascular system and a decreased production and/or bioavailability of NO is central to the development of cardiovascular disorders. NO is also important for communication in our nervous system and a critical molecule which our immune system uses to kill invading pathogens, including bacteria and cancer cells. The production of NO from L-arginine is a complex and complicated biochemical pathway involving a 5-electron oxidation with many cofactors and prosthetics groups. As a result, there are many steps and/or factors that may be altered and affect ultimate NO production. Since NO is such an important molecule in practically every organ system in our body, it is highly unlikely that Nature created such a complicated and singular pathway for NO production. In fact, most physiological systems are fraught with redundancy allowing a backup system to kick in when the primary system is not working. The inability to make NO is one of the first indicators that disease will ensue. Reduced NO availability is a hallmark of a number of disorders, including cardiovascular disease. The consequences of which are astounding. According to the World Health Organization, cardiovascular disease is the number one killer of both men and women in the United States. These deaths represent a staggering 40% of all deaths. Close to 1 million people die each year and more than 6 million are hospitalized. The cost of cardiovascular disease, in terms of health care and lost productivity, is over $270 billion and increasing as the baby boom population ages. Ischemic heart disease, as the underlying cause of most cases of acute myocardial infarction, congestive heart failure, arrhythmias, and sudden cardiac death, is the leading cause of morbidity and mortality in all industrialized nations. In the United States, ischemic heart disease causes nearly 20% of all deaths (≈600 000 deaths each year), with many of these deaths occurring before the patient arrives at the hospital. Heart disease is very likely the result of a dysfunctional endothelium and an inability to produce NO. Therefore, developing new strategies to restore and replete NO availability is of paramount importance and could potentially save millions of lives worldwide and lessen the burden on the health care system. This concept may not only lead to novel treatments for disease but may lead to strategies to prevent disease development or progression.

Nothing affects our health more than what we choose to eat. The role of diet in the prevention and control of morbidity and premature mortality due to non-communicable diseases has been well established by the vast population based epidemiological studies carried out during the last decade. Numerous epidemiological data has indicated an inverse relationship between dietary intake of fruits and vegetables and incidence of cardiovascular disease. Among the candidates that may account for these cardioprotective effects are antioxidants such as polyphenolics, ascorbate and glutathione. Although antioxidants are generally credited with improving states of oxidative stress, studies which have evaluated the efficacy of supplementation with a high dose of an antioxidant alone, such as vitamin E or Vitamin C, have shown no apparent improvement and in some cases a decrease in cardiovascular protection. Yet, when these antioxidants are consumed through the diet in the form of fruits and vegetables, there is a significant degree of protection, best represented by the decrease in mortality rates from heart disease and cancer of those consuming the popular Mediterranean diet. Epidemiological studies, such as the Seven Country Study, have led to theories describing why and how the Mediterranean diet may promote a lower incidence of coronary heart disease, and antioxidants are emerging as a key component. However, since antioxidant supplementation alone does not confer the cardiovascular benefits, there must be more to explain the protection and health benefits afforded by fruits and vegetables. Therefore there must be other bioactive food components of the Mediterranean diet that account for the protective phenotype.

Recent biomedical research has demonstrated that NO can be modulated by the diet independent of its enzymatic synthesis from L-arginine, e.g., the consumption of nitrite- and nitrate-rich foods such as fruits, leafy vegetables, and some meats along with anti-oxidants. Regular intake of nitrate-containing food such as green leafy vegetables may ensure that blood and tissue levels of nitrite and NO pools are maintained at a level sufficient to compensate for any disturbances in endogenous NO synthesis. Since low levels of supplemental nitrite and nitrate have been shown to enhance blood flow, dietary sources of NO metabolites can therefore improve circulation and oxygen delivery and protect against various cardiovascular disease states. This has led to the current belief that a healthy diet focus not only on reducing fat and caloric intake but on adding foodstuffs promoting nitric oxide bioactivity. The notion that there may be certain foods that can enrich nitric oxide within our body is revolutionary. An optimal diet may then consist of a sufficient supply of nitrite and nitrate for health and well being. This dietary pathway may not only provide essential nutrients and substrates for NO production from nitric oxide synthase but also provide a rescue or protective pathway for people at risk for cardiovascular disease. I believe this may be the redundant system for maintenance of NO homeostasis.

This book explains the connections between foods that enhance NO bioactivity—both through increased production and preserving NO bioactivity—and human health. It begins by clarifying what is nitric oxide and provides a biochemical analysis of its roles in human physiology. The book then turns to explaining nitrogen compounds in the human diet and showing how these compounds, along with related elements, affect steady state NO levels in our bodies. The book will demonstrate how specific foods and food groups enhance NO bioactivity in the human body and how this relates to normal physiology. The book then analyzes evidence regarding how NO-rich foods are linked to disease prevention and positive (healthy) modulation of human physiological functions. For example, it will review data showing how consuming foods with NO activity may prevent disease onset and progression and protect the human body from cardiovascular insult and trauma, conditions commonly associated with NO insufficiency. Research will be reviewed on therapeutic applications of NO and NO metabolites for a variety of diseases. I have invited the world's experts (from both academia and industry) in their particular discipline to contribute individual chapters. This approach will provide a fair and balance view of nitric oxide biochemistry, nitrite and nitrate chemistry in physiology and in the food sciences.

The early Roman physician Galen based his description of the vascular system on the concept of "pneuma" or spirits, a vital principle consisting of matter in a finely divided or ethereal state that flowed through the vascular and nervous systems and animate the entire organism. Many diseases were thought to owe their origin to some disturbances of these ethereal spirits. Although these ideas were fanciful, this paradigm actually prevented the advancement of medical science for centuries. Today evidence on the production and effects of such an ethereal substance, NO, exists. Nitric oxide is indeed formed in many organs and as previously mentioned has important roles in physiology and pathophysiology. The new emerging paradigm that NO is modulated by dietary nitrogen oxides and other bioactive food components is exciting. It appears that we may have identified a critical component of our diet that many people are missing. In fact certain compounds we have been taught to fear and avoid in our diet may be saving our lives from inflammatory diseases.

NATHAN S. BRYAN

Acknowledgments

I owe a debt of gratitude to all the writers of this book. In the presence of these great scientists, physicians and authors, I feel humble. Their individual contributions give credence to the content and message of this volume. During the course of creating this text, I have developed many close friendships and a new respect and admiration for each one of the contributing authors. I understand and appreciate the sacrifice and effort of each author in taking additional time from their busy schedules to help me produce such an important body of work. I want personally to thank Dr. Murad for his support, encouragement and stimulating conversations and for co-authoring the chapter on nitric oxide. There is no one better to tell the story than the Nobel Laureate credited with its discovery. I sincerely thank Dr. Matt Grisham for his contribution. Dr. Grisham first introduced me to nitric oxide and reactive oxygen species during my student years at LSU. I feel very fortunate to call him a trusted friend. Drs. Lundberg and Weitzberg are two of the pioneers in the field, who first described a dietary nitrate, nitrite pathway in humans and linked it to nitric oxide physiology. I am honored by their contributions and the friendly relationship that resulted and continues from this project. Dr. Norm Hord has become a true friend and collaborator. In these pages Dr. Hord provides a unique and balanced perspective on dietary nitrite and nitrate and thus offers more than ample reason for co-authoring several chapters. My goal was to present an unbiased, balanced, and scientific account of the scientific literature that supports bioactive food components contributing to nitric oxide's status. This could not have been accomplished without Dr. Hord's contributions and perspective. Drs. Randy Huffman, Jim Coughlin and Andy Milkowski are perhaps the most seasoned nitrite and nitrate professionals, insofar as they have been active in the meat and food industry for many years. Their expertise and perspectives on nitrite and nitric oxide chemistry in meats and foods antedates and at the same time augments the modern biomedical science literature. Collectively they have helped bridge the gap between the biomedical science community and food professionals and nutritionists. I would like to acknowledge Dr. Coughlin for his assertion that nitrite acts in many ways like a vitamin. Dr. Mark Gladwin transformed the nitrite-NO field by questioning the long-held notion that nitrite was inert and simply just a surrogate marker of NO, in contrast to a hypoxic physiological mediator. His work has moved the field to where it is today. Dr. Sruti Shiva's investigations have helped us to understand potential cellular mechanisms on how nitrite may be affecting physiological systems. I am grateful for their two contributions. Dr. Malte Kelm, a respected and world-renowned cardiologist brings enormous credibility. His insight and contribution are greatly appreciated. Dr. Tienush Rassaf, my friend and colleague for 10 years, brought a unique combined clinical and scientific perspective to the story and demonstrates the involvement of flavanols as mediators of NO bioactivity. Drs. Minshew and Grief are sufficiently removed from the NO field to provide balance and a global perspective on nutrition and health. Their individual expertise in homeopathic medicine and clinical nutrition and obesity respectively validate the enormous and profound implications the NO pathway may have on public health. Finally I must thank my wife Kristen for her patience, support and caring for our children during the nights and weekends I spent writing and editing. As scientists we all strive to make a difference through our work. We seek knowledge and understanding of human health and disease. A dietary approach to combat sickness is logical. I hope the information presented in this book will create awareness of bioactive food components that promote nitric oxide biology and ultimately may lead to novel and effective strategies to treat and/or prevent human disease.

CHAPTER 1

What is Nitric Oxide?

NATHAN S. BRYAN and FERID MURAD
Brown Foundation Institute of Molecular Medicine
The University of Texas Health Science Center
Houston, TX 77030

NITRIC OXIDE (NO) is one of the most important signaling molecules in our body. NO or nitrogen monoxide is a gaseous compound with the chemical formula NO. NO is an important messenger molecule involved in many physiological and pathological processes within the mammalian body with both beneficial and detrimental properties [1]. It is a small, relatively unstable, potentially toxic, free radical that has become one of the most studied and fascinating molecules in biological chemistry and medicine. NO is a common air pollutant, a constituent of cigarette smoke, and a toxic gas, which appears in the exhaust of motor cars, causes acid rain, and destroys the ozone layer. The realization of such a molecule being produced within our bodies and acting as an endogenous signaling molecule has revolutionized conceptual reasoning in science and medicine over the past 30 years. It is involved in virtually every organ system within our body but is known primarily for maintaining normal blood pressure and blood flow to tissues. In the cardiovascular system it can expand narrow blood vessels, eliminate dangerous clots, lower high blood pressure, and reduce artery-clogging plaque formation. It also has important properties in the immune system where it helps us fight off infections and cancer cells and in the nervous system where it helps our brain cells communicate properly.

NO should not be confused with nitrous oxide (N_2O), a general anaesthetic, or with nitrogen dioxide (NO_2) which is another poisonous air pollutant. The NO molecule is a free radical with an unshared electron, which is relevant to understanding its high reactivity. It reacts with the ozone in air to form nitrogen dioxide, signaled by the appearance of the reddish-brown color as seen in smog. NO is a fundamental player in the fields of neuroscience, physiology, and immunology, and was proclaimed "Molecule of the Year" by Science in 1992 [2].

NO is one of the few gaseous signaling molecules known which has resulted in the search for other gaseous messengers. It is a key vertebrate biological messenger, playing a role in a variety of biological processes. Nitric oxide, also known as the "endothelium-derived relaxing factor", or EDRF, is biosynthesised endogenously from the amino acid L-arginine and oxygen by various NO synthase (NOS) enzymes. NO is also formed within our body by the reduction of inorganic nitrate and nitrite. The endothelium (inner lining) of blood vessels uses NO to signal the surrounding smooth muscle to relax, thus resulting in vasodilation and increasing blood flow and oxygen delivery. NO is highly reactive (having a lifetime less than a second), yet diffuses freely across membranes and can travel 100–200 microns (about 10 to 20 cell diameters). These attributes make NO ideal for a transient signal molecule between adjacent cells and within cells. Effects of NO are widespread throughout the body including, but not limited to blood vessel dilatation, neurotransmission, host response, modulation of the hair cycle, and penile erections. Nitroglycerin, an old and effective treatment for angina for more than a century, serves as a vasodilator because it is converted to NO in the body. Sildenafil, popularly known by the trade name Viagra, stimulates erections primarily by enhancing signaling through the NO pathway in the penis. There are a number of therapeutic strategies designed to affect the NO pathway in humans and more are surely to follow as we learn and understand more about its actions.

DISCOVERY OF NO

In 1980, Furchgott and Zawadzki published an article [3] underlining the obligatory role of endothelial cells in the acetylcholine-induced relaxation of arterial smooth muscle and recognized that vasodilation by bradykinin, histamine, and ATP was due to the same relaxing substance, which they named endothelium derived relaxing factor (EDRF). Earlier in the 1970s, Ferid Murad and his colleagues demonstrated that the enzyme soluble guanylyl cyclase (sGC) was stimulated by nitrogen-containing compounds, causing an increase in the second messenger cGMP, which in turn brought about vascular relaxation [4,5]. Murad first showed that the activation of soluble guanylyl cyclase by nitrovasodilators could occur via the formation of NO. They were fascinated by the idea that a gas and free radical could regulate smooth muscle function and they proposed early on that hormones and other endogenous factors may also act through NO. NO function as a messenger was proposed for first the time [6,7]. It was Ignarro [8] who went on to conclude that EDRF from the artery and vein is either NO or a chemically related radical species in 1987 after Murad suggested [9] that EDRF was an "endogenous nitrovasodilator". Subsequently, Salvador Moncada's group revealed that NO release accounts for the biological activity of EDRF [10]. In 1982, prior to the identification of EDRF, the endogenous activator of the enzyme soluble guanylyl cyclase (sGC) in neuroblastoma cells was identified as L-arginine [11] and later it was recognized that NO is formed from L-arginine in the central nervous system [12]. Even earlier however, nitrogen oxides were emerging as a central participant in the immune response. The investigations of NO as an immunoreactive compound began with the observation that high concentrations of urinary nitrates were excreted from a patient with infectious diarrhea [13]. The source of these nitrogen compounds remained unclear until Stuehr and Marletta [14] demonstrated that serum and urinary nitrates were increased in normal mice after immunostimulation, but not in C3H/HeJ mice, which have a genetic alteration rendering their macrophages resistant to endotoxin. It was through this model that NO was identified as the intermediate compound in the L-arginine to nitrite/nitrate pathway. These observations, together with the discovery of the L-arginine:NO pathway in the vasculature, led to the investigations and subsequent discovery of the existence of this ubiquitous pathway in mammalian physiology. It was really the collective efforts of many research groups working in completely different fields that converged on a single pathway in multiple systems. On October 12, 1998, the Nobel Assembly awarded the Nobel Prize in Medicine or Physiology to scientists Robert Furchgott, Louis Ignarro, and Ferid Murad for their discoveries concerning NO as a signaling molecule in the cardiovascular system.

Since the identification of endothelial derived relaxing factor as NO [8, 10], an enormous amount of research has been devoted to unraveling the complex chemistry and biochemistry of this simple molecule. At normal atmospheric pressure and temperature, NO is a gas that is moderately stable in aqueous media and functions as a biological messenger in physiological solutions. Several research fields converged to show that NO functions as an essential signaling molecule in the cardiovascular, nervous and immune systems. Its ever expanding range of functions already include neurotransmission, blood clotting, blood pressure control, and a role in the immune systems ability to kill tumor and bacterial cells. The production of a highly reactive and diffusible free radical gas at first complicated our established concept and model of specific and targeted receptor-ligand interaction to elicit cell signaling events. However the gas as a messenger seems logical now because it can pass through biological membranes readily and reach its intracellular targets with little or no energy expenditure. NO produced in small controlled doses in the body is extraordinarily beneficial. It helps maintain blood pressure by dilating blood vessels, helps kill foreign invaders and tumor cells, is a major biochemical mediator of penile erection and a major biochemical component of long term memory and neural communication. Furthermore, NO is also implicated in the pathophysiology of many diseases, whereby either there is decreased bioavailability or production of NO, or there is an enormous prolonged over-production that exposes its toxic, noxious properties [15].

Another biologically important reaction of NO is through post-translational protein modification termed S-nitrosylation, the conversion of thiol groups, including cysteine residues in proteins, to form S-nitrosothiols (RSNOs). S-Nitrosylation is a mechanism for dynamic, post-translational regulation of most or all major classes of protein [16]. Nitrosylation thereby conveys a large part of the ubiquitous influence of NO on cellular signal transduction and provides a mechanism for redox-based physiological regulation. This signaling pathway is independent of the well characterized NO-soluble guanylyl cyclase (sGC) pathway whereby NO binds directly to the heme group of sGC which then catalyzes the conversion of guanosine triphosphate (GTP) to second messenger cyclic guanosine monophosphate (cGMP). Genetic and biochemical data demonstrate a pivotal role for RSNOs in mediating the actions of NO [17]. RSNOs serve to convey NO bioactivity and to regulate protein function [16]. This redox based signal transduction pathway is akin to phosphorylation [18] in that both exemplify dynamic regulation of protein function by reversible modification. Although mechanisms of regulation of phosphorylation have been known for years, the precise regulation of RSNO formation and degradation on specific sites on proteins to affect function is still a subject of intense research. However, Stamler and colleagues have made great strides in our understanding of the regulation of S-nitrosylation signal transduction [19]. The temporal and spatial regulation of S-nitrosylation within and between proteins allows for a redox based cell signaling pathway [17]. Most recently nitrite mediated RSNO formation has been described in physiological systems [20–22]. Thus, via direct formation of nitroso and nitrosyl products, endogenous or exogenous nitrite may account for some of the biochemistry and pharmacology previously attributed to NO. The current paradigm is that formation of nitrosothiols specifically elicits changes in protein structure and function and therefore represents a ubiquitous and fundamental form of cell signaling. Therefore restoring NO homeostasis through repletion of nitrite and nitrosothiols through dietary means is a first line of defense for diseases and conditions associated with NO insufficiency.

NO is one of the most important signaling molecules in mammalian physiology. To date there are over 100,000 published papers on NO with greater than 99% coming after the seminal discovery by Ferid Murad in 1977 [4]. A substantial knowledge of the NO signaling pathway has been gained during the past three decades. However there is a growing appreciation that there are alternative sources of NO other than the endogenous synthesis through the L-arginine pathway. A substantial portion of our total body NO may come from what we eat. Therefore individual differences in dietary habits may reflect individual susceptibility or resistance to disease. If this is the case, then there is an opportunity to intervene early on and prevent disease simply through changing and understanding our diet. In order to gain an appreciation for the complexity of production and regulation of NO through conversion of L-arginine, we will describe the known and well characterized L-arginine NO pathway.

NO GENERATION AND NO SYNTHASE

NO is perhaps best studied and characterized in the blood vessels. NO contributes to vessel homeostasis by inhibiting vascular smooth muscle contraction and growth, platelet aggregation, and blood cell adhesion to the endothelium, all processes involved in inflammation and atherosclerosis. Therefore maintaining NO homeostasis is critical for the prevention of chronic diseases such as atherosclerosis. Our understanding of the process leading to cardiovascular diseases is allowing us to adopt principles of therapy that may be more beneficial for patients. For instance, hypertension, particularly in high-risk patients, is a result of loss of balance and the absence of the ability to vasodilate normally. The interaction between the endothelial cell and the smooth muscle cell is very important in this process. The endothelium is a group of cells that produce compounds that are important in regulating vascular homeostasis by elaborating factors such as angiotensin II, NO, endothelin, and prostaglandins. Specifically, NO is produced by endothelial cells and is responsible for smooth muscle relaxation. Normal endothelium maintains vascular tone and blood viscosity, prevents abnormal blood clotting and bleeding, limits inflammation of the vasculature, and suppresses smooth muscle cell proliferation. Abnormal endothelium unable to produce NO causes increased inflammation and hypertrophy of the smooth muscle cells, promotes thrombosis and vasoconstriction, leading to the rapid growth of atherosclerotic plaques. Therefore, understanding endothelial function will be imperative as researchers develop newer compounds that may enhance NO bioavailability within the vasculature. These may include compounds that promote the production of or extend the biological half life of NO or enhancing the cellular targets of NO.

Nitric oxide synthase (NOS) enzymes produce ·NO by catalyzing a five electron oxidation of a guanidino nitrogen of L-arginine (L-Arg). Oxidation of L-Arg to L-citrulline occurs via two successive monooxygenation reactions producing N^Ghydroxy L-arginine as an intermediate. Two moles of oxygen (O_2) and 1.5 moles of NADPH are consumed per mole of ·NO formed [23] (Figure 1.1). NOS enzymes are the only enzymes known to simultaneously require five bound cofactors/prosthetic groups: flavin adenine dinucleotide (FAD), flavin mononucleotide (FMN), heme iron, tetrahydrobiopterin (BH_4) and calcium-calmodulin. There are three isoforms of NOS, the genetic sequence of each residing on three distinct chromosomes. Two types are constitutive, cytosolic, Ca^{2+}/calmodulin dependent and releases NO for short time periods in response to receptor or physical stimulation. The NO released by these enzymes act as a transduction mechanism underlying several physiological responses. The other enzyme type is induced after activation of macrophages, endothelial cells and a number of other cells by endotoxin and pro-inflammatory cytokines and once expressed, synthesizes NO for long periods of time. Furthermore, the inducible

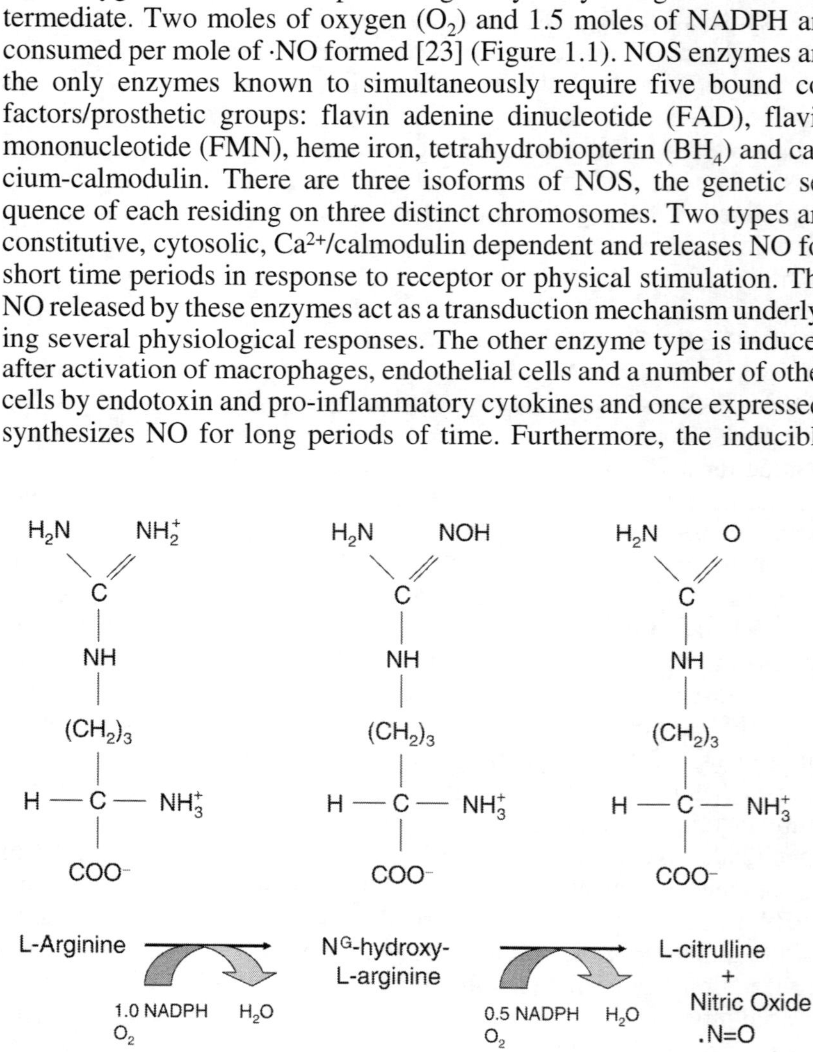

FIGURE 1.1 The L-Arginine—Nitric Oxide pathway.

form is cytosolic, Ca^{2+} independent since calmodulin is already bound to the enzyme, and its induction is inhibited by glucocorticoids [24]. It is now appreciated that eNOS is found in other cells and tissues besides the endothelium, iNOS is found constitutively in some tissues, and there are inducible forms of both eNOS and nNOS, adding confusion to the nomenclature as it was first described. In an attempt to clarify the nomenclature, the three different isoforms are now commonly referred to as NOSI, NOSII, and NOSIII for neuronal, inducible and endothelial isoforms, respectively, based on the order in which they were first purified and cloned.

All three isoforms of the enzyme function as a homodimer consisting of two identical monomers, which can be functionally and structurally divided into two major domains: a C-terminal reductase-carboxy domain, and an N-terminal oxygenase-amino domain [23,25]. The catalytically active isoforms exist as homodimers with tetrahydrobiopterin and heme serving to facilitate dimer formation [26,27]. The carboxy terminal domain has considerable homology between the isoforms, and is homologous to cytochrome P450 [28]. However, the amino terminal domain has less homology. The homology of the three isoforms is about 50 to 60% while the homology of a given isoform between species can be as great as 85 to 92%. All isoforms are catalytically self-sufficient provided all required substrates and co-factors are available. Enzyme-bound calmodulin facilitates the transfer of electrons from NADPH to the flavoprotein domain of NOS and also from the flavins to the heme domain of NOS [29]. These electrons are used to reduce the iron to the ferrous state so that it can bind oxygen, which is incorporated into the substrate, arginine, to generate NO plus citrulline. Calmodulin also facilitates NADPH dependent reduction of cytochrome *c* and ferricyanide in BH_4 and heme depleted nNOS [29,30]. If any of the co-factors become limiting, then NO production from NOS shuts down, and in many cases NOS then produces superoxide instead. This is indeed a very complex and coordinated effort to enzymatically produce NO which normally proceeds very efficiently. However, in disease characterized by oxidative stress where cofactors become oxidized, NOS uncoupling, or conditions of hypoxia where oxygen is limiting, or increased formation of asymmetric dimethyl arginine (ADMA) occurs this process can no longer maintain NO production. One consequence is "endothelial dysfunction" where blood vessels make too little NO. Therefore there has to be an alternate route to NO production. It is highly unlikely that Nature devised such a sophisticated mechanism of NO production as a sole source of a critical molecule. To better understand the local regulation and production of NO in various tissues, it is worth describing the individual isoforms of NOS that are responsible for a host of physiological actions in different organ systems.

eNOS

In the vascular endothelium, agonists such as acetylcholine and bradykinin stimulate inositol 1,4,5-triphosphate or IP3 production by activating the phosphoinositide second messenger system. IP3 binds to receptors on the endoplasmic reticulum and causes Ca^{2+} release from intracellular stores [31]. This transient elevation of intracellular Ca^{2+} promotes calcium binding to calmodulin, forming a complex that is a crucial cofactor for constitutive NOS activity [32]. eNOS produces modest amounts of NO until the calcium concentration decreases. This rapid and transient production of NO by eNOS allows NO to function in maintaining basal vascular tone [31]. NO, once produced, then diffuses into nearby target cells to interact with specific molecular targets. NO regulates protein activity by reversibly binding to available acceptor functionalities, including heme iron and thiols [33]. The interaction between NO and its primary receptor the enzyme guanylyl cyclase, which mediates target cell responses such as vascular smooth muscle relaxation and platelet inhibition, has been well characterized [34, 35]. After entering the target cell, NO binds to the heme moiety of guanylyl cyclase and activates the enzyme by inducing a conformational change that displaces iron out of the plane of the porphoryrin ring [36]. Guanylyl cyclase then catalyzes the production of cyclic GMP from GTP to elevate cyclic GMP. Cyclic GMP then triggers a cascade of intracellular events that culminate in a reduction in calcium-dependent vascular smooth muscle tone by inactivating myosin light chain kinase or MLCK [37, 38]. MLCK normally phosphorylates the regulatory set of myosin light chain. This phosphorylation event activates cross-bridge cycling and initiates contraction [39]. cGMP modulates MLCK activity by activating a cGMP-dependent protein kinase that phosphorylates MLCK [40]. Phosphorylation of MLCK diminishes its affinity for calmodulin and, as a consequence, decreases the phosphorylation of myosin light chain, which in turn stabilizes the inactive form of myosin. In this manner, cGMP may induce vasorelaxation by indirectly decreasing myosin light chain-dependent myosin activation. Infusion of a NOS inhibitor causes a sustained hypertension that is reversible by administration of excess L-arginine [41,42]. NO is now considered the endogenous nitrovasodilator. However, the physiological effects of NO extend well beyond the vascular endothelium. Radomski *et al.* [43] has shown that human platelets contain a NOS that is activated when platelets are stimulated to aggregate. Thus, platelets themselves also have the enzymatic capacity to synthesize NO with both a constitutive and inducible form of NOS identified in human megakaryoblasts [44]. NOS activity increases with platelet activation, and this response appears to modulate platelet aggregation, thereby potentially limiting the self-amplification of platelet thrombus formation *in vivo*. It was also reported early on that human neutrophils inhibit platelet aggregation by releasing an NO-like factor [45]. These anti-thrombotic properties of the endothelium may be a consequence of the synergistic action of NO and prostacyclin. Radomski *et al.* [46] has shown the synergistic antiaggregatory effects of NO and prostacyclin on platelets. NO and prostacyclin may act in concert to oppose local vasospasm or thrombus formation at sites where platelets aggregate and the coagulation cascade is activated. It has also been proposed that the antiplatelet effects of endothelial-derived NO may prevent thromboembolic events during administration of potent prostacyclin inhibitors such as aspirin [47]. In this regard NO acts as an anti-inflammatory molecule.

iNOS

NO is also generated by macrophages and neutrophils as part of the human immune response. NO is toxic to bacteria and other human pathogens. It is the inducible isoform of NOS that is responsible for macrophage NO production. Inducible NOS has been found in many cell types including macrophages [48], and neutrophils [49] and is immunologically activated by exposure to bacterial endotoxin or pro-inflammatory cytokines such as interleukin-1, or interferon-gamma [50,51] and tumor necrosis factor. Inducible NOS activity is regulated at the transcriptional level [52] and is not affected by changes in intracellular calcium concentrations nor is dependent on the cofactors NADPH and tetrahydrobiopterin. iNOS induction after cytokine exposure requires several hours and once induced, can generate far greater amounts of NO per mole of enzyme than the constitutive NOS [53]. Macrophages stimulated with interferon gamma, and lipopolysaccharide have NOS messenger ribonucleic acid present by 2 hours, and NOS protein by 4 hours. The presence of NOS-2 message or protein can serve as biomarker for inflammation in tissues. The NOS protein may remain present for several days [54]. The expression of the inducible form of NOS, but not nNOS or eNOS is specifically inhibited by glucocorticoids [55]. Although cultured macrophages can produce large amounts of NO, multiple cytokines are required to achieve maximal induction. Interferon gamma or LPS alone can induce noncytotoxic levels of NO. However, when cytokines work synergistically, they can induce cytotoxic levels of NO. Priming cell cultures with IFN-gamm prior to exposure to other agents result in enhanced NO production. The synergistic activity between IFN-gamma and microbial products is mediated by tumor necrosis factor-alpha. At these high concentrations and flux rates, NO is cytotoxic and plays a key role in the immune response of macrophages to bacteria and other pathogens. Tumor necrosis factor acts in an autocrine fashion to amplify the synthesis and release of NO by primed macrophages; however, it cannot stimulate NO synthesis by itself. Antimicrobial activity and NO production parallel tumor necrosis factor activity [56]. A strong correlation exists between antimicrobial activity and production of L-Arg-derived NO by cytokine-activated cells observed during *in vitro* studies [56,57]. The precise mechanism of NO-mediated bactericidal and tumoricidal activity is unknown, but these observations suggest that macrophage NO production contributes to nonspecific immunity [58]. NO from activated macrophages may be responsible for the profound loss of vascular tone seen in septic patients. It is this relative overproduction of NO and the subsequent vasodilation that are thought to mediate NO's pathophysiologic role during sepsis and multiorgan failure during hypovolemia and hypoxia. Because NO is known to directly or indirectly modulate the inflammatory response as well as to play an important role in pain perception, there is also an increasing interest in defining the role that NO may play in the pathogenesis of chronic inflammation and the associated chronic pain [59]. Despite the rapid progress in our understanding of the complex physiological and pathophysiological processes involving NO, uncertainties remain with regard to the critical cellular targets of NO cytotoxicity, the relative importance of different NO redox states and carrier molecules, and the importance of the NO antimicrobial system in human phagocytes. Ultimately, the immunoregulatory and vasoregulatory activities of NO may prove to be just as important as its antimicrobial properties during infection.

nNOS

In the central nervous system, NO is a neurotransmitter that underpins several functions, including the formation of memory. Recurrent as in other organ systems, this NO pathway may also play a role in the pathology of the central nervous system. The NOS isoform in the nervous system is activated by glutamate acting on N-methyl-D-aspartate receptors. In a matter of seconds the glutamate-induced increase in intracellular calcium concentration activates NOS via the calcium/calmodulin interaction as previously described. Under most circumstances, eNOS and nNOS are constitutive in the sense that their activation does not require new enzyme synthesis. However, both forms of NOS are inducible in that new enzyme synthesis occurs primarily under conditions of traumatic or pathological insult. The calcium influx that accompanies prolonged NMDA receptor activation is associated with degeneration of the neurons [60]. It is likely that excessive NMDA receptor activation, with the consequent increase in calcium, contributes to glutamate neurotoxicity by enhancing NO which reacts with superoxide and then performs its nitrosative chemistry [61]. The dichotomy of both the protective and deleterious actions of NO is again revealed in the nervous system.

In the periphery, there is a widespread network of nerves, previously recognized as nonadrenergic and non cholinergic (NANC), that operate through a NO-dependent mechanism to mediate some forms of neurogenic vasodilation and regulate various gastrointestinal, respiratory, and genitourinary tract functions as well as autonomic innervation of smooth muscle in the gastrointestinal tract, the pelvic viscera, the airways, and other systems [62]. In the stomach, a decrease in gastric mucosal blood flow has been identified as a prerequisite to the development of acute erosions and stress ulcers [63,64]. NOS has been detected in the gastric mucosa, and NO appears to play a role in protecting the gastric mucosa during physiologic stress by acting as an endogenous vasodilator and thus supporting mucosal blood flow [65]. The exact mechanism of NO's protective effect is unclear, but may relate to vasodilation, inhibition of platelet aggregation in the gastric microvasculature, or a protective effect on the epithelial cells themselves [66]. However, alternative means to enhance NO in the periphery and stomach will certainly provide benefit to a number of conditions.

THE EVOLUTION OF NO FORMATION

The pathway of NO formation may be one of the oldest bioregulatory systems controlling human and animal physiology [67]. Mammals are not the only species that benefit from NO production. Interestingly plants grown in soils also produce NO as part of their normal nitrogen cycle. This becomes an important pathway when we discuss the nitrite and nitrate content of certain foodstuff in later chapters. NO can be produced by plants by any of four routes: (i) L-arginine-dependent NOsynthase [68–70], (ii) by plasma membrane-bound nitrate reductase, (iii) by mitochondrial electron transport chain, or (iv) by non-enzymatic reactions. It is a signaling molecule in plants as well and acts mainly against oxidative stress and also plays a role in plant pathogen interactions. Nitrite and nitrate are important molecules in this pathway and are essential for plant growth. In fact, nitrate is a key component of many fertilizers. The diagram above shows an overview of the nitrogen cycle in soil or aquatic en-

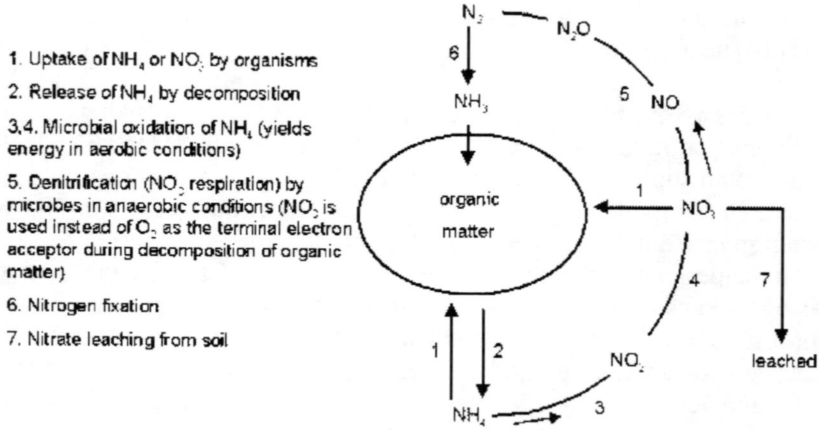

FIGURE 1.2

vironments. At any one time a large proportion of the total fixed nitrogen will be locked up in the biomass or in the dead remains of organisms (shown collectively as "organic matter"). So, the only nitrogen available to support new growth will be that which is supplied by nitrogen fixation from the atmosphere pathway 6 in the diagram) or by the release of ammonium or simple organic nitrogen compounds through the decomposition of organic matter (pathway 2). Some of the other stages in this cycle are mediated by specialized groups of microorganisms and are explained below. This will be covered in much more detail in later chapters but it is important to introduce the concept here to highlight the importance of nitrogen containing molecules in nature and the natural formation of NO, nitrite and nitrate in nature.

The superficial and cursory overview of nitric oxide has hopefully provided a sense of appreciation for the human body's ability to synthesize such a simple molecule through a complicated series of reactions in single cells. The capability of the human body to control its NO production is the premise for health and well-being. When we lose our ability to produce or control NO production, it is becoming increasingly clear that this is the earliest sign of disease. The healthy human body is amazingly adept at responding to a changing internal and external environment. In particular its ability to modulate the amount of NO produced at a given time. It is known that when we exercise we increase NO production to account for the increase blood flow and oxygen demands of working tissues [71] and plasma nitrite predicts exercise capacity in humans [72]. A recent study involving Tibetans living at 4200 meters above sea level beautifully illustrates the dynamic physiological response in humans to changes in ambient oxygen. The low barometric pressure at high altitude causes lower arterial oxygen content among Tibetan highlanders, who maintain normal levels of oxygen use as indicated by basal and maximal oxygen consumption levels that are consistent with sea level predictions. Lower levels of inhaled oxygen can be offset by increasing blood flow to improve oxygen delivery. Blood flow is determined by numbers, length, and diameter of blood vessels that in turn are largely determined by the amount of NO produced. The production of NO is elevated in populations living at high-altitudes, which helps these people avoid hypoxia and adapt to lower oxygen levels they breathe in [73]. Tibetans have roughly 100 times the amount of nitrite and nitrate circulating in their blood than do people living at sea level. The adaptive increase in steady state nitrite and nitrate is proof of principle on the benefits of nitrite and nitrate without any harmful health effects. On the contrary, those who are unable to maintain normal NO production develop disease.

The maintenance of NO homeostasis in humans is absolutely critical for good health and well being. In fact, without adequate NO many diseases ensue. The recent and emerging paradigm of restoring and enhancing NO availability through natural dietary means is revolutionary and very timely as our baby boom generation ages and reaches the critical age at which many succumb to disease, particularly cardiovascular disease. The focus of the remaining chapters will be on modulating the nitric oxide pathway through what we eat and how this can positively affect our health. We will provide compelling evidence for such a pathway. From a public health perspective, simple changes in dietary habits may have profound implications in health and disease and provide a natural low cost treatment or preventive measure against contemporary disease.

ABOUT THE AUTHORS

Nathan S. Bryan, Ph.D.

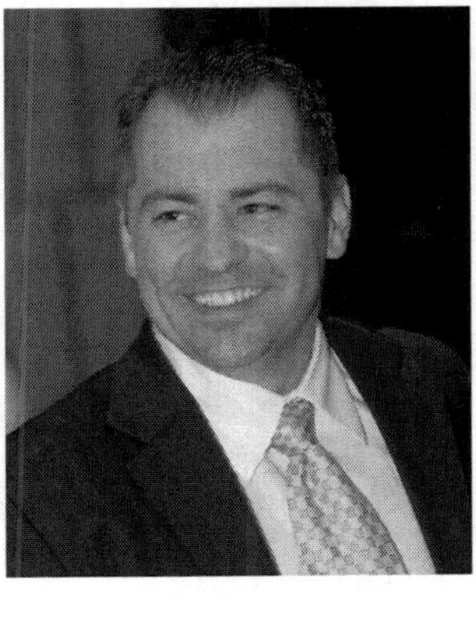

Dr. Bryan was born in Bryan Texas in November 1973. Nathan grew up in small town Texas. He spent his grade school years in Lexington (population 1000) and attended High School in Caldwell (population 3000). He earned his undergraduate Bachelor of Science degree in Biochemistry from the University of Texas at Austin and his doctoral degree from Louisiana State University School of Medicine in Shreveport where he was the recipient of the Dean's Award for Excellence in Research. He pursued his post-doctoral training as a Kirschstein Fellow at Boston University School of Medicine in the Whitaker Cardiovascular Institute. Dr. Bryan joined the Institute of Molecular Medicine, University of Texas Health Science Center in Houston, in June 2006 in the Center for Cell Signaling. He is also a faculty member of the Department of Integrative Biology and Pharmacology and Graduate School of Biomedical Sciences at the UT Houston Medical School. He is an active member of the Nitric Oxide Society, Society for Free Radical Biology and Medicine and the American Heart Association.

Dr. Bryan's research is dedicated to providing a better understanding of the interactions of nitric oxide (NO) and related metabolites with their different biological targets at the molecular and cellular level and the significance of these reactions for physiology and pathophysiology. Attempts are made to identify what particular changes in NO-related signaling pathways and reaction products occur in disease states such as endothelial dysfunction, ischemia/reperfusion, tissue/cardiac protection, diabetes, atherosclerosis and inflammation with the aim of testing their amenability as biomarkers for diagnosis and/or treatment of specific disease.

Current research is directed to understand the interactions of exogenous dietary nitrite/nitrate (NO_x) on the endogenous NO/cGMP pathway and how perturbations in each system affect cardiovascular health. This involves mechanisms of nitrite transport and cellular uptake as well as mechanism of nitrite reduction back to NO and via direct NO-independent signaling actions of nitrite. Work in Dr. Bryan's lab involves molecular biology and analytical biochemistry utilizing gas phase chemiluminescence and HPLC in multiple organ systems and blood. Much of the work involves *in vivo* characterization of NO/nitrite metabolism using a number of transgenic and knockout animal models of disease. Dr. Bryan and colleagues recently discovered that nitrite is a biologically active molecule which was previously thought to be an inert breakdown product of NO production. These findings have unveiled many beneficial effects of nitrite in the treatment and prevention of human disease. These discoveries may provide the basis for new preventive or therapeutic strategies in diseases associated with NO insufficiency and new guidelines for optimal health. Since nitrite and nitrate are common constituents of many fruits and vegetables, changes in dietary habits may have profound effects on many diseases associated with NO insufficiency. NO insufficiency is a hallmark of a number of diseases including cardiovascular disease. The notion that nitrite can recapitulate NO biochemistry and serve as an alternative and compensatory mechanism of NO production is revolutionary. It may also serve as the endocrine mediator of NO signaling. Moreover, the direct signaling actions of nitrite may represent a novel NO independent pathway for nitrite. If our current understanding is true, then an optimal diet may then consist of a sufficient supply of nitrite and nitrate for health and disease prevention. Understanding this pathway will provide the basis for new preventive or therapeutic strategies in diseases associated with NO insufficiency and new guidelines for optimal health. To date Dr. Bryan has published over 20 peer reviewed papers that have been cited over 1000 times. He has been invited to speak at a number of national and international meetings.

Dr. Bryan currently resides in Houston with his wife Kristen and their two sons Grant and Lincoln. The Bryans spend their weekends at their ranch near Caldwell where they raise cattle and horses and enjoy the great outdoors. Nathan enjoys playing golf and calf roping and team roping on his ranch and in competition.

Ferid Murad, MD, PhD

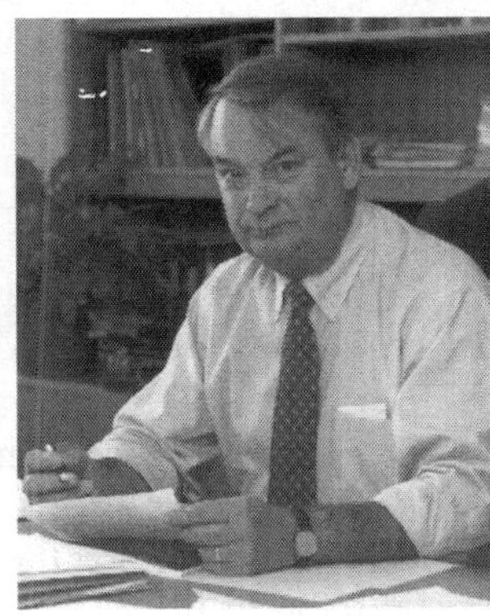

Ferid Murad, MD, PhD won the 1998 Nobel Prize in Physiology or Medicine for his work with nitric oxide as a signaling molecule in the cardiovascular system. Nitric oxide is now recognized to have applications ranging from treatment for heart disease and shock, to reducing the possibility of pulmonary hypertension in premature babies.

At the University of Texas Health Science Center at Houston, Dr. Murad is a Regental Professor in the Department of Integrative Biology and Pharmacology. He is also the Director Emeritus of the Brown Foundation Institute of Molecular Medicine for the Prevention of Human Diseases and the John S. Dunn, Sr., Distinguished Chair in Physiology and Medicine.

Dr. Murad's research focuses on the formation, metabolism, and function of nitric oxide and cyclic GMP in various cellular signaling processes. His work with nitric oxide began more than 30 years ago when he was at the University of Virginia School of Medicine. Despite initial disbelief from fellow researchers, Dr. Murad persevered in his conviction that the short-lived gas was crucially important to the body's signaling system. In the 1970s, Dr. Murad discovered that nitroglycerin relieves chest pain in heart patients by releasing nitric oxide. By 1992, Science magazine had named NO its "molecule of the year".

Subsequent research has shown that nitric oxide and/or cyclic GMP is synthesized by hormones, toxins, cytokines, growth factors, and drugs. Dr. Murad's laboratory had characterized and purified and cloned most of the guanylyl cyclases and nitric oxide syntheses. Another current research focus is on formation of peroxynitrite from nitric oxide and the nitration of various cellular proteins. He believes the protein nitration might represent another important cell signaling system, further regulating many biological processes. His laboratory also works with embryonic stem cells, cancer cells, wound healing and inflammatory diseases where NO and cyclic GMP also participate.

Dr. Murad has been active in both academic medicine and industry throughout his distinguished career with more than 400 publications. Among his many awards and honors, he received the prestigious Albert and Mary Lasker Basic Medical Research Award (1996), the American Heart Association Ciba Award (1988), and the Baxter Award for Distinguished Research in the Biomedical Sciences from the Association of American Medical Colleges (2000). He has received nine honorary degrees and is a member of the National Academy of Sciences, a member of the Institute of Medicine of the National Academy of Sciences, a Fellow of the American Academy of Arts and Sciences, and a member of the Chinese Academy of Sciences and several other foreign academies.

He earned his undergraduate degree in premedical science and chemistry from DePauw University in 1958 and received his M.D. and Ph.D. in Pharmacology from Case Western University in 1965. He completed and internship and residency in Medicine at Massachusetts General Hospital in Boston in 1967. From 1967–1970, he was a researcher at NIH. Dr Murad was on the faculty of the University of Virginia School of Medicine from 1970 to 1981, reaching the rank of professor. He was also the director of the medical school's clinical research center and of the Department of Clinical Pharmacology. Dr. Murad joined the Palo Alto Veterans Hospital, a Stanford University affiliate, in 1981 as Chief of Medicine and Associate Chairman and later Chairman of Medicine at Stanford. In 1988, he became vice president of research and development at Abbott Laboratories. He left Abbott in 1993 to found Molecular Geriatrics Corporation. In 1997, Dr. Murad became the University of Texas-Houston's first chair of the Department of Integrative Biology, Pharmacology and the Director of the Institute of Molecular Medicine in 1999. In 2006 he became the Director Emeritus of the Institute of Molecular Medicine with active research programs in Houston and Shanghai.

REFERENCES

1. Murad, F. Shattuck Lecture. Nitric oxide and cyclic GMP in cell signaling and drug development. *The New England journal of medicine* 355:2003–2011; 2006.
2. Culotta, E.; Kochland, D. E. J. NO news is good news (Molecule of the Year). *Science* 258:1862–1864; 1992.
3. Furchgott, R. F.; Zawadzki, J. V. The obligatory role of endothelial cells in the relaxation of arterial smooth muscle by acetycholine. *Nature* 288:373–376; 1980.
4. Arnold, W. P.; Mittal, C. K.; Katsuki, S.; Murad, F. Nitric oxide activates guanylate cyclase and increases guanosine 3′:5′-cyclic monophosphate levels in various tissue preparations. *Proceedings of the National Academy of Sciences of the United States of America* 74:3203–3207; 1977.
5. Katsuki, S.; Arnold, W.; Mittal, C.; Murad, F. Stimulation of guanylate cyclase by sodium nitroprusside, nitroglycerin and nitric oxide in various tissue preparations and comparison to the effects of sodium azide and hydroxylamine. *J Cyclic Nucleotide Res* 3:23–35; 1977.
6. Murad, F.; Mittal, C. K.; Arnold, W. P.; Katsuki, S.; Kimura, H. Guanylate cyclase: activation by azide, nitro compounds, nitric oxide, and hydroxyl radical and inhibition by hemoglobin and myoglobin. *Advances in cyclic nucleotide research* 9:145–158; 1978.
7. Murad, F.; Arnold, W. P.; Mittal, C. K.; Braughler, J. M. Properties and regulation of guanylate cyclase and some proposed functions for cyclic GMP. *Advances in cyclic nucleotide research* 11:175–204; 1979.
8. Ignarro, L. J.; Buga, G. M.; Wood, K. S.; Byrns, R. E.; Chaudhuri, G. Endothelium-derived relaxing factor produced and released from artery and vein is nitric oxide. *Proc. Natl. Acad Sci.* USA 84:9265–9269; 1987.
9. Murad, F. Cyclic guanosine monophosphate as a mediator of vasodilation. *The Journal of clinical investigation* 78:1–5; 1986.
10. Palmer, R. M. J.; Ferrige, A. G.; Moncada, S. Nitric oxide release accounts for the biological activity of endothelium-derived relaxing factor. *Nature* 327:524–526; 1987.
11. Deguchi, T.; Yoshioka, M. L-Arginine identified as an endogenous activator for soluble guanylate cyclase from neuroblastoma cells. *The Journal of Biological Chemistry* 257:10147–10151; 1982.
12. Knowles, R. G.; Palacios, M.; Palmer, R. M. J.; Moncada, S. Formation of nitric oxide from L-arginine in the central nervous system: A transduction mechanism for stimulation of the soluble guanylate cyclase. *Proc. Natl. Acad Sci.* USA 86:5159–5162; 1989.
13. Tannenbaum, S. R.; Fett, D.; Young, V. R.; Land, P. D.; Bruce, W. R. Nitrite and nitrate are formed by endogenous synthesis in the human intestine. *Science* 200:1487–1488; 1978.
14. Stuehr, D. J.; Marletta, M. A. Mammalian nitrate biosynthesis: mouse macrophages produce nitrite and nitrate in response to Escherichia coli lipopolysaccharide. *Proc. Natl. Acad Sci.* USA 82:7738–7742; 1985.
15. Moncada, S.; Higgs, A. The L-arginine-nitric oxide pathway. *N Engl J Med* 329:2002–2012; 1993.
16. Foster, M. W.; McMahon, T. J.; Stamler, J. S. S-nitrosylation in health and disease. *Trends in molecular medicine* 9:160–168; 2003.
17. Stamler, J. S.; Lamas, S.; Fang, F. C. Nitrosylation. The prototypic redox-based signaling mechanism. *Cell* 106:675–683; 2001.
18. Lane, P.; Hao, G.; Gross, S. S. S-nitrosylation is emerging as a specific and fundamental posttranslational protein modification: head-to-head comparison with O-phosphorylation. *Sci STKE* 2001:RE1; 2001.

19. Hess, D. T.; Matsumoto, A.; Kim, S. O.; Marshall, H. E.; Stamler, J. S. Protein S-nitrosylation: purview and parameters. *Nature reviews* 6:150–166; 2005.
20. Bryan, N. S.; Fernandez, B. O.; Bauer, S. M.; Garcia-Saura, M. F.; Milsom, A. B.; Rassaf, T.; Maloney, R. E.; Bharti, A.; Rodriguez, J.; Feelisch, M. Nitrite is a signaling molecule and regulator of gene expression in mammalian tissues. *Nature chemical biology* 1:290–297; 2005.
21. Angelo, M.; Singel, D. J.; Stamler, J. S. An S-nitrosothiol (SNO) synthase function of hemoglobin that utilizes nitrite as a substrate. *Proceedings of the National Academy of Sciences of the United States of America* 103:8366–8371; 2006.
22. Bryan, N. S.; Rassaf, T.; Rodriguez, J.; Feelisch, M. Bound NO in human red blood cells: fact or artifact? *Nitric Oxide* 10:221–228; 2004.
23. Liu, Q.; Gross, S. S. Binding sites of nitric oxide synthases. *Methods Enzymol* 268:311–324; 1996.
24. Moncada, S.; Palmer, R. M. J.; Higgs, A. Nitric oxide: physiology, pathophysiology and pharmacology. *Pharmacol Rev* 43:109–142; 1991.
25. Xia, H.; Bredt, D. S. Cloned and expressed nitric oxide synthase proteins. *Methods in enzymology* 268:427–436; 1996.
26. Marletta, M. A. Another activation switch for endothelial nitric oxide synthase: why does it have to be so complicated? *Trends in biochemical sciences* 26:519-521; 2001.
27. Bredt, D. S. Endogenous nitric oxide synthesis: biological functions and pathophysiology. *Free radical research* 31:577–596; 1999.
28. White, K. A.; Marletta, M. A. Nitric oxide synthase is a cytochrome P-450 type hemoprotein. *Biochemistry* 31:6627–6631; 1992.
29. Abu-Soud, H. M.; Yoho, L. L.; Stuehr, D. J. Calmodulin controls neuronal nitric-oxide synthase by a dual mechanism. *J Biol Chem.* 269:32047–32050; 1994.
30. Abu-Soud, H. M.; Stuehr, D. J. Nitric oxide synthases reveal a role for calmodulin in controlling electron transfer. *Proceedings of the National Academy of Sciences of the United States of America* 90:10769–10772; 1993.
31. Dinerman, J. L.; Lowenstein, C. J.; Snyder, S. H. Molecular Mechanisms of Nitric Oxide Regulation Potential Relevance to Cardiovascular Disease. *Circulation Research* 73:217–222; 1993.
32. Bredt, D. S.; Snyder, S. H. Isolation of nitric oxide synthetase, a calmodulin-requiring enzyme. *Proc. Natl. Acad Sci.* USA 87:682–685; 1990.
33. Stamler, J. S.; Singel, D. J.; Loscalzo, J. Biochemistry of Nitric oxide and its redox-activated forms. *Science* 258:1898–1902; 1992.
34. Ignarro, L. J. Haem-Dependent Activation of Guanylate Cyclase and Cyclic GMP Formation by Endogenous Nitric Oxide: A Unique Transduction Mechanism for Transcellular Signalling. *Pharmacology & Toxicology* 67:1–7; 1990.
35. Ignarro, L. J.; Adams, J. B.; Horwitz, P. M.; Wood, K. S. Activation of Soluble Guanylate cyclase by NO-Hemoproteins Involves NO-Heme Exchange. *The Journal of Biological Chemistry* 261:4997–5002; 1986.
36. Ignarro, L. J. Signal Transduction Mechanisms Involving Nitric Oxide. *Biochemical Pharmacology* 41:485–490; 1991.
37. Waldman, S. A.; Murad, F. Cyclic GMP Synthesis and Function. *Pharmacol Rev* 39:163–195; 1987.
38. Twort, C. H. C.; van Breemen, C. Cyclic Guanosine Monophosphate-Enhanced Sequestration of Ca^{2+} by Sarcoplasmic Reticulum in Vascular Smooth Muscle. *Circulation Research* 62:961–964; 1988.

39. Hathaway, D. R.; March, K. L.; Lash, J. A.; Adam, L. P.; Wilensky, R. L. Vascular Smooth Muscle: A review of the Molecular Basis of Contractility. *Circulation* 83:382–390; 1991.

40. Hathaway, D. R.; Konicki, M. V.; Coolican, S. A. Phosphorylation of Myosin Light Chain Kinase from Vascular Smooth Muscle by cAMP- and cGMP-dependent Protein Kinases. *J Mol Cell Cardiol* 17:841–850; 1985.

41. Sakuma, I.; Stuehr, D. J.; Gross, S. S.; Nathan, C.; Levi, R. Identification of arginine as a precursor of endothelium-derived relaxing factor. *Proc. Natl. Acad Sci.* USA 85:8664–8667; 1988.

42. Palmer, R. M. J.; Rees, D. D.; Ashton, D. S.; Moncada, S. L-Arginine is the physiological precursor for the formation of nitric oxide in endothelium-dependent relaxation. *Biochemical and Biophysical Research Communications* 153:1251–1256; 1988.

43. Radomski, M. W.; Palmer, R. M. J.; Moncada, S. An L-Arginine/nitric oxide pathway present in human platelets regulates aggregation. *Proc. Natl. Acad Sci.* USA 87:5193–5197; 1990.

44. Sase, K.; Michel, T. Expression of Constitutive Endothelial Nitric Oxide Synthase in Human Blood Platelets. *Life Sciences* 57:2049–2055; 1995.

45. Salvemini, D.; De Nucci, G.; Gryglewski, R. J.; Vane, J. R. Human neutrophils and mononuclear cells inhibit platelet aggregation by releasing a nitric oxide like factor. *Proc. Natl. Acad Sci.* USA 86:6328–6332; 1989.

46. Radomski, M. W.; Palmer, R. M. J.; Moncada, S. Comparative pharmacology of endothelium-derived relaxing factor, nitric oxide and prostacyclin in platelets. *Br. J. Pharmac* 92:181–187; 1987.

47. Bednar, M. M.; Gross, C. E.; Howard, D. B.; Russell, S. R.; Thomas, G. R. Nitric Oxide reverses aspririn antagonism of t-PA Thrombolysis in a rabbit model of thromboembolic stroke. *Experimental Neurology* 146:513–517; 1997.

48. Marletta, M. A.; Yoon, P. S.; Iyengar, R.; Leaf, C. D.; Wishnok, J. S. Macrophage oxidation of L-arginine to nitrite and nitrate: nitric oxide is an intermediate. *Biochemistry* 27:8706–8711; 1988.

49. Yui, Y.; Hattori, R.; Kosuga, K.; Eizawa, H.; Hiki, K.; Ohkawa, S.; Ohnishi, K.; Terao, S.; Kawai, C. Calmodulin-independent nitric oxide synthase from rat polymorphonuclear neutrophils. *The Journal of Biological Chemistry* 266:3369–3371; 1991.

50. Stuehr, D. J.; Marletta, M. A. Induction of nitrite/nitrate synthesis in murine macrophages by BCG infection, lymphokines, or interferon-gamma. *The Journal of Immunology* 139:518–525; 1987.

51. Ding, A. H.; Nathan, C. F.; Stuehr, D. J. Release of reactive nitrogen intermediates and reactive oxygen intermediates from mouse peritoneal macrophages. *The Journal of Immunology* 141:2407–2412; 1988.

52. Cho, H. J.; Xie, Q.-w. X.; Calaycay, J.; Mumford, R. A.; Swiderek, K. M.; Lee, T. D.; Nathan, C. F. Calmodulin is a subunit of nitric oxide synthase from macrophages. *J. Exp. Med* 176:599–604; 1992.

53. Welch, G.; Loscalzo, J. Nitric oxide and the Cardiovascular System. *J. Card Surg* 9:361–371; 1994.

54. Xie, Q.-w. X.; Cho, H. J.; Calaycay, J.; Mumford, R. A.; Swiderek, K. M.; Lee, T. D.; Ding, A.; Troso, T.; Nathan, C. F. Cloning and Characterization of inducible nitric oxide synthase from mouse macrophages. *Science* 256:225–228; 1992.

55. Radomski, M. W.; Palmer, R. M. J.; Moncada, S. Glucocorticoids inhibit the expression of an inducible, but not the constitutive, nitric oxide synthase in vascular endothelial cells. *Proc. Natl. Acad Sci.* USA 87:10043–10047; 1990.

56. Nathan, C. F.; Hibbs Jr, J. B. Role of Nitric Oxide synthesis in macrophage antimicrobial activity. *Current Opinion in Immunology* 3:65–70; 1991.

57. Stuehr, D. J.; Griffith, O. W. Mammalian nitric oxide synthases. *Adv Enzymol Relat Areas Mol Biol* 65:287–346; 1992.

58. Rodeberg, D. A.; Chaet, M. S.; Bass, R. C.; Arkovitz, M. S.; Garcia, V. F. Nitric Oxide: *An Overview. The American Journal of Surgery* 170:292–303; 1995.

59. Roerig, S.; Wolf, R.; Grisham, M. B. Nitric Oxide, Chronic Joint Inflammation, and Pain. In: Ignarro, L. J., ed. *Nitric Oxide Biology and Pathobiology.* San Diego: Academic Press; 2000: 873–894.

60. Garthwaite, G.; Garthwaite, J. Differential dependence on Ca^{2+} of N-methyl-D-aspartate and quisqualate neurotoxicity in young rat hippocampal slices. *Neuroscience Letters* 97:316–322; 1989.

61. Lipton, S. A.; Choi, Y.-B.; Pan, Z.-H.; Lei, S. Z.; Chen, H.-S. V.; Sucher, N. J.; Loscalzo, J.; Singel, D. J.; Stamler, J. S. A redox based mechanism for the neuroprotective and neurodestructive effects of nitric oxide and related nitroso compounds. *Nature* 364:626–632; 1993.

62. Gillespie, J. S.; Liu, X.; Martin, W. *The neurotransmitter of the non-adrenergic non-cholinergic inhibitory nerves to smooth muscle of the genital system.* Elsevier Science Publishers BV; 1990.

63. Mersereau, W. A.; Hinchey, E. J. Effect of Gastric acidity on gastric ulceration induced by hemorrhage in the rat, utilizing a gastric chamber technique. *Gastroenterology* 64:1130–1135; 1973.

64. Ritchie, W. P.; Shearburn, E. W. Influence of isoproterenol and cholestyramine on acute gastric mucosal ulcerogenesis. *Gastroenterology* 73:62–65; 1977.

65. Whittle, B. J. R.; Boughton-Smith, N. K.; Moncada, S. Biosynthesis and role of th endothelium-derived vasodilator, nitric oxide, in the gastric mucosa. *Ann NY Acad Sci* 664:126–139; 1992.

66. Stark, M. E.; Szurszewski, J. H. Role of Nitric Oxide in Gastrointestinal and Hepatic Function and Disease. *Gastroenterology* 103:1928–1949; 1992.

67. Feelisch, M.; Martin, J. F. The early role of nitric oxide in evolution. *TREE* 10:496–499; 1995.

68. Corpas, F. J.; Barroso, J. B.; Carreras, A.; Quiros, M.; Leon, A. M.; Romero-Puertas, M. C.; Esteban, F. J.; Valderrama, R.; Palma, J. M.; Sandalio, L. M.; Gomez, M.; del Rio, L. A. Cellular and subcellular localization of endogenous nitric oxide in young and senescent pea plants. *Plant physiology* 136:2722–2733; 2004.

69. Corpas, F. J.; Barroso, J. B.; Carreras, A.; Valderrama, R.; Palma, J. M.; Leon, A. M.; Sandalio, L. M.; del Rio, L. A. Constitutive arginine-dependent nitric oxide synthase activity in different organs of pea seedlings during plant development. *Planta* 224:246–254; 2006.

70. Valderrama, R.; Corpas, F. J.; Carreras, A.; Fernandez-Ocana, A.; Chaki, M.; Luque, F.; Gomez-Rodriguez, M. V.; Colmenero-Varea, P.; Del Rio, L. A.; Barroso, J. B. Nitrosative stress in plants. *FEBS Lett* 581:453–461; 2007.

71. Sessa, W. C.; Pritchard, K.; Seyedi, N.; Wang, J.; Hintze, T. H. Chronic exercise in dogs increases coronary vascular nitric oxide production and endothelial cell nitric oxide synthase gene expression. *Circ Res* 74:349–353; 1994.

72. Rassaf, T.; Lauer, T.; Heiss, C.; Balzer, J.; Mangold, S.; Leyendecker, T.; Rottler, J.; Drexhage, C.; Meyer, C.; Kelm, M. Nitric oxide synthase-derived plasma nitrite predicts exercise capacity. *British journal of sports medicine* 41:669–673; discussion 673; 2007.

73. Erzurum, S. C.; Ghosh, S.; Janocha, A. J.; Xu, W.; Bauer, S.; Bryan, N. S.; Tejero, J.; Hemann, C.; Hille, R.; Stuehr, D. J.; Feelisch, M.; Beall, C. M. Higher blood flow and circulating NO products offset high-altitude hypoxia among Tibetans. *Proceedings of the National Academy of Sciences of the United States of America* 104:17593–17598; 2007.

CHAPTER 2

Mechanisms and Physiological Implications for Nitric Oxide Insufficiency

MATTHEW B. GRISHAM and NATHAN S. BRYAN

Department of Molecular and Cellular Physiology
LSU Health Sciences Center
Shreveport, LA 71130

Brown Foundation Institute of Molecular Medicine
The University of Texas Health Science Center
Houston, TX 77030

THE production of NO from L-arginine is a critical cellular function in most if not all organ systems throughout the body. This has been described in Chapter 1. NO has been shown to be involved in and affect neurotransmission, memory, stroke, glaucoma and neural degeneration, vasodilation, blood pressure, blood flow, pulmonary hypertension, penile erection, angiogenesis, wound healing, atherogenesis, inflammation such as arthritis, nephritis, colitis, etc, cytotoxicity, invading pathogens, tumors, asthma, tissue transplantation, septic shock, hypotension, platelet aggregation, gastrointestinal motility, hormone secretion, gene regulation, hemoglobin delivery of oxygen, stem cell proliferation and differentiation and bronchodilation to name a few. One can then imagine the host of diseases or conditions that may be caused or affected by the body's inability to produce NO. Therefore maintaining NO homeostasis is critical for optimal health and disease prevention. For years physicians and scientists assumed simply feeding more substrate L-arginine would be sufficient to enhance NO production. It is becoming increasingly clear that this may not be the most effective strategy especially in patients that are insufficient in NO due to endothelial dysfunction. The effect of L-arginine on endothelial function in humans is inconsistent. Recognizing the complex pathway to make NO from L-arginine helps us understand that giving L-arginine alone is not enough to drive NO production especially in disease conditions characterized by endothelial dysfunction or oxidative stress. This chapter will illustrate the physiological mechanisms and consequence of NO insufficiency, either through inefficient oxidation of L-arginine or through rapid degradation by oxygen radicals once NO is produced. Regardless of the cause, the ultimate outcome is clear and detrimental.

Let's first begin by defining endothelial dysfunction. The endothelium is the thin layer of cells that line the interior surface of blood vessels, forming an interface between circulating blood in the lumen and the rest of the vessel wall. Endothelial cells line the entire circulatory system, from the heart to the smallest capillary. These cells reduce turbulence of the flow of blood allowing the fluid to be pumped farther. Endothelial dysfunction is a loss of normal biochemical processes carried out by the endothelium, the cells that line the inner surface of all blood vessels including arteries and veins (as well as the innermost lining of the heart and lymphatics). Endothelial dysfunction is a hallmark for vascular diseases, and often leads to atherosclerosis. This is very common in patients with diabetes mellitus, hypertension or other chronic pathophysiological conditions. One of the main mechanisms of endothelial dysfunction is the diminishing of nitric oxide, often due to high levels of asymmetric dimethylarginine, which interfere with the normal L-arginine-stimulated nitric oxide synthesis. Part of the normal function of the endothelium is to produce NO from L-arginine by the enzymes nitric oxide synthase (NOS). The inability of endothelial cells to produce NO is associated with several cardiovascular disorders, including atherosclerosis. This can be due either to decreased production or to increased degradation of NO once produced [1]. Experimental and clinical studies provide evidence that defects of endothelial NO function is not only associated with all major cardiovascular risk factors, such as hyperlipidemia, diabetes, hypertension, smoking and severity of atherosclerosis, but also has a profound predictive value for the future atherosclerotic disease progression [2–5]. Atherosclerosis is a chronic disease in which fatty substances form a deposit of plaque on the inner lining of arterial walls eventually leading to blood vessel occlusion. The dysfunctional NO pathway is considered as an early marker or a common mechanism for various cardiovascular disorders. In the presence of known atherogenic risk factors, such as essential hypertension, several forms of dyslipidemia, diabetes mellitus, cigarette smoking, aging, physical inactivity, and hyperhomocysteinemia, the normal endothelium can become dysfunctional and unable to produce NO from L-arginine. The endothelium is a direct, sensitive target for the damaging effects of atherogenic risk factors, as evidenced from the experimental introduction of risk factors into

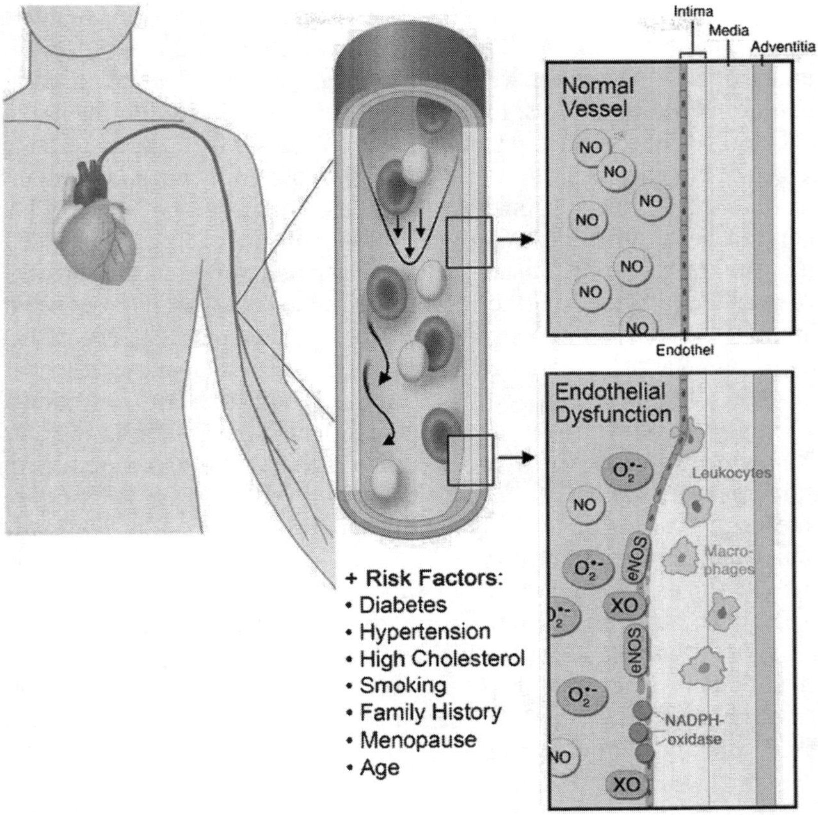

FIGURE 2.1 The innermost lining of our blood vessels is single layer of endothelial cells. Healthy endothelial cells produce nitric oxide to combat disease and regulate blood pressure. Endothelial dysfunction is defined by the inablility of the vessels to transducer NO activity, either by inability to produce from L-arginine or inactivation by superoxide ($O_2^{\bullet -}$).

healthy subjects, such as feeding with a high-fat meal leads to endothelial vasodilator dysfunction in a time span of just a few hours [6]. Central to the development of endothelial dysfunction, regardless of its cause, is a loss of bioactive endothelial NO. This is illustrated in Figure 2.1. There are 2 fundamental mechanisms for the loss of NO bioactivity: (1) reduced synthesis from L-arginine and (2) increased oxidative inactivation by reactive oxygen intermediates. Reactive oxygen species (ROS) such as superoxide are produced in abundance in the dysfunctional endothelium and limitation of ROS generation increases the availability of NO. For this reason antioxidant therapy with vitamin C and cholesterol-lowering therapy with statins (HMG-CoA reductase inhibitors) improves endothelial function. An alternative approach to increase levels of bioactive NO and to improve endothelial function is to increase the synthesis of NO. Enhanced synthesis of NO can be achieved by increased availability of agonists that stimulate release of NO from the endothelial cells like bradykinin assuming a healthy endothelium and sufficient cofactor to supply the NOS enzymes. Another straightforward approach to increase NO synthesis is to provide additional substrate to the endothelial cell. The semiessential amino acid L-arginine serves as the substrate for the NOS enzymes. Furthermore, L-arginine takes part in protein production, endocrine functions, wound healing, and erectile function. It is not regarded as an essential amino acid as the adult human is able to synthesize L-arginine *de novo* from the urea cycle. In adults the synthesis of L-arginine results from citrulline, a by-product of the glutamine metabolism in the gut and in the liver. Citrulline is excreted into the circulation and is reabsorbed in the kidney and converted to L-arginine. L-Citrulline is reformed if L-arginine is shunted through the NOS pathway. The dietetic application of L-arginine is the basic determinant of the L-arginine level in plasma, as the biosynthesis of L-arginine is not able to balance inadequate intake or deficiency. Providing supplementation substrate to individuals with inadequate NO, therefore, has been suggested as a rational approach to increase NO production by the NO synthase. We will describe the 2 fundamental mechanisms of NO insufficiency and then discuss the physiological implications.

L-ARGININE METABOLISM

As illustrated in Chapter 1 the production of NO from L-arginine is a complex and complicated biochemical pathway in which there are many steps that may be altered and affect ultimate NO production. Both acute and chronic administration of L-arginine evokes benefits in improving endothelial function. The precise molecular mechanisms by which L-arginine improves endothelial function remain puzzling. Providing the enzyme NOS with substrate because of lowered availability of L-arginine does not appear to be rate limiting since the intracellular levels of the amino acid are in the millimolar range [7], and the enzyme's Michaelis constanst (K_M) for substrate is in the micromolar range (2.9 μmol/L) [8]. In contrast, circulating L-arginine measured in plasma of healthy humans as well as in plasma of patients with vascular disorders is in the range of 45–100 μmol/L [9]. This is up to 15 to 30-fold higher than the concentration required to saturate the NOS enzyme. This biochemical discrepancy is termed as the "arginine paradox." For this reason, other possible explanations have been proposed to explain the effects of L-arginine. It is important to consider the steps to enzymatic NO production from NOS activation of cellular target to understand at which step things may become dysregulated or interrupted:

1. L-arginine production or availability which is dictated by flux through urea cycle and dietary intake as well as expression and activity of arginase, an enzyme that metabolizes L-arginine to urea,
2. Transport of L-arginine into the cell which competes with its endogenous analog asymmetric dimethyl L-arginine (ADMA),
3. Subcellular localization of L-arginine within the NOS enzyme complex,
4. Sufficient availability of NOS cofactors and prosthetic groups on the enzyme once L-arginine binds,
5. Once NO is formed it must reach its intended target. It can be quickly scavenged by reactive oxygen species and inactivated before it reaches it cellular target. These steps are illustrated in Figure 2.2. Each step in this pathway will now be discussed.

L-arginine is a naturally occurring amino acid that is necessary for the production of nitric oxide and other mediators in the inflammatory process. L-arginine is involved in and produced in the urea cycle (Figure 2.3). L-arginine is a basic amino acid and although it can be made in the body from L-citrulline in an ATP-dependent process, it appears that dietary or supplemental L-arginine is key to adequate production of nitric oxide. L-arginine can be synthesized from amphibolic intermediates and 7 enzymes, but it cannot be produced at rates sufficient to support growth and must therefore be ingested in the diet. Arginine is classified as a semi-essential or conditionally essential amino acid. L-arginine has been generally well tolerated by healthy volunteers as well as patients who have taken oral doses up 30 grams. Although the vasodilator action of L-arginine may lead to hypotension, the effects on blood pressure are usually low. Side effects are rare, mild, and dose dependent. Side effects include a bitter taste, nausea, and vomiting in about 3% of patients taking L-arginine higher doses. There are a number of genetic urea cycle disorders that result in insufficient L-arginine production such as arginosuccinate acidurea (ASA) whereby there is a genetic deletion of the arginosuccinate lyase (ASL) enzyme. A metabolic condition involving elevated arginine levels is known as hyperargininemia results from a defect in urea synthesis. This condition is characterized by increased arginine levels in cerebrospinal fluid, low erythrocyte levels of arginase and a urinary amino acid pattern similar to that seen in patients with

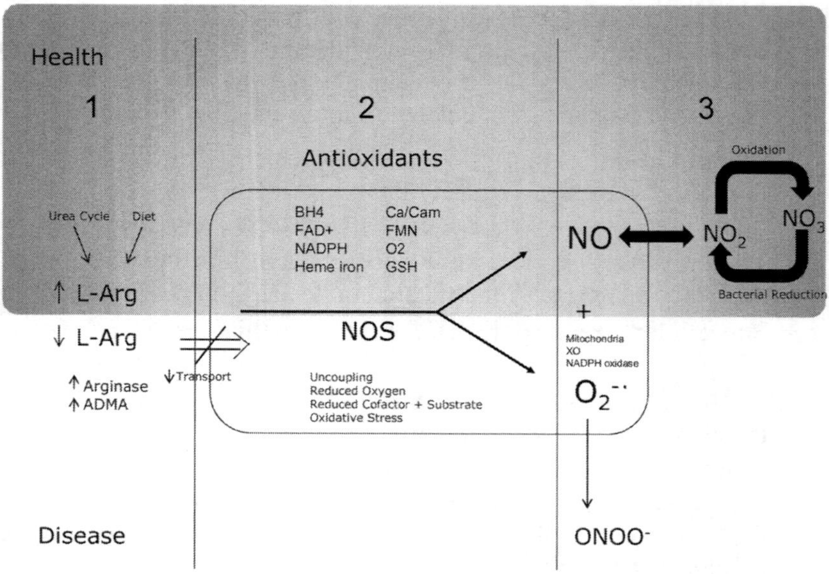

FIGURE 2.2 NOS production of NO from L-arginine is a complex stepwise biochemical reaction. NO homeostasis is determined by (1) L-arginine availability which comes from urea cycle and diet. The amount of L-arginine fed into the NOS system is determined by the activity of arginase as well as the presence of the endogenous NOS inhibitor asymmetric dimethyl L-arginine (ADMA). The transport of L-arginine into the cell can also be affected by a number of conditions. Step 2 in the scheme above represents the NOS enzyme activity and conformation. NOS requires several cofactors and proper conformation for NO production from L-arg. Under conditions of oxidative stress or uncoupling, NOS produces superoxide instead of NO. This is the early sign of endothelial dysfunction. Step 3 in the scheme represents the fate of NO once it is produced. The fate of NO is determined by te redox environment of the cell. Excess superoxide production will quickly scavenge NO and lead to NO insufficiencey despite enzymatic production.

lysine-cystinuria. Hyperargininemia is not associated with L-arginine supplements. Typical dietary intake of L-arginine is 3.5 to 5.0 grams daily and mainly derived from plant or animal foods. Small amounts of free L-arginine are found in fruits and vegetables and in some fermented foods such as miso and yogurt. Soy protein is particularly high in L-arginine, whereas other protein sources tend to be high in lysine which competes with L-arginine.

Arginase (the enzyme which converts arginine to ornithine and urea thereby diverting away from nitric oxide pathway) activity may alter the cellular levels of L-arginine, leading to decreased nitric oxide production. It has been shown in animal models that the upregulation of arginase may contribute to smooth muscle proliferation, resulting from endothelial dysfunction [10]. In the vessels of older animals, endothelial arginase activity is elevated and thus can contribute to endothelial dysfunction by further reducing cellular capacity for NO synthesis [11]. L-arginine is first converted to NG-hydroxy-L-arginine by eNOS which inhibits arginase and may hereby increase intracellular steady state levels of L-arginine [12]. Steady state levels of any given metabolite in physiology is determined by its rate of production or ingestion vs its rate of metabolism and excretion. There are multiple levels of regulation of L-arginine and thus NO production.

Another level of complexity arises from the transport of L-arginine from the circulation into the cell. A possible mechanism whereby this step is affected is that oxidized LDL and lysophosphatidylcholine have been shown to decrease L-arginine transport into endothelial cells [13,14]. This may be the reason for the beneficial effects of L-arginine in patients with hypercholesterolemia. L-arginine competes with other

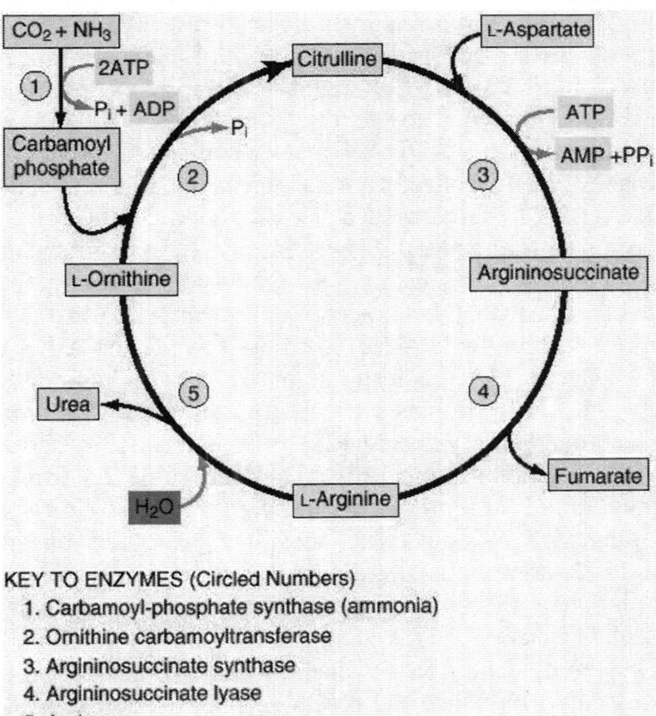

FIGURE 2.3 Urea cycle enzymes and substrates.

cationic amino acids for y+-transporter system into cells, especially L-glutamine, and increased L-arginine may increase intracellular substrate concentration by competitively enhancing cellular uptake in this setting. Another possibility could be the compartmentalization of L-arginine in the cytoplasm so that local concentrations in the vicinity of eNOS may be lower than expected from L-arginine levels in whole cell homogenates [15]. Extracellular L-arginine may be preferentially utilized by eNOS within this microenvironment.

The presence of endogenously occurring analogs of L-arginine, asymmetric dimethyl L-arginine (ADMA) and monomethylarginine (L-NMMA) exert biological activity by competitively inhibiting NOS [16]. Today we know that an elevation in plasma ADMA occurs in hypercholesterolemia and that the elevation in ADMA correlates with endothelial dysfunction [17]. A systemic infusion of ADMA in healthy humans causes temporary reduction in the cardiac output and induces a reduction of effective renal plasma flow. Systemic vascular resistance and blood pressure were increased in a dose-dependent manner [18]. ADMA is released from proteins that have been post-translationally methylated by proteinarginine methyltransferases (PRMT) and subsequently hydrolysed (see Figure 2.4). A healthy subject produces 60 mg of ADMA per day, 10 mg are excreted renally. The enzymatic metabolism is regulated by the enzyme dimethylarginine dimethylaminohydrolase (DDAH) and we could assume today that elevated ADMA plasma concentrations are caused by a reduced activity of the DDAH. Many factors, such as oxidized low-density lipoprotein cholesterol, inflammatory cytokines, hyperhomocysteinemia, hyperglycemia, infectious agents, and high doses of erythropoietin, have been shown to attenuate DDAH activity, allowing ADMA to accumulate and block NO synthesis [19–23]. Elevations in plasma ADMA have a high prevalence in hypercholesterolemia [17], hyperhomocysteinemia [24], hypertension [25], diabetes mellitus [26], peripheral arterial disease [27], coronary artery disease [28], preeclampsia [29], chronic heart failure [30], and other clinical disorders (see Table 2.1 from [31], in which circulating L-arginine concentration have been found to be in the normal range of NOS activity may be overcome by increased extracellular L-arginine/ADMA ratio through excess substrate and could explain how L-arginine improves endothelial function in patients with vascular disease [31]. Taken together, the above-mentioned results provide a lot of evidence that extracellular ADMA and L-arginine concentrations could modulate the eNOS activity. Today several studies have provided convincing data to support the hypothesis that ADMA could be a potential novel cardiovascular risk factor [28,32,33]. This im-

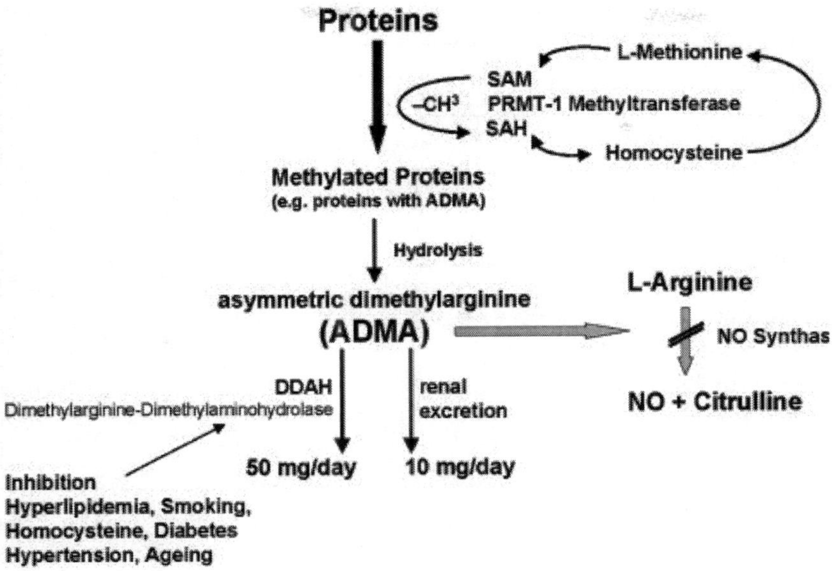

FIGURE 2.4 Simplified scheme describing ADMA main effects an dmetabolism. PRMT-1, a proteinarginine methyltransferase, methylates arginine residues within proteins utilizing S-adenosylmethionine (SAM) as a methyl donor. After hydrolysis of these proteins, free AdMA as a competitive inibitor of the NOS is present in the cytoplasm and in the blood plasma. ADMA is eliminated renally by about 20%. The main excretion route is via metabolism by the enzyme DDAH to citrulline an ddimethylamine. SAH, S-adenosylhomo-cysteine. (Taken from Bode-Boger *et al.* 114 (2007) 295–306).

plicates further therapeutic options for L-arginine supplementation along with additional anti-oxidants to preserve reduced co-factor availability. Thus, nutritional supplementation with L-arginine may be able to restore the physiological status by normalizing the extracellular L-arginine/ADMA ratio.

INCREASED INACTIVATION OF NO

Despite the complex pathway for the production of NO from L-arginine, once NO is produced it is subject to quick inactivation under certain conditions. Endothelial dysfunction in the setting of cardiovascular risk factors such as hypercholesterolemia, hypertension, diabetes mellitus, chronic smoking as well as in patients with heart failure has been shown to be at least in part dependent on the production of ROS such as superoxide and the subsequent decrease in vascular

TABLE 2.1 Clinical Conditions with Elevated ADMA.

Disease	Fold Increase versus Controls	Reference
Hypercholesterolemia	~2	Böger *et al.*, 1998a
Chronic heart failure	~2	Usui *et al.*, 1998
Impaired renal function	2–7	Kielstein *et al.*, 1999 and Zoccali *et al.*, 2001
Hypertension	~2	Goonasekera *et al.*, 1997 and Surdaki *et al.*, 1999
Peripheral arterial disease	2–3	Böger *et al.*, 1997b and Böger *et al.*, 1998b
Heart failure	2–3	Valkonen *et al.*, 2001
Diabetes mellitus	2–3	Abbasi *et al.*, 2001
Preeclampsia	2–3	Pettersson *et al.*, 1998
Hyperhomocyst(e)inemia	~2	Sydow *et al.*, 2003

Taken from Bode-Boger *et al.* 114 (2007) 295–306.

bioavailability of nitric oxide. Although the mechanisms underlying endothelial dysfunction may be multifactorial, there is a growing body of evidence that increased production of reactive oxygen species (ROS) may contribute considerably to this phenomenon. ROS production has been demonstrated to occur in the endothelial cell layer and also within the media and adventitia, all of which may impair NO signaling within vascular tissue to endothelium-dependent but also endothelium-independent vasodilators. More recent experimental but also clinical studies point to the pathophysiological importance of the xanthine oxidase, the vascular NADPH oxidase, mitochondria, and an uncoupled endothelial nitric oxide synthase as significant enzymatic superoxide sources. We will discuss each of these systems below.

The mitochondrial respiratory chain can be a major source of superoxide. During aerobic metabolism, the oxidoreduction energy of mitochondrial electron transport is converted to the high-energy phosphate bond of ATP via a multicomponent NADH dehydrogenase complex [34]. Molecular oxygen serves as the final electron acceptor for cytochrome (Cyt)-c oxidase (complex IV), the terminal component of the respiratory chain, and is ultimately reduced to water (H_2O). Up to 1–4% of O_2 even under normal physiological conditions may be incompletely reduced, resulting in $O_2^{-\bullet}$ formation, mainly at complex I (NADH coenzyme Q reductase) and complex III (ubiquinol Cyt c reductase). Increased mitochondrial $O_2^{-\bullet}$ generation can be enhanced in certain conditions such as conditions of metabolic perturbation, hypoxia-reoxygenation and ischemia-reperfusion, where the enhanced $O_2^{-\bullet}$ is at least partially responsible for an increase in endothelial permeability [35].

XO. Xanthine oxidoreductase (XOR) is a ubiquitous metalloflavoprotein found as one of two interconvertible yet functionally distinct forms, namely xanthine dehydrogenase (XD), which is constitutively expressed *in vivo*, and XO, which is generated by the posttranslational modification of XD [36]. Functionally, both XD and XO catalyze oxidation of hypoxanthine to xanthine and xanthine to urate. However, whereas XD requires NAD+ as an electron acceptor, XO instead requires the reduction of molecular O_2, thereby generating $O_2^{-\bullet}$. The conversion of XD to XO occurs either through reversible thiol oxidation of sulfhydryl residues on XD or via irreversible proteolytic cleavage of a segment of XD during hypoxia, ischemia, or in the presence of various proinflammatory mediators [e.g., tumor necrosis factor-α (TNF-α)] [36].

Dysfunctional or uncoupled NOSs are a source of oxygen radicals. Even the enzyme that makes NO can produce oxygen radicals instead. NOSs are complex homodimeric oxidoreductases that shuttle electrons from the reductase domain of one monomer (a CYP-like region containing the cofactors FAD, FMN, and NADPH) to the oxidase domain in the other subunit that contains the heme active site. In view of this enzymatic structure, it is not surprising that NOS can become "uncoupled," leading to the generation of $O_2^{-\bullet}$ rather than NO. The essential NOS cofactor tetrahydrobiopterin (BH_4) appears to have a key role in regulating NOS function by "coupling" the reduction of molecular O_2 to L-arginine oxidation as well as maintaining the stability of NOS dimers [37]. Thus BH_4 availability may be a crucial factor in the balance between NO and $O_2^{-\bullet}$ generation by eNOS. Furthermore, BH_4 itself is highly susceptible to oxidative degradation, and the initial oxidative loss of BH_4 in response to increased ROS production by NADPH oxidases has been shown to amplify oxidative stress through the resulting loss of NO production and increased NOS-dependent $O_2^{-\bullet}$ generation [38]. In addition to increased catabolism or degradation, another reason for BH_4 depletion may be its reduced synthesis.

NADPH oxidases. In recent years, it has become apparent that endothelial cells and other nonphagocytic cells constitutively express an $O_2^{-\bullet}$-generating enzyme analogous to the phagocyte NADPH oxidase of neutrophils [39]. All the classical neutrophil oxidase components are expressed in endothelial cells, but the enzyme nevertheless exhibits several major differences from the neutrophil oxidase for example it continuously generates a low level of $O_2^{-\bullet}$ even in unstimulated cells, although its activity can be further increased by several agonists and a substantial proportion of the $O_2^{-\bullet}$ generated by the enzyme is produced intracellularly, whereas neutrophil oxidase $O_2^{-\bullet}$ generation occurs mainly in the extracellular compartment.

Normal physiological processes are continuously generating superoxide and other oxygen radicals that can quickly and effectively inactivate NO. Fortunately there are a number of antioxidant systems, both enzymatic and non-enzymatic that help to limit the amount of ROS produced to preserve NO activity. It appears the production of NO is a war of attrition. There are many circumstances in the production pathway that can diminish its output but there are also many physiological factors that can quickly inactivate NO once it has been successfully produced.

ENDOTHELIAL DYSFUNCTION AND CARDIOVASCULAR RISK FACTORS

It is well known that endothelial dysfunction is frequently encountered in the presence of cardiovascular risk factors. This has been shown for chronic smokers, patients with increased low-density lipoprotein (LDL) levels, for patients with diabetes Type I and II, for hypertensive patients, and for patients with the metabolic syndrome. It is important to note that cardiovascular risk factors synergistically impair endothelial function. Chronic smoking, defined as 20 pack years, have comparable negative effects for endothelial function to high LDL levels. The combination of both risk factors drastically impairs NO dependent forearm blood flow [40]. What is the key mechanism underlying endothelial dysfunction in patients with cardiovascular risk factors or established coronary artery disease? As described above it is the changes in the activity and/or expression of the eNOS, decreased sensitivity of vascular smooth muscle cells to NO, or increased degradation of NO via its interaction with ROS such as superoxide.

ASSESSMENT OF NITRIC OXIDE AVAILABILITY

The major pathway for NO metabolism is the stepwise oxidation to nitrite and nitrate [41]. In plasma or other physiological fluids or buffers NO is oxidized almost completely to nitrite, where it remains stable for several hours [42,43]. NO and nitrite are rapidly oxidized to nitrate in whole blood. The half life of nitrite (NO_2^-) in human blood is about 110 seconds [44]. Nitrate (NO_3^-) on the other hand has a circulating half life of 5–8 hours [45,46]. For years both nitrite and nitrate have been used as surrogate markers of NO production in biological tissues. During fasting conditions with low intake of nitrite/nitrate, enzymatic NO formation from NOS accounts for the majority of nitrite [47]. On the basis of these studies, it was believed that NO is acutely terminated by oxidation to nitrite and nitrate. However, it is now appreciated that nitrite or nitrate can recapitulate NO physiology.

A report by Kleinbongard *et al.* [48] demonstrates that plasma nitrite levels progressively decrease with increasing cardiovascular risk load indicating a reduction in nitric oxide produced. Risk factors considered include age, hypertension, smoking, and hypercholesterolemia, conditions all known for reduced bioavailability of NO. Although a correlation exists in the plasma, it is not known whether the situation is mirrored in the heart or other tissue at risk for ischemic injury or disease. If so, tissue nitrite may serve as an index of risk and restoring tissue nitrite may act as a first line of defense for protecting organs from ischemic and/or I/R injury. Since a substantial portion of steady state nitrite concentrations in blood and tissue are derived from dietary sources [49,50], modulation of nitrite intake may provide a first line of defense for cardiovascular disease [51].

CLINICAL CONSEQUENCES OF NO INSUFFICIENCY

The inability of our body to produce nitric oxide is the earliest indication that disease will ensue. Physical or biochemical injury to the endothelium impairs production and/or function of endothelium-derived vasoprotective mediators of vascular health, such as NO, resulting in increased vascular contractions to vasoconstrictors such as endothelin-1, thromboxanes and serotonin [52], enhanced thrombus formation and exacerbated SMC proliferation and migration [53]. It is, therefore, not surprising that loss of endothelial NO function is associated with several cardiovascular disorders, including atherosclerosis, which is due either to decreased production or to increased degradation of NO [1]. Decreased production may be the result of oxidized LDL mediated displacement of eNOS from plasmalemmal caveolae thereby inhibiting acetylcholine induced activation of the enzyme [54]. Moreover, decreased NO increases the tendency for lesion progression by enhancing vascular smooth muscle proliferation and migration, augmenting platelet activation and thrombosis, possibly participating in intravascular neovascularization, and favoring adverse lipid modification [55]. Once lesions have developed, endothelial dysfunction may exacerbate development of clinical events. Impaired endothelium may abnormally reduce vascular perfusion, produce factors that decrease plaque stability, and augment the thrombotic response to plaque rupture [56]. Augmentation of NO or restoration of NOS function seems a logical means to inhibit atherosclerosis. However, overexpression of endothelial NOS accelerates lesion formation in apoE-deficient mice [57] demonstrating that enhanced NOS derived NO may not always be beneficial. Supplementation with tetrahydrobiopterin (BH_4) reduced the lesion size to those seen in Apo E knockout mice revealing the requirement of enzyme cofactors. Even with BH_4 supplementation there was still no effect on lesion development.

Atherosclerosis involves several highly interrelated processes, including lipid disturbances, platelet activation, thrombosis, endothelial dysfunction, inflammation, oxidative stress, vascular smooth cell activation, altered matrix metabolism, remodeling, and genetic factors [58]. There is now a consensus that atherosclerosis represents a state of heightened oxidative stress characterized by lipid and protein oxidation in the vascular wall [59]. Production of reactive oxygen and nitrogen species by vascular cell as well as oxidative modification to proteins contribute to important clinical manifestations of coronary artery disease such as endothelial dysfunction and plague disruption. Experimental and clinical studies provide evidence that defects of endothelial NO function is not only associated with all major cardiovascular risk factors, such as hyperlipidemia, diabetes, hypertension, smoking and severity of atherosclerosis, but also has a profound predictive value for the future atherosclerotic disease progression [2–5]. Therefore, the dysfunctional eNOS/NO pathway is considered as an early marker or a common mechanism for various cardiovascular disorders and therefore provides an ideal target for therapeutic or preventive intervention once NO homeostasis is better understood in atherosclerosis.

Our ability to produce NO from the classical L-arginine pathway is complex and requires normal blood flow and oxygen and substrate delivery. One of the most important clinical conditions that affect public health today is ischemia-reperfusion injury. Ischemia and reperfusion (I/R)-induced injury and inflammation represents a major clinical problem associated with hemorrhagic or endotoxin shock and thermal injury as well as transplantation and resectional surgery, stroke, heart attack and sickle cell disease. Ischemia is defined by as a disruption or deficiency in blood flow either due to vessel constriction or physical obstruction of the vessel as in atherosclerosis. Reperfusion is the restoration of blood flow to ischemic tissue. schemic heart disease, including myocardial infarction, remains the leading cause of morbidity and mortality in all industrialized nations [60]. There are two distinct components of damage to the heart or brain in patients who experience acute myocardial infarction or ischemic stroke: ischemic injury and reperfusion injury. The myocardium or brain is able to tolerate brief periods of ischemia as activation of inherent, adaptive mechanisms can preserve energy levels and prevent injury. These include switching metabolism to anaerobic glycolysis and fatty acid utilization, increasing glucose uptake, and decreasing contractility. If ischemia persists however, the myocardium will develop a severe ATP deficit, resulting in irreversible injury and culminating in cell death. Although reperfusion of ischemic tissues provides oxygen and metabolic substrates necessary for the recovery and survival of reversibly injured cells, reperfusion itself paradoxically results in the acceleration of cellular necrosis [61]. Reperfusion is characterized by the formation of oxygen radicals upon reintroduction of molecular oxygen to ischemic tissues, resulting in widespread lipid and protein oxidative modifications, mitochondrial injury, as well as tissue apoptosis and necrosis [62,63]. NO has been shown to be a critical molecule in limiting I/R injury. However the L-arginine:NO pathway is not functional during ischemia due to insufficient oxygen, substrate delivery and reduced co-factors. A growing body of experimental data suggests that an important initiating event in the pathophysiology of I/R-induced tissue injury is the decrease steady production of NO concomitant with increased generation of reactive oxygen species. There is evidence supporting the hypothesis that this redox imbalance induced in post-ischemic tissue creates a more oxidative environment within inflammatory cells and the parachyma. Production of these inflammatory mediators may injure tissue directly as well as induce chemokine and endothelial cell adhesion molecule expression thereby promoting leukocyte infiltration into the post-ischemic tissue and amplifying inflammatory tissue damage. Emerging evidence reveals very impressive protective properties of nitrite and nitrate in ischemia reperfusion injury that can be modulated by dietary changes. We will reveal those protective properties in the coming chapters.

Risk factors for Endothelial Dysfunction:

- Smoking
- Physical inactivity
- High cholesterol
- Diabetes
- Hypertension
- Family history
- Menopause
- Age

ABOUT THE AUTHORS

Nathan S. Bryan, Ph.D.

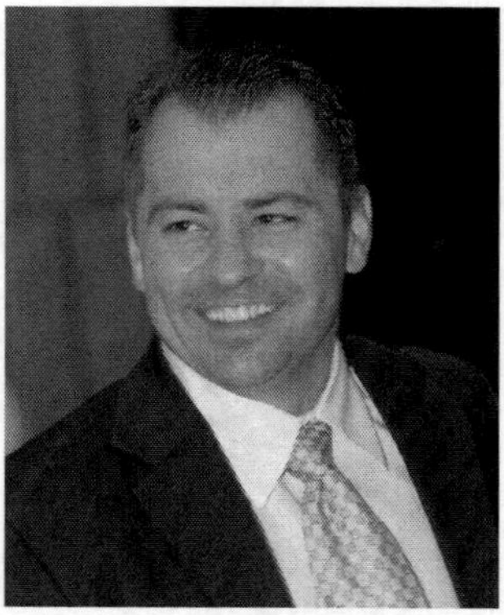

Dr. Bryan was born in Bryan Texas in November 1973. Nathan grew up in small town Texas. He spent his grade school years in Lexington (population 1000) and attended High School in Caldwell (population 3000). He earned his undergraduate Bachelor of Science degree in Biochemistry from the University of Texas at Austin and his doctoral degree from Louisiana State University School of Medicine in Shreveport where he was the recipient of the Dean's Award for Excellence in Research. He pursued his post-doctoral training as a Kirschstein Fellow at Boston University School of Medicine in the Whitaker Cardiovascular Institute. Dr. Bryan joined the Institute of Molecular Medicine, University of Texas Health Science Center in Houston, in June 2006 in the Center for Cell Signaling. He is also a faculty member of the Department of Integrative Biology and Pharmacology and Graduate School of Biomedical Sciences at the UT Houston Medical School. He is an active member of the Nitric Oxide Society, Society for Free Radical Biology and Medicine and the American Heart Association.

Dr. Bryan's research is dedicated to providing a better understanding of the interactions of nitric oxide (NO) and related metabolites with their different biological targets at the molecular and cellular level and the significance of these reactions for physiology and pathophysiology. Attempts are made to identify what particular changes in NO-related signaling pathways and reaction products occur in disease states such as endothelial dysfunction, ischemia/reperfusion, tissue/cardiac protection, diabetes, atherosclerosis and inflammation with the aim of testing their amenability as biomarkers for diagnosis and/or treatment of specific disease.

Current research is directed to understand the interactions of exogenous dietary nitrite/nitrate (NOx) on the endogenous NO/cGMP pathway and how perturbations in each system affect cardiovascular health. This involves mechanisms of nitrite transport and cellular uptake as well as mechanism of nitrite reduction back to NO and via direct NO-independent signaling actions of nitrite. Work in Dr. Bryan's lab involves molecular biology and analytical biochemistry utilizing gas phase chemiluminescence and HPLC in multiple organ systems and blood.

Much of the work involves *in vivo* characterization of NO/nitrite metabolism using a number of transgenic and knockout animal models of disease. Dr. Bryan and colleagues recently discovered that nitrite is a biologically active molecule which was previously thought to be an inert breakdown product of NO production. These findings have unveiled many beneficial effects of nitrite in the treatment and prevention of human disease. These discoveries may provide the basis for new preventive or therapeutic strategies in diseases associated with NO insufficiency and new guidelines for optimal health. Since nitrite and nitrate are common constituents of many fruits and vegetables, changes in dietary habits may have profound effects on many diseases associated with NO insufficiency. NO insufficiency is a hallmark of a number of diseases including cardiovascular disease. The notion that nitrite can recapitulate NO biochemistry and serve as an alternative and compensatory mechanism of NO production is revolutionary. It may also serve as the endocrine mediator of NO signaling. Moreover, the direct signaling actions of nitrite may represent a novel NO independent pathway for nitrite. If our current understanding is true, then an optimal diet may then consist of a sufficient supply of nitrite and nitrate for health and disease prevention. Understanding this pathway will provide the basis for new preventive or therapeutic strategies in diseases associated with NO insufficiency and new guidelines for optimal health. To date Dr. Bryan has published over 20 peer reviewed papers that have been cited over 1000 times. He has been invited to speak at a number of national and international meetings.

Dr. Bryan currently resides in Houston with his wife Kristen and their two sons Grant and Lincoln. The Bryans spend their weekends at their ranch near Caldwell where they raise cattle and horses and enjoy the great outdoors. Nathan enjoys playing golf and calf roping and team roping on his ranch and in competition.

Matthew B. Grisham, Ph.D.

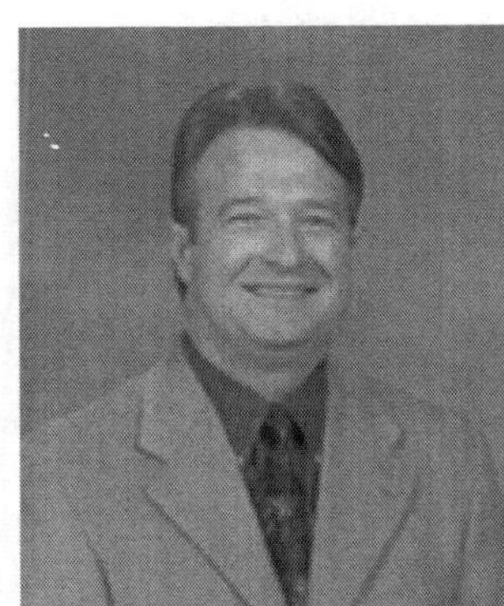

Dr. Grisham is a Boyd Professor in the Department of Molecular and Cellular Physiology and the Associate Director of Research for the Center of Excellence for Arthritis and Rheumatology at LSU Health Sciences Center in Shreveport, Louisiana. Dr. Grisham is currently an Associate Editor of the journals Inflammatory Bowel Disease, American Journal of Physiology and Free Radical Biology and Medicine.

He has served or is currently serving on the editorial boards of the Journal of Immunology, Inflammatory Bowel Disease and the American Journal of Physiology. Dr. Grisham is an active member of the Grants Review Committee for the Crohn's and Colitis Foundation of America (CCFA) and for the National Institute of Digestive Diseases and Kidney at the National Institutes of Health. He has held the position of President of the Society for Free Radical Biology and Medicine as well as served as Councilor for the Immunology, Microbiology and Inflammatory Bowel Disease section of the American Gastroenterological Association. In addition, Dr. Grisham served as Chair of the Gastrointestinal and Liver Section of the American Physiological Society. Dr. Grisham's research focuses on T-cell trafficking and regulation of chronic inflammation. His research has been continuously funded for the past 20 years by NIH and has been awarded several research grants from the CCFA and Broad Foundation. He has published more than 266 peered-reviewed journal articles, 85 book chapters, edited two books and written one book all related to the immuno-pathological mechanisms responsible for acute and chronic inflammation.

REFERENCES

1. Davignon, J. and P. Ganz, Role of endothelial dysfunction in atherosclerosis. *Circulation,* 2004. 109(23 Suppl 1): p. III27–32.
2. Schachinger, V., M.B. Britten, and A.M. Zeiher, Prognostic impact of coronary vasodilator dysfunction on adverse long-term outcome of coronary heart disease. *Circulation,* 2000. 101(16): p. 1899–906.
3. Halcox, J.P., et al., Prognostic value of coronary vascular endothelial dysfunction. *Circulation,* 2002. 106(6): p. 653–8.
4. Bugiardini, R., et al., Endothelial function predicts future development of coronary artery disease: a study of women with chest pain and normal coronary angiograms. *Circulation,* 2004. 109(21): p. 2518–23.
5. Lerman, A. and A.M. Zeiher, Endothelial function: cardiac events. *Circulation,* 2005. 111(3): p. 363–8.
6. Esposito, K., et al., Effect of dietary antioxidants on postprandial endothelial dysfunction induced by a high-fat meal in healthy subjects. *Am J Clin Nutr,* 2003. 77(1): p. 139–43.
7. Gold, M.E., P.A. Bush, and L.J. Ignarro, Depletion of arterial L-arginine causes reversible tolerance to endothelium-dependent relaxation. *Biochem Biophys Res Commun,* 1989. 164(2): p. 714–21.
8. Bredt, D.S. and S.H. Snyder, Isolation of nitric oxide synthetase, a calmodulin-requiring enzyme. *Proc Natl Acad Sci U S A*, 1990. 87(2): p. 682–5.
9. Boger, R.H. and S.M. Bode-Boger, The clinical pharmacology of L-arginine. Annu Rev Pharmacol Toxicol, 2001. 41: p. 79–99.
10. Wei, L.H., et al., IL-4 and IL-13 upregulate arginase I expression by cAMP and JAK/STAT6

pathways in vascular smooth muscle cells. *Am J Physiol Cell Physiol,* 2000. 279(1): p. C248–56.

11. Berkowitz, D.E., et al., Arginase reciprocally regulates nitric oxide synthase activity and contributes to endothelial dysfunction in aging blood vessels. *Circulation,* 2003. 108(16): p. 2000–6.
12. Buga, G.M., et al., Arginase activity in endothelial cells: inhibition by NG-hydroxy-L-arginine during high-output NO production. *Am J Physiol,* 1996. 271(5 Pt 2): p. H1988–98.
13. Jay, M.T., et al., Modulation of vascular tone by low density lipoproteins: effects on L-arginine transport and nitric oxide synthesis. *Exp Physiol,* 1997. 82(2): p. 349–60.
14. Kikuta, K., et al., High-affinity arginine transport of bovine aortic endothelial cells is impaired by lysophosphatidylcholine. *Circ Res,* 1998. 83(11): p. 1088–96.
15. McDonald, K.K., et al., A caveolar complex between the cationic amino acid transporter 1 and endothelial nitric-oxide synthase may explain the "arginine paradox". *J Biol Chem,* 1997. 272(50): p. 31213–6.
16. Vallance, P., et al., Accumulation of an endogenous inhibitor of nitric oxide synthesis in chronic renal failure. *Lancet,* 1992. 339(8793): p. 572–5.
17. Boger, R.H., et al., Asymmetric dimethylarginine (ADMA): a novel risk factor for endothelial dysfunction: its role in hypercholesterolemia. *Circulation,* 1998. 98(18): p. 1842–7.
18. Kielstein, J.T., et al., Cardiovascular effects of systemic nitric oxide synthase inhibition with asymmetrical dimethylarginine in humans. *Circulation,* 2004. 109(2): p. 172–7.
19. Stuhlinger, M.C., et al., Homocysteine impairs the nitric oxide synthase pathway: role of asymmetric dimethylarginine. *Circulation,* 2001. 104(21): p. 2569–75.
20. Stuhlinger, M.C., et al., Relationship between insulin resistance and an endogenous nitric oxide synthase inhibitor. *Jama,* 2002. 287(11): p. 1420–6.
21. Stuhlinger, M.C., et al., Endothelial dysfunction induced by hyperhomocyst(e)inemia: role of asymmetric dimethylarginine. *Circulation,* 2003. 108(8): p. 933–8.
22. Lin, K.Y., et al., Impaired nitric oxide synthase pathway in diabetes mellitus: role of asymmetric dimethylarginine and dimethylarginine dimethylaminohydrolase. *Circulation,* 2002. 106(8): p. 987–92.
23. Weis, M., et al., Cytomegalovirus infection impairs the nitric oxide synthase pathway: role of asymmetric dimethylarginine in transplant arteriosclerosis. *Circulation,* 2004. 109(4): p. 500–5.
24. Sydow, K., et al., ADMA and oxidative stress are responsible for endothelial dysfunction in hyperhomocyst(e)inemia: effects of L-arginine and B vitamins. *Cardiovasc Res,* 2003. 57(1): p. 244–52.
25. Goonasekera, C.D., et al., Nitric oxide synthase inhibitors and hypertension in children and adolescents. *J Hypertens,* 1997. 15(8): p. 901–9.
26. Abbasi, F., et al., Plasma concentrations of asymmetric dimethylarginine are increased in patients with type 2 diabetes mellitus. *Am J Cardiol,* 2001. 88(10): p. 1201–3.
27. Boger, R.H., et al., Biochemical evidence for impaired nitric oxide synthesis in patients with peripheral arterial occlusive disease. *Circulation,* 1997. 95(8): p. 2068–74.
28. Valkonen, V.P., et al., Risk of acute coronary events and serum concentration of asymmetrical dimethylarginine. *Lancet,* 2001. 358(9299): p. 2127–8.
29. Pettersson, A., T. Hedner, and I. Milsom, Increased circulating concentrations of asymmetric dimethyl arginine (ADMA), an endogenous inhibitor of nitric oxide synthesis, in preeclampsia. *Acta Obstet Gynecol Scand,* 1998. 77(8): p. 808–13.

30. Usui, M., et al., Increased endogenous nitric oxide synthase inhibitor in patients with congestive heart failure. *Life Sci,* 1998. 62(26): p. 2425–30.
31. Bode-Boger, S.M., F. Scalera, and L.J. Ignarro, The l-arginine paradox: Importance of the l-arginine/asymmetrical dimethylarginine ratio. *Pharmacol Ther,* 2007. 114(3): p. 295–306.
32. Miyazaki, H., et al., Endogenous nitric oxide synthase inhibitor: a novel marker of atherosclerosis. *Circulation,* 1999. 99(9): p. 1141–6.
33. Zoccali, C., et al., Plasma concentration of asymmetrical dimethylarginine and mortality in patients with end-stage renal disease: a prospective study. *Lancet,* 2001. 358(9299): p. 2113–7.
34. Lenaz, G., Role of mitochondria in oxidative stress and ageing. *Biochim Biophys Acta,* 1998. 1366(1-2): p. 53–67.
35. Pearlstein, D.P., et al., Role of mitochondrial oxidant generation in endothelial cell responses to hypoxia. *Arterioscler Thromb Vasc Biol,* 2002. 22(4): p. 566–73.
36. Meneshian, A. and G.B. Bulkley, The physiology of endothelial xanthine oxidase: from urate catabolism to reperfusion injury to inflammatory signal transduction. *Microcirculation,* 2002. 9(3): p. 161–75.
37. Vasquez-Vivar, J., B. Kalyanaraman, and P. Martasek, The role of tetrahydrobiopterin in superoxide generation from eNOS: enzymology and physiological implications. *Free Radic Res,* 2003. 37(2): p. 121–7.
38. Landmesser, U., et al., Oxidation of tetrahydrobiopterin leads to uncoupling of endothelial cell nitric oxide synthase in hypertension. *J Clin Invest,* 2003. 111(8): p. 1201–9.
39. Griendling, K.K., D. Sorescu, and M. Ushio-Fukai, NAD(P)H oxidase: role in cardiovascular biology and disease. *Circ Res,* 2000. 86(5): p. 494–501.
40. Heitzer, T., et al., Cigarette smoking potentiates endothelial dysfunction of forearm resistance vessels in patients with hypercholesterolemia. Role of oxidized LDL. *Circulation,* 1996. 93(7): p. 1346–53.
41. Yoshida, K., et al., Biotransformation of nitric oxide, nitrite and nitrate. *Int Arch Occup Environ Health,* 1983. 52: p. 103–115.
42. Grube, R., et al., *The Biology of Nitric Oxide, in Enzymology, Biochemistry, and Immunology,* S. Moncada, et al., Editors. 1994, Portland Press: London. p. 201–204.
43. Kelm, M., et al., *The Biology of nitric oxide. Physiological and Clinical Aspects, S. Moncada,* et al., Editors. 1992, Portland Press: London. p. 319–322.
44. Kelm, M., Nitric oxide metabolism and breakdown. *Biochim Biophys Acta,* 1999. 1411: p. 273–289.
45. Tannenbaum, S.R., Nitrate and nitrite: origin in humans. *Science,* 1994. 205: p. 1333–1335.
46. Kelm, M. and K. Yoshida, Metabolic Fate of Nitric Oxide and Related N-oxides, in *Methods in Nitric Oxide Research,* M. Feelisch and J.S. Stamler, Editors. 1996, John Wiley and Sons: Chichester. p. 47–58.
47. Rhodes, P., et al., The L-arginine:nitric oxide pathway is the major source of plasma nitrite in fasted humans. *Biochem Biophys Res Commun,* 1995. 209: p. 590–596.
48. Kleinbongard, P., et al., Plasma nitrite concentrations reflect the degree of endothelial dysfunction in humans. *Free Radic Biol Med,* 2006. 40(2): p. 295–302.
49. Bryan, N.S., et al., Dietary nitrite restores NO homeostasis and is cardioprotective in endothelial nitric oxide synthase-deficient mice. *Free Radic Biol Med,* 2008. 45(4): p. 468–74.
50. Bryan, N.S., et al., Nitrite is a signaling molecule and regulator of gene expression in mammalian tissues. *Nat Chem Biol,* 2005. 1(5): p. 290–7.

51. Bryan, N.S., Nitrite in nitric oxide biology: Cause or consequence? A systems-based review. *Free Radic Biol Med,* 2006. 41(5): p. 691–701.

52. Lamping, K. and F. Faraci, Enhanced vasoconstrictor responses in eNOS deficient mice. *Nitric Oxide,* 2003. 8(4): p. 207–13.

53. Moncada, S., R.M.J. Palmer, and A. Higgs, Nitric oxide: physiology, pathophysiology and pharmacology. *Pharmacol Rev,* 1991. 43(2): p. 109–142.

54. Blair, A., et al., Oxidized low density lipoprotein displaces endothelial nitric-oxide synthase (eNOS) from plasmalemmal caveolae and impairs eNOS activation. *J Biol Chem,* 1999. 274(45): p. 32512–9.

55. Loscalzo, J., Nitric oxide insufficiency, platelet activation, and arterial thrombosis. *Circ Res,* 2001. 88(8): p. 756–62.

56. Faxon, D.P., et al., Atherosclerotic Vascular Disease Conference: Writing Group III: pathophysiology. *Circulation,* 2004. 109(21): p. 2617–25.

57. Ozaki, M., et al., Overexpression of endothelial nitric oxide synthase accelerates atherosclerotic lesion formation in apoE-deficient mice. *J Clin Invest,* 2002. 110(3): p. 331–40.

58. Libby, P., Inflammation in atherosclerosis. *Nature,* 2002. 420(6917): p. 868–74.

59. Stocker, R. and J.F.J. Keaney, Role of Oxidative Modifications in Atherosclerosis. *Physiol Rev,* 2004. 84: p. 1381–1478.

60. Myerburg, R.J., Sudden cardiac death: exploring the limits of our knowledge. *J Cardiovasc Electrophysiol,* 2001. 12(3): p. 369–81.

61. Braunwald, E. and R.A. Kloner, Myocardial reperfusion: a double-edged sword? *J Clin Invest,* 1985. 76(5): p. 1713–9.

62. McCord, J.M., R.S. Roy, and S.W. Schaffer, Free radicals and myocardial ischemia. The role of xanthine oxidase. *Adv Myocardiol,* 1985. 5: p. 183–9.

63. Nayler, W.G., The role of calcium in the ischemic myocardium. *Am J Pathol,* 1981. 102(2): p. 262–70.

CHAPTER 3

The Nitrate-Nitrite-Nitric Oxide Pathway

JON O LUNDBERG and EDDIE WEITZBERG

Karolinska Institutet

NOW that we have an appreciation for complexity of nitric oxide production and cell signaling in health and disease, we will begin now with an introduction to an alternative pathway to make nitric oxide independent of the L-arginine pathway that involves a symbiotic relationship with commensal bacteria that reside on and in our body as well as the bacteria that reside in the soil. This chapter will describe the transformation of atmospheric nitrogen in the environment to assimilation into nitrogen oxide metabolites in the plants and animals we eat. We will then reveal how the anions nitrite and nitrate affect nitric oxide homeostasis and how changes in these metabolites function in our body. This will provide the critical link between our dietary habits and NO homeostasis in our body. We first begin with a description of the nitrogen cycle.

Earth's atmosphere is about 78% nitrogen, making it the largest pool of nitrogen. Nitrogen is essential for many biological processes; and is crucial for any life here on Earth. It is in all amino acids, is incorporated into proteins, and is present in the bases that make up nucleic acids, such as DNA and RNA. In plants, much of the nitrogen is used in chlorophyll molecules which are essential for photosynthesis and further growth [1]. Processing, or fixation, is necessary to convert gaseous nitrogen into forms usable by living organisms. The nitrogen cycle in nature involves a process in which the abundant supply of atmospheric nitrogen (N_2) is fixed into forms usable by living organisms. The nitrogen cycle is the biogeochemical cycle that describes the transformations of nitrogen and nitrogen-containing compounds in nature. Nitrogen in the air becomes a part of biological matter mostly through the actions of bacteria and algae in a process known as nitrogen fixation. Legume plants such as clover, alfalfa, and soybeans form nodules on the roots where nitrogen fixing bacteria take nitrogen from the air and convert it into ammonia, NH_3. These bacteria have the nitrogenase enzyme that combines gaseous nitrogen with hydrogen to produce ammonia, which is then further converted by the bacteria in the soil to make its own organic compounds. Some nitrogen fixing bacteria, such as *Rhizobium,* live in the root nodules of legumes (such as peas or beans). Here they form a mutualistic relationship with the plant, producing ammonia in exchange for carbohydrates. Nutrient-poor soils can be planted with legumes to enrich them with nitrogen. During the nitrogen cycle ammonia is converted by bacteria first into nitrite ions, NO_2^-, and then into nitrate ions, NO_3^-. Plants utilize the nitrate ions as a nutrient or fertilizer for growth. In the denitrification part of the nitrogen cycle, nitrate is converted back to N_2 again in a series of reductions catalysed by anaerobic bacteria. In this pathway nitric oxide is an obligate intermediate [2] (see Figure 3.1). All nitrogen obtained by animals can be traced back to the eating of plants at some stage of the food chain.

During anaerobic (low oxygen) conditions, denitrification by bacteria occurs. Denitrification is the reduction of nitrites back into the largely inert nitrogen gas (N_2), completing the nitrogen cycle. This process is performed by bacterial species such as Pseudomonas and Clostridium in anaerobic conditions. They use the nitrate as an electron acceptor in the place of oxygen during respiration. This results in nitrates being converted to nitrogen gases (NO, N_2O, N_2) and returned to the atmosphere. Nitrate can also be reduced to nitrite and subsequently combine with ammonium in the anaerobic ammonium oxidation process, which also results in the production of dinitrogen gas. This is all part of nitrogen fixation. The conversion of nitrogen (N_2) from the atmosphere into a form readily available to plants and hence to animals and humans is an important step in the nitrogen cycle, that determines the supply of this essential nutrient. This process is illustrated in Figure 3.1.

Plants can absorb nitrate or ammonium ions from the soil via their root hairs. If nitrate is absorbed, it is first reduced to nitrite ions and then ammonium ions for incorporation into amino acids, nucleic acids, and chlorophyll. This is referred to as assimilation. In plants which have a mutualistic relationship with rhizobia, some nitrogen is assimilated in the form of ammonium ions directly from the nodules. Animals, fungi, and other heterotrophic organisms absorb nitrogen as amino acids, nucleotides and other small organic molecules. The amount of nitrite and nitrate contained in a plant depends on its developmental stage.

When a plant or animal dies, or an animal excretes, the initial form of nitrogen is organic. Bacteria, or in some cases, fungi, convert the organic

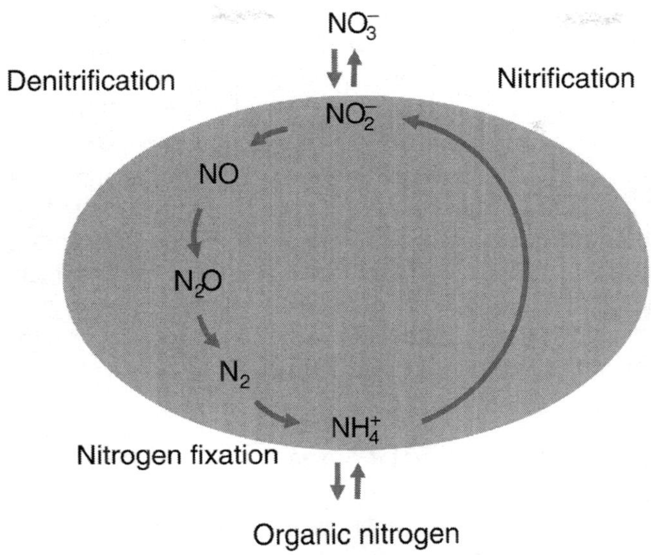

FIGURE 3.1 A highly simplified version of the nitrogen cycle in nature. Nitrogen is crucial for all living cells as it forms an essential part of amino acids and DNA. Nitrogen (N_2) is the major component of earth's atmosphere (about 78%) but gaseous nitrogen is extremely stable and virtually inert. Therefore, processing, or fixation is necessary to convert gaseous nitrogen into forms usable by living organisms. Nitrogen fixation is mainly performed by specific bacteria in the soil and root nodules of certain legumes. The ammonia then formed can be taken up directly by plants. However, much of the ammonia produced by decay is oxidized into nitrite and nitrate by other types of bacteria in a process termed nitrification. Many vegetables naturally accumulate great amounts of nitrate in their leaves and roots. Nitrate is extremely water soluble and reaches the soil through leaching and when the plants shed their leaves. The nitrogen cycle is completed by denitrification in which anaerobic bacteria stepwise reduce nitrate and nitrite, again forming gaseous nitrogen which is released into the atmosphere (modified from reference 2).

nitrogen within the remains back into ammonia, a process called ammonification or mineralization. The conversion of ammonia to nitrates is performed primarily by soil-living bacteria and other nitrifying bacteria. The primary stage of nitrification, the oxidation of ammonia (NH_3) is performed by bacteria such as the Nitrosomonas species, which converts ammonia to nitrites (NO_2^-). Other bacterial species, such as the Nitrobacter, are responsible for the oxidation of the nitrites into nitrates (NO_3^-). It is important for the nitrites to be converted to nitrates because accumulated nitrites are toxic to plant life.

While bacteria generate NO anaerobically via reductions, mammals instead utilize oxidation reactions to produce the same gas. As stated in Chapter 1, NO synthases catalyze an oxygen-dependent 5-electron oxidation of the amino acid L-arginine to form NO and L-citrulline. Until recently, this was thought to be the only way by which NO can be formed in humans and other mammals. However, this has turned out not to be true. Here we discuss a previously unknown mammalian nitrogen cycle, in which the inorganic anions nitrate and nitrite are converted back to NO and other bioactive nitrogen oxides in blood and tissues. Again, bacteria play a central role in this cycle, but in this case it's the commensal bacteria that inhabit our body surfaces and our gastrointestinal system. In addition, a number of mammalian enzymes and proteins participate in the formation of NO from nitrate and nitrite.

NO GENERATION WITHOUT NO SYNTHASE

In 1994 two groups independently presented evidence for generation of NO in the stomach resulting from the acidic reduction of inorganic nitrite [3,4]. Benjamin and colleagues demonstrated that the antibacterial effects of acid alone was markedly enhanced by addition of nitrite which is present in saliva whereas Lundberg and colleagues could measure high levels of NO in expelled air from the stomach in humans. These levels were abolished after pretreatment with a proton pump inhibitor and markedly increased after ingestion of nitrate, showing the importance of both luminal pH and the conversion of nitrate to nitrite for stomach NO generation. These were the first reports of NO synthase-independent formation of NO *in vivo*. In the classical NO synthase pathway NO is formed by oxidation of the guanidino nitrogen of L-arginine with molecular oxygen as the co-substrate [5]. This complex reaction is catalysed by specific heme-containing enzymes; the NO synthases, and the reaction requires several co-factors. The alternative pathway was fundamentally different; instead of L-arginine it used the simple inorganic anions nitrate (NO_3^-) and nitrite (NO_2^-) as substrates in a stepwise reduction process that did not require NO synthase or multiple co-factors. The biochemical pathway and biological effects of nitrate reduction to nitrite and further on to NO in the gastrointestinal tract have now been further characterized [2] (Figure 3.2). Oral commensal bacteria are essential for the first step in the nitrate-nitrite-NO pathway since they are responsible for the reduction of the higher nitrogen oxide nitrate to form nitrite. It was known from the literature that the salivary glands extract nitrate from plasma but the reason for this active process was not explained. This active process leads to levels of salivary nitrate that are 10–20 fold

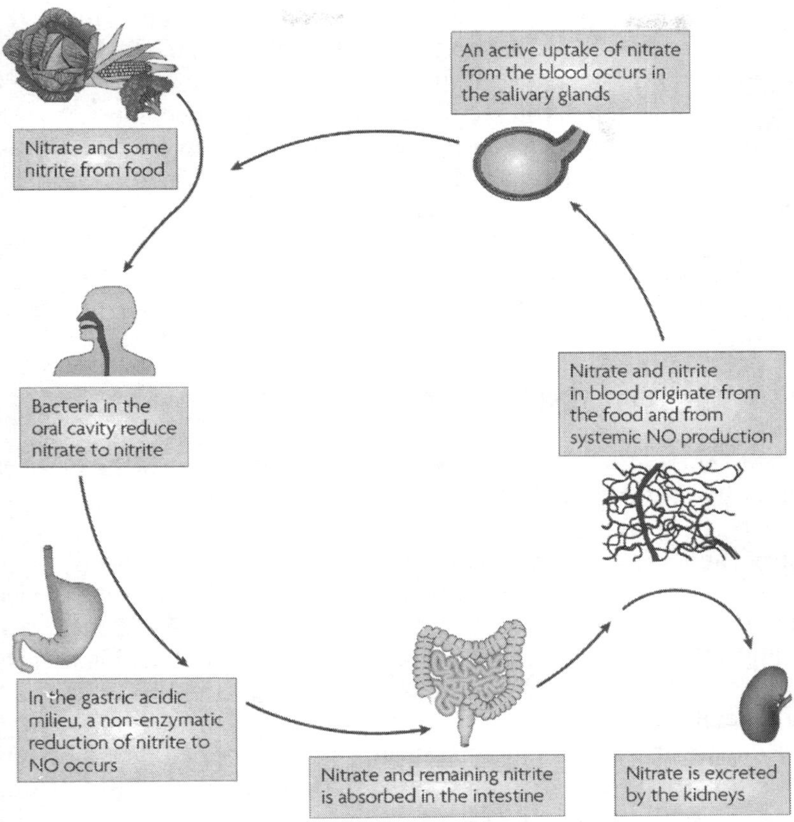

FIGURE 3.2 Ingested inorganic nitrate from dietary sources is rapidly absorbed in the small intestine. Although much of the circulating nitrate is eventually excreted in the urine, up to 25% is actively extracted by the salivary glands and concentrated in saliva. In the mouth, commensal facultative anaerobic bacteria effectively reduce nitrate to nitrite by the action of nitrate reductase enzymes. Nitrate reduction to nitrite requires the presence of these bacteria, as mammalian cells cannot effectively metabolize this anion. In the acidic stomach, nitrite is spontaneously decomposed to form nitric oxide (NO) and other bioactive nitrogen oxides, which regulate important physiological functions. Nitrate and remaining nitrite is absorbed from the intestine into the circulation and can convert to bioactive NO in blood and tissues under physiological hypoxia. (reproduced with permission from Lundberg et al *Nat Rev Drug Discov.* 2008 Feb; 7(2): 156–67).

higher than in plasma. Oral facultative anaerobic bacteria residing mainly in the crypts of the tongue, then reduce nitrate to nitrite by the action of nitrate reductase enzymes [6,7]. These bacteria use nitrate as an alternative electron acceptor to gain ATP in the absence of oxygen.

This highly effective bacterial nitrate reduction results in salivary levels of nitrite that are > 1000-fold higher than those found in plasma [8]. When nitrite-rich saliva meets the acidic gastric juice, nitrite is protonated to form nitrous acid (HNO_2) which then decomposes to NO and a variety of other nitrogen oxides [3,4]. It is now established that oral commensal bacteria are pivotal in gastric NO formation, and gastric NO levels are consistently low in animals reared under complete germ-free conditions [9]. If the oral flora is selectively removed by topical treatment with an antibacterial mouthwash, the gastric NO levels decrease drastically [10].

WHAT IS NO DOING IN THE STOMACH?

With regards to the biochemistry of nitrate and nitrite in the stomach, until 1994 when gastric NO was discovered, the entire research community had been focusing on one single issue; the formation of nitrosamines from nitrite and its possible role in carcinogenesis, in particular gastric cancer. At the time however, it was becoming very clear that NO synthase-derived NO was playing vital roles in a great variety of physiological processes. So, researchers started to study if gastric nitrite-derived NO instead of promoting carcinogenesis in fact could be beneficial.

Knowing that NO is used by activated white blood cells to kill bacteria and virus, Benjamin and coworkers first focused on host-defense. Indeed, NO and other nitrite-derived nitrogen oxides turned out to be toxic to microorganisms, including a variety of human pathogens [11–13]. Benjamin's lab elegantly showed that *E. coli*, *Salmonella*, *Shigella* and other potential pathogens are remarkably resistant in vitro when exposed to acid alone but are killed if exposed to a mixture of nitrite and acid [12]. Thus, gastric juice in combination with saliva might form an important part of our first line of defense against pathogens entering via the oral route. In addition to acting on luminal bacteria, nitrite-derived NO also affects the host mucosa. We now know that it stimulates gastric mucosal blood flow and mucus formation, and it reduces epithelial leakage; the three dominant mucosal defense mechanisms against luminal aggressors [14,15]. In animal experiments it has been shown that stimulation of gastric NO via ingestion of nitrate provides strong protection against ulcers caused by non-steroidal anti-inflammatory drugs [16] and other ulcerogenic stress [17,18].

In aggregate, it is becoming clear that the active extraction of nitrate from plasma by the salivary glands is not one of nature's flaws, but instead this energy-consuming process might serve important physiological purposes. In fact, this seems to be a beautiful example of symbiosis where the bacteria receive from the host a substrate (nitrate) necessary for its own respiration and in return give us nitrite, a substrate used for the production of NO.

INTERACTIONS BETWEEN NITRITE AND OTHER DIETARY COMPOUNDS

In one sense the stomach can be regarded as a bioreactor where different dietary compounds mix and react to form novel compounds, some of which are bioactive. Figure 3.3 highlights some reactions that specifically relate to nitrogen oxide chemistry under gastric conditions. In this example the focus is on vegetables, olive oil and wine which constitute a central part of the typical Mediterranean diet. As will be discussed in subsequent chapters, many vegetables including

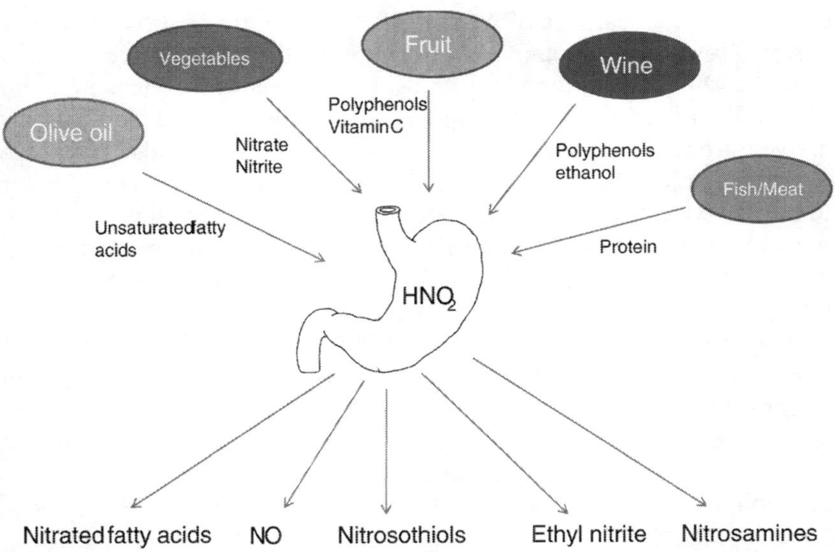

FIGURE 3.3 The stomach as a bioreactor for Chemical Interactions Between nitrate, nitrite and other dietary components. Nitrite-containing saliva is continuously swallowed into the acidic stomach where it immediately forms nitrous acid (HNO_2). From nitrous acid a variety of reactive nitrogen oxides (RNIs) are generated, and these can react with other dietary constituents to form novel biologically active compounds that act locally in the stomach, or systemically after absorption.

spinach, lettuce and beetroot are very rich in inorganic nitrate (NO_3^-). After ingestion, nitrate rapidly accumulates in saliva where it is reduced by commensal bacteria to form nitrite (NO_2^-). Nitrite is then swallowed into the acidic stomach and forms HNO_2. As described above, HNO_2 spontaneously yields NO via disproportionation, and this reduction is greatly enhanced in the presence of dietary polyphenols [19,20] and ascorbic acid [21]. An example is red wine in which the anthocyanin fraction and wine catechol (caffeic acid) greatly enhance NO generation from nitrite [19]. Interestingly, the ethanol in wine also reacts with nitrite under gastric conditions, thereby forming ethyl nitrite, another bioactive compound [22]. Ethyl nitrite is a potent vasodilator and it forms rapidly via O-nitrosation, when HNO_2 reacts with ethanol. Ethyl nitrite is also a potent nitrosating compound that can give rise to S-nitrosothiols and N-nitrosamines.

S-nitrosylation reactions give rise to nitrosothiols [23], and clearly these highly bioactive compounds are formed intragastrically from acidified nitrite [14]. Many of the NO-like effects of nitrite described in the stomach such as stimulation of mucosal blood flow and mucus generation, might proceed via intermediate formation of nitrosothiols which can act as stable carriers of NO. In addition, S-nitrosylation of critical cysteine residues in proteins, is also important in regulation of protein function [23]. Unsaturated fatty acids (e.g. linoleic and oleic acid) from olive oil or other oils may undergo nitration following reaction with reactive nitrogen intermediates (in particular the NO_2 radical) giving rise to nitrated lipids [24]. Although the existence of this latter reaction, is yet to be proven in vivo, the acidic nitrite-containing stomach is indeed an ideal milieu for nitration. Interestingly, nitrated lipids have anti-inflammatory effects and act as potent agonists of PPAR-gamma, a key regulator of the inflammatory cascade [25,26].

In aggregate, NO, nitrosothiols, ethyl nitrite and nitrated lipids are readily formed from dietary constituents when they react with nitrite under acidic conditions in the stomach. These can all act as transducers of NO-like bioactivity including vasodilation, stimulation of mucus generation, antimicrobial and anti-inflammatory effects. Many of the compounds formed intragastrically from acidified nitrite are fairly stable and readily absorbed which likely allows also for systemic effects. It is interesting that most nutrients highlighted in the figure may divert the chemistry in the stomach away from nitrosamine formation and instead favor the formation of other chemically related bioactive compounds. Future studies will clarify if the well-known heath promoting effects of a Mediterranean diet is related to this alternative chemical fate of dietary nitrate.

NITRITE REDUCTION TO NO IN BLOOD AND TISSUE

One year after the discovery of gastric NO, Zweier et al showed that the same reaction could occur also systemically [27]. They noted NO generation in the ischemic heart that was not inhibited by NO synthases, and through a series of experiments they could show that nitrite was the substrate. Today it is clear that nitrite can be reduced in vivo via numerous pathways to form bioactive NO. These include deoxyhemoglobin [28,29], deoxymyoglobin [30,31], xanthine oxidase [32–35], mitochondrial respiratory chain enzymes [36,37], cytochrome P-450 [38] and even NO synthase [39]. It seems clear that nitrite can induce vasodilation *in vitro* [40] and *in vivo* [28] at near physiological concentrations, and nitrite also has therapeutic effects, most notably in models of ischemia-reperfusion injury [41]. These interesting aspects of nitrite biology are discussed in more detail in Chapters 6 and 12. In the following we will focus on how the more stable nitrate anion, surprisingly also can have systemic NO-like effects.

SYSTEMIC EFFECT OF INORGANIC NITRATE

Nitrate is by far the dominating final oxidation product of NO and circulates in levels up to 1000-fold higher than nitrite [42]. In addition, our diet is a major provider of nitrate [2]. In all the experimental therapeutic studies mentioned above, nitrite has been used but the more stable anion nitrate has never been considered to have effects outside of the oral cavity or stomach where bacteria can reduce it to nitrite. In 2004 however, it was shown that inorganic nitrate indeed can be a major source of circulating nitrite [8]. In healthy subjects ingesting nitrate, a sustained 4–5 fold increase in plasma nitrite was noted. Intriguingly, these nitrite levels are similar to those that are tissue protective in animal models of I/R injury [43]. It turns out that much of the nitrite entering the stomach from saliva in fact survives intact and reaches the systemic circulation. This made researchers suggest that inorganic nitrate can be a substrate for systemic NO formation, a statement that seemed highly provocative considering the fact that nitrate is universally considered to be completely inert. Nevertheless, through numerous studies it now seems clear that nitrate indeed is bioactive. A reduction in blood pressure was demonstrated in healthy volunteers after three days oral treatment with inorganic nitrate [44], and the year after it was shown that dietary nitrate decreases whole body oxygen consumption in humans during submaximal exercise [45]. This latter finding is remarkable but the mechanism is still to be elucidated. Webb and colleagues showed that blood pressure also decreases if healthy volunteers ingest a natural nitrate source (beetroot juice). They could convincingly show that it was the nitrate in the juice that had the effect and it occurred via reduction to nitrite [46]. In this study, the dietary nitrate load also prevented endothelial dysfunction induced by an acute ischemic insult in the human forearm and significantly attenuated ex vivo platelet aggregation in response to collagen and ADP. In addition to this, Bryan et al could show recently that oral treatment with nitrate also protects against myocardial infarction in a mouse model [47].

Nitrate itself is very stable and is not believed to have any major direct effects on cellular processes. Thus, it first needs to be bioactivated and this involves its initial reduction to the more reactive nitrite anion. Once nitrite is formed there are several pathways for its further reduction to bioactive NO in blood and tissues [41]. In addition, nitrite effects might proceed via intermediate formation of nitrosothiols. As mentioned above oral commensal bacteria play a key role in this process as they very effectively reduce nitrate, and in fact, after a dietary nitrate load (5–10 mg/kg), salivary nitrite levels can easily reach several millimolar [8]. Moreover, if the oral flora is depressed by an antibacterial mouthwash solution, the rise in plasma nitrite after a nitrate-load is markedly attenuated [48]. Clearly, facultative anaerobic oral bacterial are highly effective nitrate reduces but a recent study unexpectedly shows that also mammalian cells can reduce nitrate, and even more surprisingly, this takes place in vivo under normoxic conditions [49]. Although the physiological and therapeutic importance of a mammalian nitrate reductase activity is yet to be elucidated, preliminary results indeed suggest nitrite-mediated bioactivity arising from this newly-described pathway [49].

DIETARY NITRATE AND CARDIOVASCULAR DISEASE

Hypertension affects approximately 1 billion individuals worldwide and remains the most common risk factor for cardiovascular morbidity and mortality [50]. A diet rich in fruits and vegetables is associated with a lower blood pressure and reduced risk of cardiovascular events. Yet, despite extensive research the active ingredient(s) responsible for these effects has not been pinpointed and trials with single nutrients have been largely unsuccessful. Remarkably, in our recent study in healthy volunteers [44] the blood pressure-lowering effect of dietary nitrate supplementation was similar to that seen in the healthy control group in the DASH project, a classical vegetable/fruit diet trial [51], indicating that nitrate could be an important active ingredient of this diet [52–54]. It should be noted that the dose of nitrate used in our study (0.1 mmol/kg/day) is readily achievable through a diet rich in vegetables. Moreover, in the Webb study mentioned above, 0.5 liters of fresh beetroot juice decreased systolic blood pressure as much as 10 mmHg, and blood pressure was still significantly reduced when measured 24 h later [46]. If these results can be reproduced in clinical trials in hypertensives, and if we can show that the effect is sustained over time, it will open the door to entirely new strategies for prevention and treatment of this disorder. It is not unlikely that dietary nitrate may affect also other cardiovascular disorders, including atherosclerosis and ischemic heart disease, conditions in which a decreased NO bioavailability is thought to be central.

In summary, it is ironic that of all the natural constituents of vegetables, it is only one that is believed to have detrimental health effects - the nitrate anion. Yet, this particular nutrient is now emerging as a prime candidate for mediating cardioprotective effects of a vegetarian diet.

ABOUT THE AUTHORS

Jon O. Lundberg MD, PhD

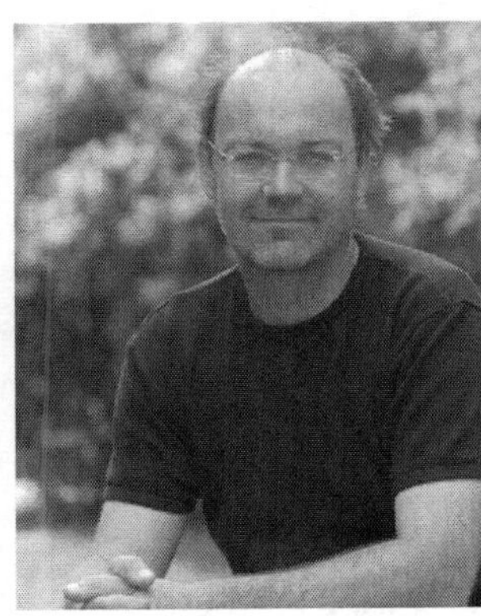

Jon Lundberg serves as Professor in the Department of Physiology and Pharmacology at Karolinska Institutet, Stockholm, Sweden. He received his Medical Degree from Karolinska Institutet in 1993 and his PhD at the same University in 1996. Jon Lundberg became Associate Professor in 1999 and full Professor of Pharmacology in 2004.

His interest is in the biology of nitric oxide (NO) and related nitrogen oxides. In 1994 he and his colleagues discovered an NO-synthase-independent pathway for NO generation in humans resulting from the reduction of inorganic nitrite and nitrate. His main focus is on characterizing NO-synthase-independent NO generation from nitrate and nitrite and clarifying its role in health and disease. He is also particularly interested in the nutritional aspects of nitrate and nitrite research.

Eddie Weitzberg, MD, PhD

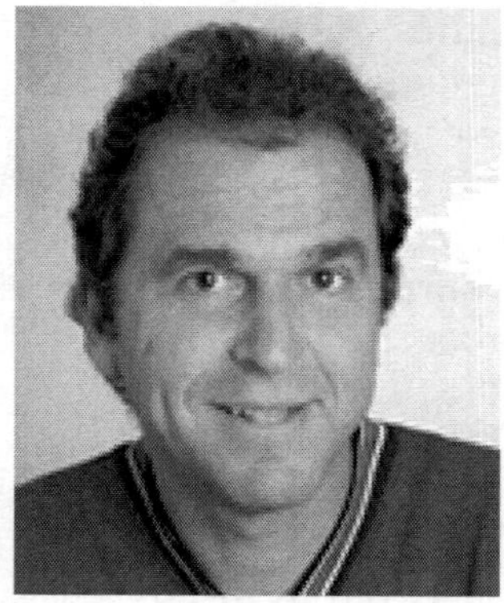

Department of Physiology and Pharmacology, Section for Anesthesiology and Intensive Care, Karolinska Institutet, Stockholm, Sweden.

Dr Weitzberg received his medical degree from Uppsala University in 1982 and did graduate work at the Karolinska Institute from 1990 to 1993. He has been a Full Professor of Anesthesiology and Intensive Care since 2003 and has published more than 120 articles.

Dr Weitzberg's research interests include the roles of endothelin and nitric oxide in various inflammatory conditions, such as gastroenteritis, endotoxin shock, urinary tract infections, and pulmonary hypertension. The main focus is now to explore the nitrate-nitrite-NO pathway in relation to normal physiology as well as in disease states. Special attention is given to the role of this pathway in the Intensive Care setting.

REFERENCES

1. Smil V. *Cycles of LIfe*. New York: Scientific American Library, 2000.
2. Lundberg JO, Weitzberg E, Cole JA, Benjamin N. Nitrate, bacteria and human health. *Nat Rev Microbiol* 2004;2:593–602.
3. Benjamin N, O'Driscoll F, Dougall H, et al. Stomach NO synthesis. *Nature* 1994;368:502.
4. Lundberg JO, Weitzberg E, Lundberg JM, Alving K. Intragastric nitric oxide production in humans: measurements in expelled air. *Gut* 1994;35:1543-6.
5. Moncada S, Higgs A. The L-arginine-nitric oxide pathway. *N Engl J Med* 1993;329:2002–12.
6. Spiegelhalder B, Eisenbrand G, Preussman R. Influence of dietary nitrate on nitrite content of human saliva: possible relevance to in vivo formation of N-nitroso compounds. *Food Cosmet Toxicol* 1976;14:545–548.
7. Duncan C, Dougall H, Johnston P, et al. Chemical generation of nitric oxide in the mouth from the enterosalivary circulation of dietary nitrate [see comments]. *Nat Med* 1995;1:546–51.
8. Lundberg JO, Govoni M. Inorganic nitrate is a possible source for systemic generation of nitric oxide. *Free Radic Biol Med* 2004;37:395–400.
9. Sobko T, Reinders C, Norin E, Midtvedt T, Gustafsson LE, Lundberg JO. Gastrointestinal nitric oxide generation in germ-free and conventional rats. *Am J Physiol Gastrointest Liver Physiol* 2004;287:G993–7.
10. Petersson J., Carlstrom, M., Schreiber, D., et al., Gastroprotective and blood pressure lowering effects of dietary nitrate are abolished by an antiseptic mouthwash. *Free Radic Bio Med* 2009; 46:1068–1075.
11. Duncan C, Li H, Dykhuizen R, et al. Protection against oral and gastrointestinal diseases: im-

portance of dietary nitrate intake, oral nitrate reduction and enterosalivary nitrate circulation. *Comp Biochem Physiol A Physiol* 1997;118:939–48.

12. Dykhuizen RS, Frazer R, Duncan C, et al. Antimicrobial effect of acidified nitrite on gut pathogens: importance of dietary nitrate in host defense. *Antimicrob Agents Chemother* 1996;40:1422–5.
13. Bjorne H, Weitzberg E, Lundberg JO. Intragastric generation of antimicrobial nitrogen oxides from saliva—physiological and therapeutic considerations. *Free Radic Biol Med* 2006;41:1404–12.
14. Bjorne HH, Petersson J, Phillipson M, Weitzberg E, Holm L, Lundberg JO. Nitrite in saliva increases gastric mucosal blood flow and mucus thickness. *J Clin Invest* 2004;113:106–14.
15. Petersson J, Phillipson M, Jansson EA, Patzak A, Lundberg JO, Holm L. Dietary nitrate increases gastric mucosal blood flow and mucosal defense. *Am J Physiol Gastrointest Liver Physiol* 2007;292:G718–24.
16. Jansson EA, Petersson J, Reinders C, et al. Protection from nonsteroidal anti-inflammatory drug (NSAID)-induced gastric ulcers by dietary nitrate. *Free Radic Biol Med* 2007;42:510–8.
17. Miyoshi M, Kasahara E, Park AM, et al. Dietary nitrate inhibits stress-induced gastric mucosal injury in the rat. *Free Radic Res* 2003;37:85–90.
18. Larauche M, Bueno L, Fioramonti J. Effect of dietary nitric oxide on gastric mucosal mast cells in absence or presence of an experimental gastritis in rats. *Life Sci* 2003;73:1505–16.
19. Gago B, Lundberg JO, Barbosa RM, Laranjinha J. Red wine-dependent reduction of nitrite to nitric oxide in the stomach. *Free Radic Biol Med* 2007;43:1233–42.
20. Peri L, Pietraforte D, Scorza G, Napolitano A, Fogliano V, Minetti M. Apples increase nitric oxide production by human saliva at the acidic pH of the stomach: a new biological function for polyphenols with a catechol group? *Free Radic Biol Med* 2005;39:668–81.
21. Carlsson S, Wiklund NP, Engstrand L, Weitzberg E, Lundberg JO. Effects of pH, nitrite, and ascorbic acid on nonenzymatic nitric oxide generation and bacterial growth in urine. *Nitric Oxide* 2001;5:580–6.
22. Gago B, Nystrom T, Cavaleiro C, et al. The potent vasodilator ethyl nitrite is formed upon reaction of nitrite and ethanol under gastric conditions. *Free Radic Biol Med* 2008;45:404–12.
23. Stamler JS, Lamas S, Fang FC. Nitrosylation. the prototypic redox-based signaling mechanism. *Cell* 2001;106:675–83.
24. O'Donnell VB, Eiserich JP, Chumley PH, et al. Nitration of unsaturated fatty acids by nitric oxide-derived reactive nitrogen species peroxynitrite, nitrous acid, nitrogen dioxide, and nitronium ion. *Chem Res Toxicol* 1999;12:83–92.
25. Cui T, Schopfer FJ, Zhang J, et al. Nitrated fatty acids: Endogenous anti-inflammatory signaling mediators. *J Biol Chem* 2006;281:35686–98.
26. Coles B, Bloodsworth A, Clark SR, et al. Nitrolinoleate inhibits superoxide generation, degranulation, and integrin expression by human neutrophils: novel antiinflammatory properties of nitric oxide-derived reactive species in vascular cells. Circ Res 2002;91:375–81.
27. Zweier JL, Wang P, Samouilov A, Kuppusamy P. Enzyme-independent formation of nitric oxide in biological tissues. *Nature Med* 1995;1:804–809.
28. Cosby K, Partovi KS, Crawford JH, et al. Nitrite reduction to nitric oxide by deoxyhemoglobin vasodilates the human circulation. *Nat Med* 2003;9:1498–505.
29. Nagababu E, Ramasamy S, Abernethy DR, Rifkind JM. Active nitric oxide produced in the red cell under hypoxic conditions by deoxyhemoglobin-mediated nitrite reduction. *J Biol Chem* 2003;278:46349–56.

30. Shiva S, Huang Z, Grubina R, et al. Deoxymyoglobin is a nitrite reductase that generates nitric oxide and regulates mitochondrial respiration. *Circ Res* 2007;100:654–61.

31. Rassaf T, Flogel U, Drexhage C, Hendgen-Cotta U, Kelm M, Schrader J. Nitrite reductase function of deoxymyoglobin: oxygen sensor and regulator of cardiac energetics and function. *Circ Res* 2007;100:1749–54.

32. Millar TM, Stevens CR, Benjamin N, Eisenthal R, Harrison R, Blake DR. Xanthine oxidoreductase catalyses the reduction of nitrates and nitrite to nitric oxide under hypoxic conditions. *FEBS Lett* 1998;427:225–8.

33. Li H, Samouilov A, Liu X, Zweier JL. Characterization of the magnitude and kinetics of xanthine oxidase-catalyzed nitrite reduction. Evaluation of its role in nitric oxide generation in anoxic tissues. *J Biol Chem* 2001;276:24482–9.

34. Godber BL, Doel JJ, Sapkota GP, et al. Reduction of nitrite to nitric oxide catalyzed by xanthine oxidoreductase. *J Biol Chem* 2000;275:7757–63.

35. Zhang Z, Naughton DP, Blake DR, et al. Human xanthine oxidase converts nitrite ions into nitric oxide (NO). *Biochem Soc Trans* 1997;25:524S.

36. Kozlov AV, Staniek K, Nohl H. Nitrite reductase activity is a novel function of mammalian mitochondria. *FEBS Lett* 1999;454:127–30.

37. Castello PR, David PS, McClure T, Crook Z, Poyton RO. Mitochondrial cytochrome oxidase produces nitric oxide under hypoxic conditions: implications for oxygen sensing and hypoxic signaling in eukaryotes. *Cell Metab* 2006;3:277–87.

38. Kozlov AV, Dietrich B, Nohl H. Various intracellular compartments cooperate in the release of nitric oxide from glycerol trinitrate in liver. *Br J Pharmacol* 2003;139:989–97.

39. Vanin AF, Bevers LM, Slama-Schwok A, van Faassen EE. Nitric oxide synthase reduces nitrite to NO under anoxia. *Cell Mol Life Sci* 2007;64:96–103.

40. Modin A, Bjorne H, Herulf M, Alving K, Weitzberg E, Lundberg JO. Nitrite-derived nitric oxide: a possible mediator of 'acidic-metabolic' vasodilation. *Acta Physiol Scand* 2001;171:9–16.

41. Lundberg JO, Weitzberg E, Gladwin MT. The nitrate-nitrite-nitric oxide pathway in physiology and therapeutics. *Nat Rev Drug Discov* 2008;7:156–67.

42. Lundberg JO, Weitzberg E. NO generation from nitrite and its role in vascular control. *Arterioscler Thromb Vasc Biol* 2005;25:915–22.

43. Duranski MR, Greer JJ, Dejam A, et al. Cytoprotective effects of nitrite during in vivo ischemia-reperfusion of the heart and liver. *J Clin Invest* 2005;115:1232–1240.

44. Larsen FJ, Ekblom B, Sahlin K, Lundberg JO, Weitzberg E. Effects of dietary nitrate on blood pressure in healthy volunteers. *N Engl J Med* 2006;355:2792–3.

45. Larsen FJ, Weitzberg E, Lundberg JO, Ekblom B. Effects of dietary nitrate on oxygen cost during exercise. *Acta Physiol (Oxf)* 2007;191:59–66.

46. Webb AJ, Patel N, Loukogeorgakis S, et al. Acute Blood Pressure Lowering, Vasoprotective, and Antiplatelet Properties of Dietary Nitrate via Bioconversion to Nitrite. *Hypertension* 2008;51:784–90.

47. Bryan NS, Calvert JW, Elrod JW, Gundewar S, Ji SY, Lefer DJ. Dietary nitrite supplementation protects against myocardial ischemia-reperfusion injury. *Proc Natl Acad Sci U S A* 2007;104:19144–9.

48. Govoni M, Jansson EA, Weitzberg E, Lundberg JO. The increase in plasma nitrite after a dietary nitrate load is markedly attenuated by an antibacterial mouthwash. *Nitric Oxide* 2008; 19: 333–7.

49. Jansson EA, Huang L, Malkey R, et al. A mammalian functional nitrate reductase that regulates nitrite and nitric oxide homeostasis. *Nat Chem Biol* 2008; 4: 411–7.

50. Chobanian AV, Bakris GL, Black HR, et al. The Seventh Report of the Joint National Committee on Prevention, Detection, Evaluation, and Treatment of High Blood Pressure: the JNC 7 report. *JAMA* 2003;289:2560-72.

51. Appel LJ, Moore TJ, Obarzanek E, et al. A clinical trial of the effects of dietary patterns on blood pressure. DASH Collaborative Research Group. *N Engl J Med* 1997;336:1117–24.

52. Classen HG, Stein-Hammer C, Thoni H. Hypothesis: the effect of oral nitrite on blood pressure in the spontaneously hypertensive rat. Does dietary nitrate mitigate hypertension after conversion to nitrite? *J Am Coll Nutr* 1990;9:500–2.

53. Lundberg JO, Feelisch M, Bjorne H, Jansson EA, Weitzberg E. Cardioprotective effects of vegetables: is nitrate the answer? *Nitric Oxide* 2006;15:359–62.

54. Tsuchiya K, Takiguchi Y, Okamoto M, et al. Malfunction of Vascular Control in Lifestyle-Related Diseases: Formation of Systemic Hemoglobin-Nitric Oxide Complex (HbNO) From Dietary Nitrite. *J Pharmacol Sci* 2004;96:395–400.

CHAPTER 4

Dietary Nitrates and Nitrites: The Physiological Context for Potential Health Benefits

NATHAN S. BRYAN and NORMAN G. HORD

Brown Foundation Institute of Molecular Medicine, The University of Texas Health Science Center, Houston, TX 77030

Department of Food Science and Human Nutrition, Michigan State University, East Lansing, MI

THE preceding chapters have clearly defined the pathways to form NO from nitrate and nitrite and began to describe some of the beneficial effects on physiology. In order to understand how modest changes in our diet and lifestyle can enhance NO formation, we must recognize food sources rich in NO active compounds and demonstrate a link between certain diets and foods and improved health compared to foods that lead to a deficiency in NO. NO is the most important molecule in regulating blood pressure and maintaining vascular homeostasis. Therefore repleting this molecule through diet will have beneficial effects primarily on the heart and vessels.

The increase in cardiovascular complications among Americans along with a diet consisting primarily of fast food illustrates the importance of investigating the correlation between cardiovascular disease and diet. Although there are clear reports on certain foods and diets that have shown benefit in terms of preventing cancer and cardiovascular disease, the specific nature of the active constituent(s) responsible for the cardioprotective effects of certain foods is still unknown although fiber, minerals, and antioxidants have all been proposed as viable candidates. A number of large epidemiological studies have attempted to address this issue [1–4]. Joshipura *et al.* [3,5] found that a high intake of fruits and vegetables was indeed associated with a reduced risk for coronary heart disease and ischemic stroke. The large study population also allowed for analysis of the protection afforded by specific types of foods, and the strongest protection against coronary heart disease was seen with high intake of green leafy vegetables. In another study, Appel *et al.* [6] looked at the effects of dietary supplementation with vegetables on blood pressure in subjects with borderline hypertension. They found that intake of vegetables decreased blood pressure almost to the same extent as monotherapy with a standard antihypertensive drug.

On the contrary, there has been a well known connection with increased risk for cardiovascular disease and poor diet, often involving high intake of saturated fat and limited fruit and vegetable intake, characteristic of a contemporary Western diet. Whereas, traditional dietary habits of the Mediterranean area have been consistently associated with lower incidence of cardiovascular disease and cancer [7–10]. The health effects of dietary consumption of vegetables and fruits have been attributed to constituents including vitamins, minerals, fiber and so-called non-nutritive substances such as flavonoids, glucosinolates among many others [11–13]. Dietary supplements containing food components such as β-carotene and antioxidant vitamins like vitamin A and E have been employed in secondary prevention trials for the prevention of lung cancer [14,15]. These trials found that β-carotene, alone or in combination with vitamin E or retinyl palmitate, increased the incidence of lung cancers and the total cardiovascular mortality rates [16]. Indeed, meta-analyses of primary and secondary cancer prevention trials of dietary antioxidant supplements consistently demonstrate lack of efficacy and increased risk of mortality [17]. Most recently the use of antioxidants in clinical trials have consistently failed to provide benefit in terms of the prevention of cardiovascular disease [18]. Clearly more research is needed to identify nutrients and food components of vegetables and fruits associated with decreased risk of cardiovascular disease and cancer.

Clearly there are healthy choices of certain foods that can improve our health but identifying and understanding the active molecules which confer the benefits has been challenging. While the health benefits of vegetables and fruits may derive from combinations of food components rather than individual components [19–21], recent research has found specific foods associated with decreased risk of cardiovascular disease. Recent prospective epidemiologic studies show that high intake of green leafy vegetables are among the most protective foods against coronary heart disease and ischemic stroke risk [3,5]. The Dietary Approaches to Stop Hypertension (DASH) studies found that diets rich in vegetables (i.e., 8–10 servings) and low fat dairy products could lower blood pressure to an extent similar to single hypotensive medications [6,22]. The blood pressure lowering effect of this diet was hypothesized to be attributable to the high calcium, potassium, polyphenols and fiber content and low in sodium and animal protein content [23]. These and other findings also point to a less widely acknowledged but highly plausible hypothesis: the content of inorganic nitrate (NO_3^-) in certain vegetables provides a physiologic substrate for reduction to nitrite (NO_2^-), nitric oxide (NO) and other metabolic products (NO_x) that produce vasodilation, decrease blood pressure and support cardiovascular function [24–26]. This pathway was described in Chapter 3. Interestingly, both potassium nitrite, in 1880, and potassium nitrate, in 8th century China, were known to mediate hypotensive and anti-anginal actions, respectively [27,28]. As often occurs in nutrition and medicine, the past is prescient. The goal of this chapter is to provide a physiological context for the potentially health benefits of dietary nitrite and nitrate in our food supply.

The necessity for regulating nitrate and nitrite concentrations in drinking water to limit toxic exposure levels in infants has unduly suppressed investigation of the role of food sources of nitrates and nitrites in supporting optimal health. Despite historical use of nitrates and nitrites as medicinal agents and demonstration of physiological roles for nitrate and nitrite in vascular and immune function, food sources of nitrates and nitrites as healthful dietary components has received little attention. In fact the public perception is that these are harmful substances in our food supply. Approximately 80% of dietary nitrates are derived from vegetable consumption; nitrites may be consumed from vegetables, fruits and processed meats or produced endogenously by oxidation of nitric oxide (NO), and by reduction of salivary nitrate by commensal bacteria in the mouth and gastrointestinal tract. The World Health Organization's Acceptable Daily Intake (ADI) for the nitrate ion is set at 3.7 mg/kg body weight and for the nitrite ion at 0.06 mg/kg body weight. This translates into an exposure limit of 222 mg nitrate and 3.6 mg nitrite for a 60 kg adult.

DIETARY SOURCES OF NITRATE AND NITRITE

Dietary nitrate and nitrite intake is determined by the type of food consumed and our individual dietary habits, i.e. the levels of nitrate in the vegetables, the amount of vegetables consumed and the level of nitrate in the water supply [29]. The primary determinants of nitrite consumption are the levels of nitrites in cured, processed meats and the consumption level of these products. A recent survey of vegetable nitrate concentra-

TABLE 4.1 Nitrate and Nitrite Content of Edible Components of Vegetables [32].

Vegetable Types	Vegetable Varieties	NO_2^- (mg/kg FW)	NO_3^- (mg/kg FW)
Root Vegetables	Carrot	0.02–0.23	921–1956
	Mustard leaf	0.12–0.64	709–956
Green Vegetables	Lettuce	0.08–2.15	123–2678
	Spinach	0–0.73	239–3872
Cabbage	Chinese cabbage	0–0.65	429–1610
	Bok choy	0.09–2.42	1023–3098
	Cabbage	0–0.41	259–1250
	Cole	3.64–5.35	766–1365
Melon	Wax gourd	0.01–0.06	358–680
	Cucumber	0–0.11	12–143
Nightshade	Eggplant	0.07–0.49	250–424

tions in European Union (EU) States and Norway based on ~42,000 submitted analytical results showed a variation ranging from a low of 1 mg/kg (peas and Brussels sprouts) to a high of 4,800 mg/kg (rucola or rocket) [30]. The nitrate and nitrite content of edible vegetable components are listed in Table 4.1 from [31].

Table 4.2 contains a list of vegetable varieties grouped in ascending order of nitrate content from [33]. In terms of plant anatomy, the nitrate content of vegetable organs can be listed in descending order (most to least) as petiole > leaf > stem > root > inflorescence > tuber > bulb > fruit

TABLE 4.2 Classification of Vegetables According to Nitrate Content (mg/kg FW) [33].

Nitrate Content	Vegetable Varieties
Very low (< 200)	Artichoke, asparagus, broad bean, eggplant, garlic, onion, green bean, mushroom, pea, pepper, potato, summer squash, sweet potato, tomato, watermelon
Low (200–500)	Broccoli, carrot, cauliflower, cucumber, pumpkin, chicory
Middle (500–1,000)	Cabbage, dill, turnip, savoy cabbage
High (1,000–2,500)	Celeriac, Chinese cabbage, endive, fennel, kohlrabi, leek, parsley
Very high (> 2,400)	Celery, cress, chervil, lettuce, red beetroot, spinach, rocket (rucola)

> seed [34]. Accumulation of nitrate is subject to factors including genotype, soil conditions, growth conditions (i.e., nitrate uptake, nitrate reductase activity and growth rate) as well as storage and transport conditions [29,35]. For example, average nitrate content of spinach collected from three different markets in Delhi, India varied from 71 to 4293 mg/kg fresh weight (FW) [36]. These data dictate that caution be observed in linking biological effects of leafy vegetables (and other nitrate-containing vegetables and fruits) to specific health effects, particularly in observational epidemiologic studies. They also demonstrate wide variation in nitrate content based on a number of different conditions. This is more easily understood from the discussion of the nitrogen cycle in the previous chapter.

DIETARY NITRATE AND NITRITE INTAKE ESTIMATES

The mean intake estimates for nitrate and nitrite in the U.S. and Europe varies by investigator but are consistent and comparable. International estimates of nitrate intakes from food are 50–140 mg/day in Europe and in the US about 40–100 mg/day [37]. Nitrite intakes vary from 0 to 20 mg/day [29]. Nitrate intakes from sources other than vegetables, including drinking water and cured meats, has been estimated to average 35–44 mg/person per day for a 60 kg human [30]. Based upon a conservative recommendation to consume 400 grams of different fruits and vegetables per day at median nitrate concentrations, dietary intake of nitrate would be ~157 mg/day [30]. In the European union (EU) population, where fruit consumption (nitrate content averaging < 10 mg/kg FW) constitutes over half the 400 gram intake recommendation, actual nitrate intakes would approximate 81–106 mg/day before additional nitrate losses are taken into consideration based on washing, peeling and/or cooking. Depending on individual habits, dietary intake and exposure to nitrite and nitrate can vary significantly per person.

A CASE STUDY IN NITRATE AND NITRITE INTAKE ESTIMATES BASED ON A CONVENIENCE SAMPLE

In order to help us understand which foods may be enriched in nitrite and nitrate we recently used more conventional and contemporary analytical methods for the quantification of nitrite and nitrate in foods [38]. We conducted nitrate and nitrite analyses on a convenience sample of vegetables, a commercial vegetable juice beverage (V8®, Campbell Soup Co.), fruits, fruit juices as well as fresh and processed meats. Vegetables with the highest nitrate concentrations in our sample include spinach (7410 mg/kg FW), collard greens (3170 mg/kg FW), mustard greens (1160 mg/kg), broccoli (395 mg/kg FW) and tomato (392 mg/kg FW). Banana, apple sauce, and oranges had nitrate/nitrite concentrations (mg/kg and mg/kg FW, respectively) of 55/0.09, 3.0/0.08, and 8.0/0.15, respectively. Vegetable and fruit juices had nitrate/nitrite concentrations (mg/L FW) of 825/0.35 (carrot juice), 427/0.21 (V8® juice), 66.3/0.06 (pomegranate juice) and 470/2.09 (cranberry juice). Whereas the government regulates the amount of nitrite and nitrate in our drinking water, there appears to be no oversight on the NO_x content of commercially available juices. As shown above, these juices exceed the amount allowed in drinking water. Many red wines analyzed contain in the range of 1–10 mg/liter nitrate and 0.5–1 mg/liter nitrite. It is noteworthy that a dessicated vegetable dietary supplement (Nature's Way Garden Veggies) had the highest nitrate and nitrite concentration (mg/g and μg/g FW, respectively) of any food tested at 279/105 respectively. Each capsule contains 900 mg and it is recommended to take 2 capsules daily with water. This equates to over 500 mg nitrate and 0.2 mg nitrite exposure per day based on a single daily supplement. Hot dog, ham, pork tenderloin and bacon had nitrate/nitrite concentrations (mg/kg and mg/kg FW, respectively) of 90/0.53, 9.0/8.9, 33/0, and 55/3.8 respectively. There is an enormous effort in the processed meat industry to produce a nitrite free product based primarily on unwarranted health concerns. Analysis of bacon labeled as nitrite and nitrate free for comparison revealed this product contained over twice as much nitrite as the traditionally cured product with 30 mg/kg nitrate and 6.78 mg/kg nitrite. Although no nitrite was added, the "natural" process used for these nitrate/nitrite free products are actually quite effective at producing nitrite for the curing process and remains as residual nitrite. This will be discussed in more detail in the following chapter. These data are in press in The American Journal of Clinical Nutrition (Hord et al., 2009).

MODELING NITRATE AND NITRITE INTAKES BASED ON THE VEGETABLE AND FRUIT CONTENT IN THE DASH DIET PATTERN

Emerging data, considered together with data in Tables 4.1, 4.2 and 4.3, make it plain that, due to the wide variation in nitrate and nitrite content of vegetables, fruits and their juices, practicing the oft-quoted dietary recommendation "Eat your fruits and vegetables" may not always translate into high nitrate/nitrite concentrations in the diet. We set out to model this variation by utilizing the vegetable and fruit components of the DASH dietary pattern [39] that employed high and low nitrate vege-

TABLE 4.3 Analysis of Foodstuff using Contemporary Technologies (HPLC).

	Nitrite µg/L (ppb)	Nitrate mg/L (ppm)
Cranberry juice	144.800	9.11
Acai juice	13.600	0.56
Pomegranate	69.130	12.93
Green tea	0.710	0.230
Carrot juice5	36.130	27.5
V8®	92.520	26.17
Red wine (merlot)	375.361	0.47
	Nitrite mg/kg (ppm) Average	**Nitrate mg/kg (ppm) Average**
Mustard greens	0.032	1160.0
Spinach	0.182	7410.0
Hot dog	0.529	90.0
Ham	8.900	9.0
Bacon	3.790	55.0
Nitrite free bacon	6.780	30.0
Pork tenderloin	0.000	33.0
Collard greens	0.885	3170.0
Carrots	0.062	1.0
Vegetable soup	0.011	209.0
Apple sauce	0.081	3.0
Brocolli	0.744	395.0
Banana	0.092	45.0
Cole slaw	0.706	559.0
Salad	1.330	821.0
Tomato	0.299	392.0
Orange	0.149	8.0
Fruit mix	0.796	9.0
French fries	1.690	20.0
Ketchup	1.300	1.0
Veggie supplement	104.700	278900.0

table and fruit choices. Table 4.4 lists two vegetable and fruit consumption patterns based on the DASH diet (1 cup raw leafy vegetable, 1/2 cup cut-up raw or cooked vegetable, 1/2 cup vegetable juice, 1 medium fruit, 1/4 cup dried fruit, 1/2 cup fresh, frozen, or canned fruit and 1/2 cup fruit juice) that contain choices that are low or high in nitrate and nitrite. The high nitrate/nitrite DASH diet would result in consumption of 1222 mg

TABLE 4.4 Hypothetical Dietary Nitrate/Nitrite Intakes Based on Food and Juice Serving Recommendations for Vegetables and Fruit Based on the DASH Dietary Pattern.[1,2]

Food Pattern	Serving Size	Nitrate Content (mg/serving)	Nitrite Content (mg/serving)
DASH food pattern with high nitrate/nitrite food choices (4–5 servings each of vegetables and fruit)	1 cup raw spinach	926	0.027
	1/2 cup cooked collard greens	198	0.06
	1/2 cup V8® juice	42.5	0.02
	1 medium banana	6.75	0.014
	1/4 cup raisins	1	–
	1 medium orange	1	0.02
	1/2 cup cranberry juice	47	0.21
	Total	**1222**	**0.351**
DASH food pattern with low nitrate/nitrite food choices (4–5 servings each of vegetables and fruit)	1 cup raw leaf lettuce	103	0.17
	1/2 cup broccoli	25	0.09
	1/2 cup V8® juice	42.5	0.02
	1 medium apple	0.40	0.01
	1/4 cup raisins	1	–
	1/2 cup canned fruit cocktail	1	0.1
	1/2 cup orange juice	1	0.02
	Total	**174**	**0.41**

[1]Analysis of foods reflects the mean value from triplicate or quadruplicate analyses.
[2]Analysis of juices assumes a density of 1 gram/liter.
1 cup liquid = 236 ml
1 cup solid = 125 g

nitrate and 0.351 mg nitrite compared to the low nitrate/nitrite DASH diet that yields 174 mg nitrate and 0.41 mg nitrite. These analyses make evident that consuming a dietary pattern such as the DASH diet can yield differences in nitrate intake that vary by 700% for nitrate and ~50% for nitrite. With these wide variations in intake based on dietary choices, one can speculate that the health disparities between the Mediterranean and Western populations can be attributed to better food choices primarily by their nitrite/nitrate content. This also illustrates one of the reasons many clinical trials using antioxidants found in foods have failed to account for the beneficial properties of vegetables. One may wish to consider the nitrite and nitrate content in prospective clinical trials.

MEDITERRANEAN DIET VS WESTERN DIET: A PROOF OF PRINCIPLE COMPARISON IN NITRITE/NITRATE CONSUMPTION

There has been a well known connection with increased risk for cardiovascular disease (CVD) and poor diet, often involving high intake of saturated fat and limited fruit and vegetable intake. The constituent(s) of fruits and vegetables that affords protection from CVD has and continues to be debated. Although there may be many components which may have cardioprotective effects, antioxidants appear to be one of the phytochemicals that play a significant role. One group of antioxidants present in fruits and vegetables is known as "polyphenols" or "polyphenolics" and is believed to neutralize free radicals thus preventing damage to cell membranes and other cell structures. These compounds will be discussed in subsequent chapters. There are numerous sources of polyphenols in the diet in addition to fruits and vegetables, including drinks such as coffee, tea, and red wine. Although antioxidants are generally credited with improving states of oxidative stress, studies which have evaluated the efficacy of supplementation with a high dose of an antioxidant alone, such as vitamin E, have shown no apparent improvement and in some cases a decrease in cardiovascular protection [18]. Yet, when these antioxidants are consumed through the diet in the form of fruits and vegetables, there is a significant degree of cardioprotection, best represented by the decrease in mortality rates from CVD of those consuming the popular Mediterranean diet [10]. Although Mediterranean diets vary by country, seasonal availability of ingredients and traditional cooking habits, they all tend to be rich in fruits, vegetables, olive oil, wines and monounsaturated fatty acids while low in saturated fat and meat. Epidemiological studies, such as the Seven Country Study [40], have led to theories describing why and how the Mediterranean diet may promote a lower incidence of coronary heart disease, and antioxidants are emerging as a key component. However, since antioxidant supplementation alone does not confer the cardiovascular benefits, there must be more to explain the cardioprotection afforded by certain foods. As noted above certain foods are enriched with nitrate and nitrite while others are lacking. Thus, the combination of antioxidants and nitrite/nitrate may in fact be responsible for the cardioprotective attributes of fruits and vegetables.

Diets typical of Mediterranean countries have been credited with significantly lower rates of CVD when compared with the US. Therefore, in order to directly compare the relative nitrite and nitrate consumption based on two vastly different diets, two typical 'fast food' eateries were chosen which are representative examples of foods eaten in the Mediterranean area as well as what is commonly consumed in the US. Table 4.5 illustrates the foods chosen for the respective diets. In order to reveal potential differences in nitrite and nitrate content based on the food choices, NOx (nitrite + nitrate) content as well as polyphenolic, glutathione, and ascorbic acid (antioxidant) content of both diets were analyzed (data are from H.Garg Masters Thesis [41]).

The results from the entire day food selection are illustrated in Figure 4.1. As shown in Figure 4.1(a), the nitrite and nitrate content of the Mediterranean type foods were almost 20 times higher than what was contained in the

TABLE 4.5 Comparison Between Foods Commonly Eaten by Western Populations Compared to a More Healthy Mediterranean Diet.

	Exemplary Western Menu	Exemplary Mediterranean Menu
Breakfast	Bagel w/ Cream Cheese Black Coffee (12 oz)	Toast w/ Jam and Butter Cappuccino (Espresso+Milk)
Morning Snack	Carrot Nut Muffin Diet Coke (12 oz)	Yogurt (Strawberry) Carrot Juice (12 oz)
Lunch	Big Mac Large French Fries Diet Coke (12 oz)	Mediterranean Wrap Garden Vegetable Soup Mineral Water (12 oz)
Afternoon Snack	Snickers Black Coffee (12 oz)	Trail Mix Orange Juice (12 oz)
Dinner	Cheese Pizza (4 slices) Diet Coke (12 oz)	Salmon (Smoked) Red Wine (12 oz)

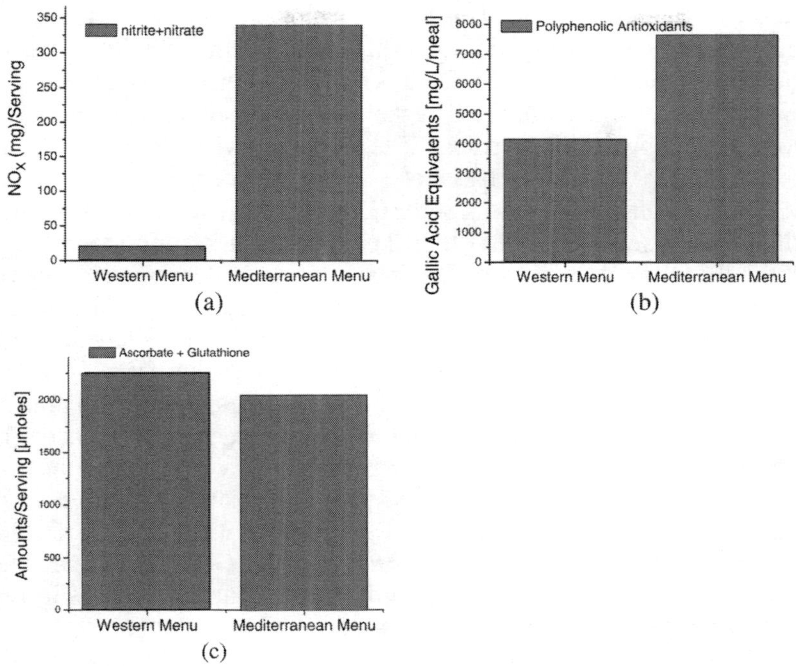

FIGURE 4.1 (a), (b), and (c) show by far the most profound difference between the two diets pertained to the content of nitrite and nitrate (NO_X). The Western diet contained only approximately 6% of the amount of nitrite and nitrate than that found in the Mediterranean menu. Additionally, the polyphenolic content of the Mediterranean menu nearly doubled the amount of the Western menu. Panel C These results may suggest that a sufficient supply of nitrite and nitrate along with antioxidant molecules such as polyphenolics are responsible for the established health benefits of certain diets. Although these food samples were contrived to represent extremes, they are intended only to demonstrate that our daily consumption of foods rich in NO activity can vary substantially based on individual habits. It is exactly this disparity that may explain individual health and susceptibility to disease based on individual dietary habits.

Western type foods. The Mediterranean type foods also contained twice as much polyphenols, Figure 4.1(b), and roughly the same ascorbic acid and glutathione, Figure 4.1(c). By far the most profound difference we evaluated between the two diets pertained to the content of nitrite and nitrate and polyphenols. The Western meals contained only approximately 6% of the amount of combined nitrite and nitrate in the Mediterranean meals. These results may suggest that nitrate/nitrite and polyphenolics can account for the many known health benefits of a mediterranean type diet. Although the total amount of glutathione and ascorbic acid were similar between the two menus it is interesting to point out that the majority of both of these antioxidant molecules was in the oxidized form in the western foods. These particular food items were chosen for a specific demonstration of potential differences in nitrite and nitrate intake and obviously other food choices would have shown different results. The purpose however is to demonstrate the potential for differences based on our daily food choices.

A comprehensive analysis of some of the beverages consumed together with meals or snacks are likely to make a significant contribution to daily NO_x and, in some cases, antioxidant intake. This will depend on the type of beverage and amounts consumed over the day. An array of different beverages was also analyzed. The types of drinks analyzed include: mineral waters, sodas, juices, alcoholic beverages, nutrient enhance drinks, coffee, tea, and milk. We found surprisingly high quantities of nitrate in mineral waters, particularly the Perrier brand which originates from France. The majority of the sodas such as Coke or Pepsi had very little if any nitrite or nitrate. The fruit and vegetable juices had significant quantities of both nitrite/nitrate and antioxidants. Bolthouse Carrot Juice contained a remarkably high level of nitrate as well as nitrite. Welch's Grape Juice contained elevated levels of polyphenolics and the Pomegranate Juice was loaded with both ascorbate and polyphenols as well as high levels of nitrite and nitrate. As expected, high levels of polyphenols was found in the homebrewed coffee and significantly less in the commercially prepared brands. The milk evaluated was also used in preparing the chocolate milk, which elevated the nitrate level substantially. This suggests that the powder used to prepare the milk contained substantial nitrate.

New beverages which have been appearing on the market are termed 'Nutrient Enhanced' Sodas. We chose to evaluate some of these to see what possible contribution to nitrite and nitrate and antioxidant content they may provide. The nitrate content of most of the sodas was comparable to those of the mineral waters. There were also elevated levels of polyphenolics in the Acai juice, iced teas and the Rockstar energy drink. Consuming several cups of coffee, expresso or red bull can translate into a consumption of several milligrams of both nitrite and nitrate. These levels are not reported on the label. Overall, these analyses showed the significant contribution that beverages provide in the daily intake of nitrite, nitrate and polyphenols. Notably vegetable juices, mineral waters and red wines were major contributors to the elevated levels present in samples representing the Mediterranean style diet.

Although these diets were contrived to demonstrate a point, when considering the differences in the composition of the two types of diets we assessed, one parameter which has not been assessed previously is the content of inorganic nitrite and nitrate. As shown in the food sample

TABLE 4.6

Food Pattern	Brand/Source	Nitrate (μM)	Nitrite (μM)	Total Ascorbate (μM)	Total Glutathione (μM)	Polyphenolic Concentration (GAE mg/L)
Coffee/Teas						
Milk (Full Milk)	Garelick Farms	2.19	7.52	92.06	5.08	522.33
Coffee	Homebrew	10.82	7.69	61.54	6.64	1216.11
Chocolate Milk	Garelick Farms	40.31	8.28	0.00	3.51	298.89
Espresso + Cream (Doubleshot)	Starbucks	11.59	6.75	0.00	4.94	548.89
Iced Tea (Lemon)	Snapple	36.65	1.15	615.64	4.59	302.89

Food Pattern	Brand/Source	Nitrate (μM)	Nitrite (μM)	Total Glutathione (μM)	Polyphenolic Concentration (GAE mg/L)
Nutrient Enhanced Sodas					
Rx Stress (Herbal Iced Tea)	Arizona	28.78	4.96	6.13	235.33
Green Tea with Ginseng + Honey	Arizona	19.34	3.20	5.51	286.67
Acai Juice (Mango)	Bossa Nova	26.58	5.52	2.56	714.00
Red Bull (Energy Drink)	Red Bull	23.70	4.43	3.24	34.89
Immune (Tangerine Lime, airforce)	Immune	14.04	0.94	5.15	0.00
Rockstar (Energy Drink)	Rockstar	8.12	0.00	6.67	209.78

analysis, there is a tremendous difference in the nitrite nitrate exposure through our individual dietary habits. New findings continue to negate the prevailing thought that nitrite and nitrate are potentially dangerous and support the possibility that both may be a significant promoter of health. In addition to the beneficial effects of nitrite and nitrate, we cannot be so naïve to believe these are solely responsible. It is likely that combined with various antioxidants, nitrite and nitrate may promote or enhance nitric oxide availability and account for the health benefits. It is intriguing to speculate that antioxidants may have multiple roles, not only as free radical quenchers, but also as facilitators of nitrite reduction to NO. This concept will be discussed in Chapter 7.

The following chapters will present an abundance of published data on the biomedical effects of nitrite and nitrate that can easily be achieved through dietary means. An optimal diet may then consist of a sufficient supply of nitrite and nitrate for health and disease prevention. Regular intake of nitrite and nitrate-containing food such as green leafy vegetables may ensure that blood and tissue levels of nitrite and NO pools are maintained at a level sufficient to compensate for any disturbances in endogenous NO synthesis (135). As you will learn low levels of supplemental nitrite have been shown to enhance blood flow (67) so dietary sources of NO metabolites could therefore improve circulation and oxygen delivery. This dietary pathway may not only provide essential nutrients for NO production but also provide a rescue or protective pathway for people at risk for cardiovascular disease (22). Moreover, any intervention, which increases blood and tissue concentrations of nitrite, may have profound outcomes on health and disease prevention. Including foods rich in nitrite, nitrate and antioxidants combined with L-arginine may provide the optimal combination of nutrients to improve nitric oxide production and homeostasis.

ABOUT THE AUTHORS

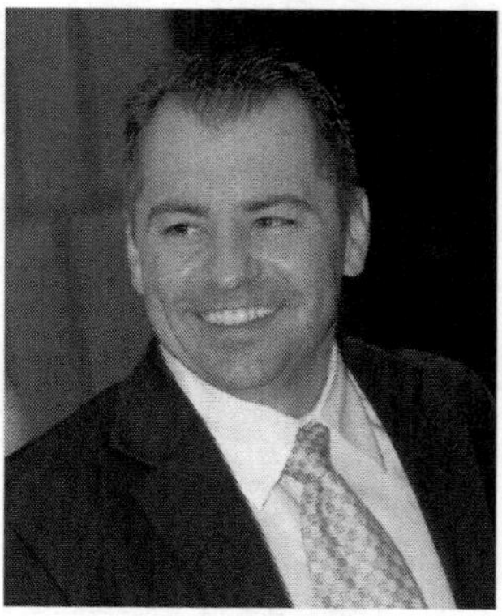

Nathan S. Bryan, Ph.D.

Dr. Bryan was born in Bryan Texas in November 1973. Nathan grew up in small town Texas. He spent his grade school years in Lexington (population 1000) and attended High School in Caldwell (population 3000). He earned his undergraduate Bachelor of Science degree in Biochemistry from the University of Texas at Austin and his doctoral degree from Louisiana State University School of Medicine in Shreveport where he was the recipient of the Dean's Award for Excellence in Research. He pursued his post-doctoral training as a Kirschstein Fellow at Boston University School of Medicine in the Whitaker Cardiovascular Institute. Dr. Bryan joined the Institute of Molecular Medicine, University of Texas Health Science Center in Houston, in June 2006 in the Center for Cell Signaling. He is also a faculty member of the Department of Integrative Biology and Pharmacology and Graduate School of Biomedical Sciences at the UT Houston Medical School. He is an active member of the Nitric Oxide Society, Society for Free Radical Biology and Medicine and the American Heart Association.

Dr. Bryan's research is dedicated to providing a better understanding of the interactions of nitric oxide (NO) and related metabolites with their different biological targets at the molecular and cellular level and the significance of these reactions for physiology and pathophysiology. Attempts are made to identify what particular changes in NO-related signaling pathways and reaction products occur in disease states such as endothelial dysfunction, ischemia/reperfusion, tissue/cardiac protection, diabetes, atherosclerosis and inflammation with the aim of testing their amenability as biomarkers for diagnosis and/or treatment of specific disease.

Current research is directed to understand the interactions of exogenous dietary nitrite/nitrate (NOx) on the endogenous NO/cGMP pathway and how perturbations in each system affect cardiovascular health. This involves mechanisms of nitrite transport and cellular uptake as well as mechanism of nitrite reduction back to NO and via direct NO-independent signaling actions of nitrite. Work in Dr. Bryan's lab involves molecular biology and analytical biochemistry utilizing gas phase chemiluminescence and HPLC in multiple organ systems and blood. Much of the work involves *in vivo* characterization of NO/nitrite metabolism using a number of transgenic and knockout animal models of disease. Dr. Bryan and colleagues recently discovered that nitrite is a biologically active molecule which was previously thought to be an inert breakdown product of NO production. These findings have unveiled many beneficial effects of nitrite in the treatment and prevention of human disease. These discoveries may provide the basis for new preventive or therapeutic strategies in diseases associated with NO insufficiency and new guidelines for optimal health. Since nitrite and nitrate are common constituents of many fruits and vegetables, changes in dietary habits may have profound effects on many diseases associated with NO insufficiency. NO insufficiency is a hallmark of a number of diseases including cardiovascular disease. The notion that nitrite can recapitulate NO biochemistry and serve as an alternative and compensatory mechanism of NO production is revolutionary. It may also serve as the endocrine mediator of NO signaling. Moreover, the direct signaling actions of nitrite may represent a novel NO independent pathway for nitrite. If our current understanding is true, then an optimal diet may then consist of a sufficient supply of nitrite and nitrate for health and disease prevention. Understanding this pathway will provide the basis for new preventive or therapeutic strategies in diseases associated with NO insufficiency and new guidelines for optimal health. To date Dr. Bryan has published over 20 peer reviewed papers that have been cited over 1000 times. He has been invited to speak at a number of national and international meetings.

Dr. Bryan currently resides in Houston with his wife Kristen and their two sons Grant and Lincoln. The Bryans spend their weekends at their ranch near Caldwell where they raise cattle and horses and enjoy the great outdoors. Nathan enjoys playing golf and calf roping and team roping on his ranch and in competition.

Norman Hord, Ph.D., M.P.H., R.D.

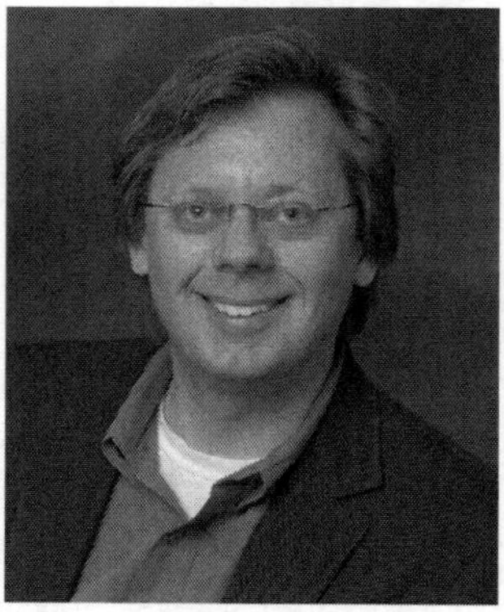

Norman Hord serves as an Associate Professor in Department of Food Science and Human Nutrition at Michigan State University (MSU), East Lansing, MI (USA). He received bachelor of science degree from Michigan State University, M.S. in nutrition from Clemson University, Ph.D. in nutrition from Purdue University, Master of Public Health degree from the Bloomberg School of Public Health from Johns Hopkins University and postdoctoral training as a Cancer Prevention Fellow at the National Cancer Institute. Dr. Hord is Chair of the Diet and Cancer Research Interest section of the American Society for Nutritional Sciences.

Dr. Hord supervises a research program that focuses on the role of dietary factors on phenotypes in colon epithelial cells related to colorectal cancer risk. His laboratory uses non-tumorigenic colon epithelial cell models to study dietary factor- and adipokine-induced cell behavior related to cancer risk. His laboratory is also characterizing the ability of probiotic bacteria to ameliorate the production of proinflammatory mediators caused by foodborne bacterial pathogens. Dr. Hord has received grant support from the USDA Higher Education Challenge Grant program, the National Cancer Institute (R03 grant program), the Kellogg Company, The J.F. Bell Institute for Health and Nutrition and various intramural funding sources. He has published research in nutrition, cancer research, cell biology and dietetics journals. He has served as a panel member of National Institutes of Health grant reviews, USDA NRI grant panel ad hoc reviewer and manuscript reviewer for cancer, cell biology, nutrition and dietetics journals.

Dr. Hord teaches courses in the undergraduate dietetics program and lectures in the Colleges of Human and Osteopathic Medicine as well as the Department of Epidemiology at MSU. He has served on the faculty of the Division of Cancer Prevention's Summer Curriculum in Cancer Prevention for the past ten years. He developed the MSU Dietetic Internship Program and currently serves as faculty coordinator for this program. This program recently received 10 year accreditation from The American Dietetic Association.

Dr. Hord advises forty undergraduate and two graduate students as well as two postdoctoral research associates. He serves on numerous theses and dissertation committees as well as on departmental, college and university committees.

REFERENCES

1. Willett, W. C. Diet and health: what should we eat? *Science* 264:532–537; 1994.
2. Hung, H. C.; Joshipura, K. J.; Jiang, R.; Hu, F. B.; Hunter, D.; Smith-Warner, S. A.; Colditz, G. A.; Rosner, B.; Spiegelman, D.; Willett, W. C. Fruit and vegetable intake and risk of major chronic disease. *Journal of the National Cancer Institute* 96:1577–1584; 2004.
3. Joshipura, K. J.; Ascherio, A.; Manson, J. E.; Stampfer, M. J.; Rimm, E. B.; Speizer, F. E.; Hennekens, C. H.; Spiegelman, D.; Willett, W. C. Fruit and vegetable intake in relation to risk of ischemic stroke. *Jama* 282:1233–1239; 1999.
4. Hu, F. B.; Willett, W. C. Optimal diets for prevention of coronary heart disease. *Jama* 288:2569–2578; 2002.
5. Joshipura, K. J.; Hu, F. B.; Manson, J. E.; Stampfer, M. J.; Rimm, E. B.; Speizer, F. E.; Colditz, G.; Ascherio, A.; Rosner, B.; Spiegelman, D.; Willett, W. C. The effect of fruit and vegetable intake on risk for coronary heart disease. *Annals of internal medicine* 134:1106–1114; 2001.
6. Appel, L. J.; Moore, T. J.; Obarzanek, E.; Vollmer, W. M.; Svetkey, L. P.; Sacks, F. M.; Bray, G. A.; Vogt, T. M.; Cutler, J. A.; Windhauser, M. M.; Lin, P. H.; Karanja, N. A clinical trial of the effects of dietary patterns on blood pressure. DASH Collaborative Research Group. *The New England journal of medicine* 336:1117–1124; 1997.
7. Willett, W. C.; Sacks, F.; Trichopoulou, A.; Drescher, G.; Ferro-Luzzi, A.; Helsing, E.; Trichopoulos, D. Mediterranean diet pyramid: a cultural model for healthy eating. *The American journal of clinical nutrition* 61:1402S–1406S; 1995.
8. Visioli, F.; Grande, S.; Bogani, P.; Galli, C. The role of antioxidants in the mediterranean diets: focus on cancer. *Eur J Cancer Prev* 13:337–343; 2004.
9. Trichopoulou, A.; Critselis, E. Mediterranean diet and longevity. *Eur J Cancer Prev* 13:453–456; 2004.

10. Visioli, F.; Bogani, P.; Grande, S.; Galli, C. Mediterranean food and health: building human evidence. *J Physiol Pharmacol* 56 Suppl 1:37–49; 2005.
11. Nothlings, U.; Schulze, M. B.; Weikert, C.; Boeing, H.; van der Schouw, Y. T.; Bamia, C.; Benetou, V.; Lagiou, P.; Krogh, V.; Beulens, J. W.; Peeters, P. H.; Halkjaer, J.; Tjonneland, A.; Tumino, R.; Panico, S.; Masala, G.; Clavel-Chapelon, F.; de Lauzon, B.; Boutron-Ruault, M. C.; Vercambre, M. N.; Kaaks, R.; Linseisen, J.; Overvad, K.; Arriola, L.; Ardanaz, E.; Gonzalez, C. A.; Tormo, M. J.; Bingham, S.; Khaw, K. T.; Key, T. J.; Vineis, P.; Riboli, E.; Ferrari, P.; Boffetta, P.; Bueno-de-Mesquita, H. B.; van der, A. D.; Berglund, G.; Wirfalt, E.; Hallmans, G.; Johansson, I.; Lund, E.; Trichopoulo, A. Intake of vegetables, legumes, and fruit, and risk for all-cause, cardiovascular, and cancer mortality in a European diabetic population. *The Journal of nutrition* 138:775–781; 2008.
12. Van Duyn, M. A.; Pivonka, E. Overview of the health benefits of fruit and vegetable consumption for the dietetics professional: selected literature. *Journal of the American Dietetic Association* 100:1511–1521; 2000.
13. Hasler, C. M. Functional foods: benefits, concerns and challenges-a position paper from the american council on science and health. *The Journal of nutrition* 132:3772–3781; 2002.
14. Albanes, D.; Heinonen, O. P.; Taylor, P. R.; Virtamo, J.; Edwards, B. K.; Rautalahti, M.; Hartman, A. M.; Palmgren, J.; Freedman, L. S.; Haapakoski, J.; Barrett, M. J.; Pietinen, P.; Malila, N.; Tala, E.; Liippo, K.; Salomaa, E. R.; Tangrea, J. A.; Teppo, L.; Askin, F. B.; Taskinen, E.; Erozan, Y.; Greenwald, P.; Huttunen, J. K. Alpha-Tocopherol and beta-carotene supplements and lung cancer incidence in the alpha-tocopherol, beta-carotene cancer prevention study: effects of base-line characteristics and study compliance. *Journal of the National Cancer Institute* 88:1560–1570; 1996.
15. Omenn, G. S.; Goodman, G. E.; Thornquist, M. D.; Balmes, J.; Cullen, M. R.; Glass, A.; Keogh, J. P.; Meyskens, F. L., Jr.; Valanis, B.; Williams, J. H., Jr.; Barnhart, S.; Cherniack, M. G.; Brodkin, C. A.; Hammar, S. Risk factors for lung cancer and for intervention effects in CARET, the Beta-Carotene and Retinol Efficacy Trial. *Journal of the National Cancer Institute* 88:1550–1559; 1996.
16. Omenn, G. S. Chemoprevention of lung cancers: lessons from CARET, the beta-carotene and retinol efficacy trial, and prospects for the future. *Eur J Cancer Prev* 16:184–191; 2007.
17. Bjelakovic, G.; Nikolova, D.; Gluud, L. L.; Simonetti, R. G.; Gluud, C. Mortality in randomized trials of antioxidant supplements for primary and secondary prevention: systematic review and meta-analysis. *Jama* 297:842–857; 2007.
18. Sesso, H. D.; Buring, J. E.; Christen, W. G.; Kurth, T.; Belanger, C.; MacFadyen, J.; Bubes, V.; Manson, J. E.; Glynn, R. J.; Gaziano, J. M. Vitamins E and C in the prevention of cardiovascular disease in men: the Physicians' Health Study II randomized controlled trial. *Jama* 300:2123–2133; 2008.
19. Byers, T. Nutrition and lung cancer: lessons from the differing effects of foods and supplements. *American journal of respiratory and critical care medicine* 177:470–471; 2008.
20. de Lorgeril, M.; Salen, P.; Martin, J. L.; Monjaud, I.; Boucher, P.; Mamelle, N. Mediterranean dietary pattern in a randomized trial: prolonged survival and possible reduced cancer rate. *Archives of internal medicine* 158:1181–1187; 1998.
21. Ibiebele, T. I.; van der Pols, J. C. Dietary pattern predicts breast cancer risk—evidence from the EPIC—Potsdam study. *The British journal of nutrition*:1–2; 2008.
22. Sacks, F. M.; Svetkey, L. P.; Vollmer, W. M.; Appel, L. J.; Bray, G. A.; Harsha, D.; Obarzanek, E.; Conlin, P. R.; Miller, E. R., 3rd; Simons-Morton, D. G.; Karanja, N.; Lin, P. H. Effects on blood pressure of reduced dietary sodium and the Dietary Approaches to Stop Hypertension

(DASH) diet. DASH-Sodium Collaborative Research Group. *The New England journal of medicine* 344:3–10; 2001.

23. Most, M. M. Estimated phytochemical content of the dietary approaches to stop hypertension (DASH) diet is higher than in the Control Study Diet. *Journal of the American Dietetic Association* 104:1725–1727; 2004.
24. Lundberg, J. O.; Feelisch, M.; Bjorne, H.; Jansson, E. A.; Weitzberg, E. Cardioprotective effects of vegetables: is nitrate the answer? *Nitric Oxide* 15:359–362; 2006.
25. L'hirondel, J. L.-L. *Nitrate and man: Toxic, Harmless or Beneficial?* Wallingford, UK: CABI Publishing; 2001.
26. McKnight, G. M.; Duncan, C. W.; Leifert, C.; Golden, M. H. Dietary nitrate in man: friend or foe? *The British journal of nutrition* 81:349–358; 1999.
27. Lo EY, C. C., eds. *Medieval Chinese Medicine.* The Dunhuang Medical Manuscripts Routledge, London, UK; 2004.
28. Reichert ET, M. S. On the physiological action of potassium nitrite. *American Journal of Medical Science* 156:158–180; 1880.
29. Pennington, J. Dietary exposure models for nitrates and nitrites. *Food Control* 9:385–395; 1998.
30. Authority, E. F. S. Nitrate in vegetables: scientific opinion of the panel on contaminants in the food chain. *The EFSA Journal* 689:1–79; 2008.
31. Hambridge, T. Nitrate and nitrite: intake assessment. *WHO Food Additive Series, World Health Organization, Geneva* 50:1053–1071; 2003.
32. Wang ZH, T. X., Wei YS, Li SX. Nitrate accumulation and its regulation by nutrient management in vegetables. In: *Balanceable Fertilization and High Quality Vegetables* China Agricultural University Press, Beijing.; 2000.
33. Santamaria, P. Nitrate in vegetables: toxicity, content, intake and EC regulation, *Journal of the science of food and agriculture* 86:10–17; 2006.
34. Santamaria, P. Ways of reducing rocket salad nitrate content. *Acta Horticulturae* 548:529–537; 2001.
35. Santamaria, P. Nitrate in vegetables: toxicity, content, intake and EC regulation, *J Sci Food Agric* 86:10–17; 2006.
36. Anjana SU, I. M., Abrol YP. Are nitrate concentrations in leafy vegetables within safe limits? *Current Science* 92:355–360; 2007.
37. Mensinga, T. T.; Speijers, G. J.; Meulenbelt, J. Health implications of exposure to environmental nitrogenous compounds. *Toxicological reviews* 22:41–51; 2003.
38. Bryan, N. S.; Grisham, M. B. Methods to detect nitric oxide and its metabolites in biological samples. *Free Radic Biol Med* 43:645–657; 2007.
39. Lin, P. H.; Aickin, M.; Champagne, C.; Craddick, S.; Sacks, F. M.; McCarron, P.; Most-Windhauser, M. M.; Rukenbrod, F.; Haworth, L. Food group sources of nutrients in the dietary patterns of the DASH-Sodium trial. *Journal of the American Dietetic Association* 103:488–496; 2003.
40. Fidanza, F.; Puddu, V.; Imbimbo, A. B.; Menotti, A.; Keys, A. Coronary heart disease in seven countries. VII. Five-year experience in rural Italy. *Circulation* 41:I63–75; 1970.
41. Garg, H. *Diet and Cardiovascular Disease: The role of antioxidants and nitrite.* School of Medicine. Boston: Boston University; 2006: 1–54.

CHAPTER 5

Nitrite and Nitrate in the Meat Industry

RANDY HUFFMAN and NATHAN S. BRYAN

Maple Leaf Foods, Toronto, Canada

Brown Foundation Institute of Molecular Medicine, The University of Texas Health Science Center, Houston, TX 77030

DESPITE the many published reports on the beneficial properties of nitrite and nitrate in physiology, nitrite and nitrate in cured and processed meats continues to be perceived as harmful. The previous chapter revealed that certain foods, particularly green leafy vegetables are naturally enriched in nitrite and nitrate from growing in soil. However, enriching meats with nitrite or nitrate during curing is perceived as harmful and advocated by some groups to be eliminated completely. The use of pure sodium nitrate in curing is now only a minor practice in the United States. The ingoing levels of sodium nitrite have been tightly controlled by the Food Safety and Inspection Service (FSIS) of the U.S. Department of Agriculture. To satisfy consumer demands for no added nitrite processed meats, efforts have recently been taken to creatively adjust the meat curing process by employing "nitrite free" organic vegetable powders instead of directly adding sodium nitrite salts. Although the end result is production of nitrite from the nitrate contained in the vegetable powders, a more "natural" or "organic" approach seems to appeal to consumers. This is primarily due to the public perception of nitrite and nitrate. Reports about methemoglobinemia in infants (blue baby syndrome) caused by drinks or food prepared with nitrate-rich (and bacterially contaminated) well water and vegetables, intentional and occupational intoxications in adults, increasing nitrate levels in soil and lakes as a result of fertilizer overuse, and the formation of potentially carcinogenic N-nitrosamines all contribute to the negative image that nitrite and nitrate have held in recent years. As a result, major efforts have been made to remove as much nitrite and nitrate as possible from our drinking water, to advocate replacement of nitrite by other (often less effective) food preservatives, and to establish cultivation conditions that result in crops with reduced levels of nitrate. We feel it prudent at this juncture to discuss the history and use of nitrite and nitrate in meat products and compare to what is contained in vegetables to hopefully dispel the fear of health concerns and the public perception of nitrite in meats.

HISTORY OF NITRITE

Documents dating to around 800 AD suggest that nitrite and nitrate were used by the Chinese medicinally to relieve "acute heart pains, and cold in the hands and feet" [1]. Inorganic nitrite and nitrate have been in use for as long as 5000 years in the preservation of food. The use of salt plus nitrite and/or nitrate in the manufacturing of meat products is commonly expressed as "curing". To cure means to correct, restore or treat so in most cases curing is thought as something positive one could do to meat. Long before the advent of refrigeration, curing and preserving foods from microbial growth was essential and commonplace. In ancient time, curing preserved the meat and fish from spoilage. It was thought in the beginning that the use of salt lowered the water activity and inhibited growth of microorganisms. In the 19th century people realized that some salts were better preservatives than others. Saltpetre (potassium nitrate) was recognized as a contaminant of the salt which enhanced its preserving action and gave meat a red color [2]. Later it was realized that the mechanism underlying food preservation was actually the conversion of nitrate to nitrite by bacteria [3]. This provided the rationale for the use of nitrite rather than nitrate in the meat preservation industry in the early 1900s. Its use is critical for both food safety and palatability. Nitrite in meat greatly delays the out growth of the obligate anaerobe *C. botulinum* and thus development of botulinum toxin, develops cured meat flavor and color, retards development of rancidity during storage, inhibits development of warmed-over flavor and preserves flavors of spice and smoke [3]. Nitrite in food controls and stabilizes the oxidative state of lipids in meat products [4], thus preventing lipid oxidation. Ascorbic acid or dehydroascorbate is also a common meat preservative. It was demonstrated very early on that the chemical basis for the nice red color and appearance of cured meat was the reaction of nitrite with oxymyoglobin to form S-nitrosomyoglobin [5]. It was later realized that free sulfhydryl groups were necessary for this effect [6]. The process was shown to involve intermediate formation of S-nitrosothiols to ultimately produce nitrosylmyoglobin [7]. In the early 20th century meat preservation regulations in the United States for the first time allowed nitrite to be used as a curative salt. According to the Meat Inspections Regulations, the maximum amount of nitrite that can be used for the curing process is one ounce per 100 pounds of meat (dry cured) or 1/4 ounce per 100 pounds chopped meat and/or meat by-product [8]. Nitrite has since become a common dietary nutrient in those who consume cured meats.

In the 1970s, there became a major public health concern regarding nitrite, when there was indication of endogenous formation of N-nitrosamines from nitrite and nitrate and its relevance to human cancer. The first report in the 1950s on the hepatocarcinogenic effects of N-nitrosodimethylamine (NDMA) [9], and the suggestion that low molecular weight N-nitrosamines (RNNOs) can be formed following nitrosation of various amines [10] ignited an enormous interest in N-nitrosamines and their association with cancer. Proof that nitrosation reactions by nitrite can occur was provided by Ender *et al.* [11] who identified NDMA in nitrite preserved fish, and by Sander and Sief [12] who demonstrated the *in vivo* formation of a nitrosamine in the acidic conditions of the human stomach. Because of the potent carcinogenicity of some low molecular weight N-nitrosamines and the ability of nitrite to form these compounds, considerable effort was made to determine the levels of nitrite and nitrate in the external and internal human environment, and to assess exposure in order to correlate it with human cancer at specific sites [13]. The deductive reasoning from this data concluded that since nitrite can form N-nitrosamines and some N-nitrosamines can cause cancer, then nitrite must cause cancer. Since the early 1980s there have been numerous reports on a possible association of N-nitrosamines and human cancers [13,14] but a causative link between nitrite or nitrate exposure and cancer is still missing [15]. The deductive reasoning does not hold true. In fact, the National Toxicology Program (NTP) which was established by the Secretary of Health and Human Services in 1978 is obligated to provide Congress a biennial report on carcinogens. The NTP consists of the relevant toxicological activities of: National Institute of Environmental Health Sciences (NIH/NIEHS), National Institute for Occupation Safety and Health (CDC/NIOSH) and National Center for Toxicological Research (FDA/NCTR). NTP cancer bioassays are the gold standard which utilize standard protocols, multiple doses of the test compound, extensive tissue pathology and statistical analysis and then draft a report prepared for peer review committee. Their results and recommendations affect regulatory action by the government. The Food and Drug Administration nominated nitrite to be tested by NTP as a carcinogen. Studies were initiated in 1989 looking at long-term carcinogenicity of nitrite. This was a two year study in rats and mice dosed with massive amounts of nitrite in their drinking water [sodium nitrite doses:

750, 1500, or 3000 ppm; (35–150 mg/kg/day in rats and 45–220 mg/kg/day in mice)]. These doses are far greater than one could ever consume through diet. The in-life portion of the study was completed in 1997 with extensive histopathology and statistical evaluation. Draft Technical Report No. 495 was issued in April 2000 for peer review. The results from the report was a unanimous decision of "no evidence" of carcinogenicity in male or female rats and male mice and "equivocal evidence" in female mice. Strongest statistical finding was $p < 0.001$ decrease in "all organs' mononuclear cell leukemia" in male and female rats. To summarize the current state of the art, nitrite, due to its inherent nitrosative chemistry has the ability to nitrosate amines. Some low molecular weight nitrosamines have been shown to be carcinogenic but to date there have been no causal relationship between nitrite and carcinogenicity. It is important to make this distinction as we go forward.

Public awareness was also brought to industrial settings and exposure of workers to nitrite. Not only is nitrite used as a color fixative and preservative in meats and fish but it is also used in manufacturing diazo dyes, in nitroso compounds, in the textile industry, in photography and in the manufacture of rubber chemicals. Nitrite is also a common clinical and laboratory chemical that is used as a vasodilator [16], bronchodilator [17], intestinal relaxant [18] and even as an antidote for cyanide poisoning [19]. Considering its widespread use, there have been many toxicological studies on acute and chronic exposure to nitrite. The fatal dose of nitrite is in the range of 22–23 mg/kg body weight (from USFDA Generally Recognized as Safe Food Ingredient: Nitrates and Nitrites (Including Nitrosamines) 1972 by Battele-Columbus Laboratories and Department of Commerce, Springfield VA). Lower doses of either nitrite or nitrate have caused acute methemoglobinemia, particularly in infants where a high nitrite or nitrate intake has been associated with "blue baby syndrome" caused by methemoglobinemia [20–22]. These negative connotations of nitrite and nitrate have led the government to regulate and restrict the levels in food and drinking water.

In the late 1970s, despite all the fear and paranoia surrounding nitrite exposure, our appreciation and understanding of nitrite took a drastic turn. Studies on nitrogen balance in humans and analyses of fecal and ileostomy samples indicated that nitrite and nitrate are formed *de novo* in the intestine. These early findings by Tannenbaum *et al.* [23] significantly altered our conceptions of human exposure to exogenous nitrite and nitrate and represented the original observations that would eventually lead to the discovery of the L-arginine:NO pathway. Prior to these studies it was thought that steady-state levels of nitrite and nitrate originated solely from the diet and from nitrogen fixing enteric bacteria.

THE CHEMISTRY OF CURING MEAT

Whereas the biomedical community was initially excited about the recently described biochemistry of nitrite, this underlying chemistry has been known and exploited for centuries in the meat industry. Polenske in 1891 [24] from the German Imperial Health Office published experiments where he proved that by adding nitrate only to a pickling solution, nitrite was formed due to the action of microorganisms in the brine. Haldane demonstrated that redox reactions occurred in meats during curing and extracted NO-myoglobin as the substance responsible for the bright pink color of cured meat [25]. It was later revealed that nitrous acid (HNO_2) or a metabolite like NO was the molecule responsible for reacting with myoglobin. This was the first demonstration of the coloring of meat by nitrogen compounds but at the turn of the 20th century the antimicrobial action was still thought to be due to sodium chloride concentrations and not nitrite or nitrate. Color formation and stability are amongst the most critical quality traits of processed meat products. It is

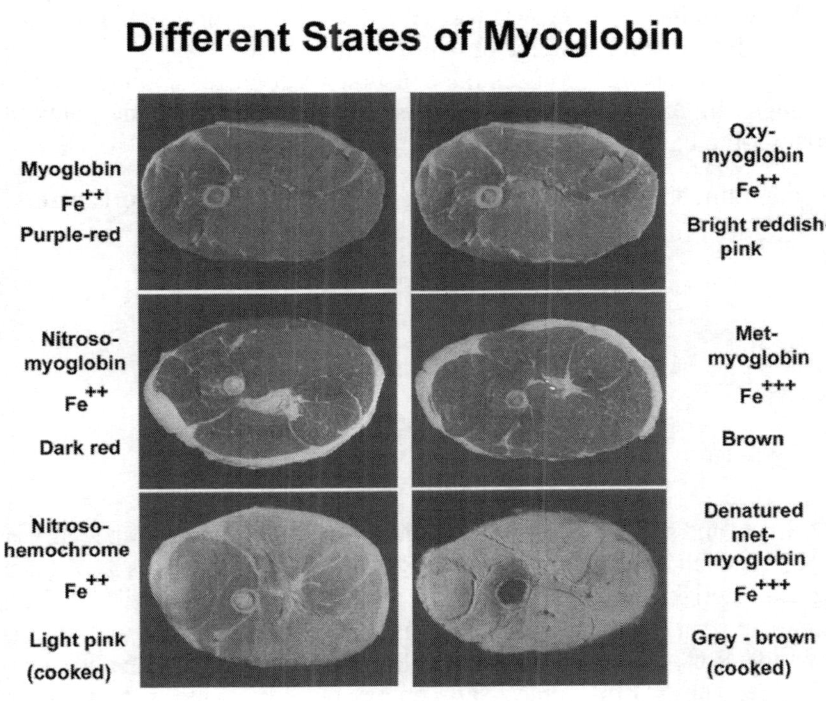

FIGURE 5.1 Scheme of the mechanism of action of nitrate in cured meats.

now known that the characteristic cured color can be derived from the concentration of heme pigments (myoglobin and hemoglobin), their chemical states and additives such as nitrogen oxides and reducing agents. The cured color is a result of the chemical reaction between compounds derived from nitrite/nitrate and the naturally occurring red myoglobin leading to the simultaneous formation of the bright red nitrosylmyoglobin whereby an axial ligand NO is coordinated to the central heme iron [26]. In the last decade ascorbic acid or ascorbate (erythorbate) began to be used in cured meats. Ascorbate reacts with nitrite to form nitrous acid or NO [27]. Ascorbate is also added to inhibit the formation of nitrosamines. By reducing enzymes or chemical reactions with a reducing agent like ascorbic acid the Fe^{3+} is reduced to Fe^{2+}. The NO formed from nitrous acid or N_2O_3 can bind to the myoglobin (Fe^{2+}) and forms a heat stable NO-myoglobin. Oxymyoglobin is not heat stable and dissociates turning the meat grey or brown. On heating NO-myoglobin, the protein moiety is denatured but the pink NO-porphyrin ring system (often called nitroso-hemochrome) still exists and is found in meat products cooked to 120°C. This heat stable pink color will change to brown ("fade") due to oxidation which can be caused by bacterial spoilage or exposure to light and oxygen. The color changes are advantageous as the consumer recognizes spoilage due to changes in color. The figure above illustrates the different states of myoglobin based on nitrite addition.

$$\text{Potassium Nitrate } KNO_3 \text{ (saltpeter)} \rightarrow \text{reduction by microorganisms} \rightarrow \text{nitrite } (KNO_2)$$

$$KNO_2 + H^+ \leftrightarrow HNO_2 + K^+$$

$$2HNO_2 \leftrightarrow N_2O_3 + H_2O$$

$$N_2O_3 \leftrightarrow NO + NO_2$$

$$NO + \text{myoglobin} \rightarrow \text{NO-myoglobin}$$

Nitrite and nitrate are highly soluble in aqueous solutions especially at pH 5.5 which is the pH of raw meat. Since the pKa of nitrite is 3.37 it can be expected that about 99% of the nitrite exist as an anion at pH 5.5. The small amount of undissociated nitrous acid is in equilibrium with its anhydride N_2O_3 which again is in equilibrium with nitric oxide and nitric dioxide. The NO molecule itself can easily be oxidized to NO_2 in the presence of oxygen. Therefore the oxygen sequestering activity of nitrite renders it as an antioxidant in meat. Due to the lack of oxygen the development of rancidity or a warmed over flavor are retarded. The antioxidant effect of nitrite in meats can be attributed to several mechanisms. (1) Fixing a Fe^{2+} heme moiety avoids having a very potent pro-oxidant Fe^{3+} heme present to initiate and promote lipid peroxidation. (2) Nitrite and its equilibrium nitrogen oxides act as free radical scavengers and also prevent lipid peroxidation. (3) The reaction with oxygen scavenges oxygen so it cannot participate in lipid peroxidation. The addition of ascorbate also can result in this antioxidant effect. The oxidation of nitrite to nitrate in meat also explains why nitrate is found in meat products to which only nitrite has been added. In fact nitrite is in some cases found at lower concentrations of nitrate in the finished product (Bryan unpublished observations).

ANTIBACTERIAL PROPERTIES OF NITRITE—AN INGREDIENT CRITICAL TO FOOD SAFETY

The anti-botulinal properties of nitrite have long been recognized. The use of nitrite to preserve meat has been employed either indirectly or directly for thousands of years. In the last 20 years however, the role of nitrite in protecting public health with respect to other pathogens has begun to be better recognized. Nitrite excreted in saliva has significant antimicrobial benefits when it is swallowed and converted to nitrous acid and other nitrogen oxides in the gut. This pathway was described in the preceding chapters. The bacteriocidal effects of gastric fluids are significantly enhanced by the presence of ingested nitrite. This has been demonstrated for known food borne pathogens such as *Escherichia coli* O157:H7 [28,29]. Nitrite and nitric oxide are also effective bacteriocidal agents against other microorganisms associated with diseases such as *Helicobacter pylori* [30], organisms associated with dental caries, [31] and skin pathogens [32,33].

As a food additive, nitrite is a key in controlling potential growth of *Listeria monocytogenes* in processed meats. Models that estimate the effects of ingredients on microbial growth show dramatic reductions when nitrite is included [34–40]. The use of such models have enabled formulations of nitrite cured processed meat products that will not support growth of *Listeria monocytogenes.* To date, this has not been achieved for uncured counterparts where the only ingredient difference is nitrite. The USDA Agricultural Research Service has done extensive research to develop models to predict growth of pathogens under a variety of conditions. In these models incorporation of nitrite at currently used levels significantly inhibits growth of *Listeria, E.coli,* and *Salmonella.*

NITROSAMINE FORMATION

The public health concerns are not related to the molecules nitrite and nitrate but their propensity to form N-nitrosamines in the stomach once swallowed. N-Nitrosamines are a large group of potent carcinogens. Approximately 300 different N-nitrosamines are carcinogenic. At least 30 animal species are responsive to their effects [41]. Human exposure to preformed N-nitrosamines occurs through the diet, in certain occupational settings, and through the use of tobacco products, cosmetics, pharmaceutical products, and agricultural chemicals. Diminishing human exposure to these carcinogens is one approach to prevention of cancer, and this has been accomplished in many instances, although exposure to N-nitrosamines in tobacco products is still unacceptably high. In the 1970s discussion began about the potential formation of nitrosamines in cured meat products, especially fried bacon. Nitrosamines are formed by amines reacting with nitrogen oxide products at very high temperatures or in an acid environment where nitrosative chemistry is predominant. It should be noted that bacon seems to be the only cured meat where this was ever deemed a practical problem due to the temperatures that can be reached during bacon frying. While there have been reports of measurable nitrosamines in other cured meats, they were generally situations not reflecting commercially produced cured meat products made since the late 1970's in the US. Many of the early reports on the formation of nitrosamines by nitrite were in artificial systems co-administering low molecular weight amines with nitrite. Due to the inherent nitrosative chemistry of nitrite in the acid environment of the stomach it is not surprising that such reactions occur. Human exposure to N-nitrosamines occurs by nitrosation of amines in the body, via their acid or bacterial catalyzed reaction with nitrite, or by reaction with products of nitric oxide generated during inflammation or infection. N-Nitrosamines undergo a simple cytochrome P450-mediated metabolic activation step, which is critical for their carcinogenicity. One of the most potent inhibitors of nitrosation reactions is ascorbic acid or vitamin C [42,43]. Substantial reductions in the formation of nitrosamines have been achieved with ascorbic acid and other nitrite scavengers. Ascorbic acid is now routinely added to cured and processed meats in addition to nitrite. There are important considerations to appreciate and understand when discussing the dietary nitrite and nitrate and formation of nitroamines in the stomach. Firstly, amines must be present. In fresh meat there are very minute amounts of amines present. They are creatine, creatinine and the free amino acids proline and hyroxyproline and some of the decarboxylation products of other amino acids. During aging and fermentation more amines will be formed. Secondly, only secondary amines form stable nitrosamines. Primary amines are immediately degraded to alcohol and nitrogen. Tertiary amines cannot react. Most amines in meats are primary amines derived from α-amino acids. Thirdly, the pH must be low enough to produce NO^+ or metal ions must be engaged to form NO^+ [2]. In products heated above 130°C nitrosamines can be formed. Bacon frying, cured sausage grilling or frying of such cured meat products as pizza toppings are conditions that may lead to formation of nitrosamines. This can be avoided by proper frying, grilling and preparation. It should be noted that even though temperatures of frying/grilling may be high, the evaporative cooling that occurs limits the formation in most products. Bacon is the notable exception because of its high fat content.

NITRITE AND NITRATE IN CONTEXT

The concern about nitrite and nitrate and their potential to react with secondary amines to form carcinogenic nitrosamines resulted in intensive nutritional, biochemical and metabolic research in the 1970's and 1980's. One of the basic approaches in these studies was to measure consumption and excretion of nitrite and nitrate. The results produced an anomaly. Excretion always seemed to exceed consumption [44–46]. This implied synthesis of these compounds in the body and led to a search for the pathways. In 1987, nitric oxide was identified as the transient factor that caused smooth muscle relaxation [47]. It was determined that synthesis of nitric oxide was synthesized from the amino acid arginine as a substrate and that it was degraded into nitrite and nitrite for excretion as a biological control mechanism [48–50]. Typically endogenous nitric oxide is produced at about 1milligram per kilogram of weight per day in humans. Being a very reactive molecule it is quickly bound to heme and oxidized to nitrite and nitrate. The nitrate is circulated in the blood and can be excreted in the urine, sweat or saliva of the individual. The following chapter will reveal evidence indicating that nitrite itself has a biological function as a signaling molecule independent of nitric oxide [51]. Curiously this function involves nitrosyl and s-nitroso heme species—the very same compounds involved in production of cured meat pigments. In a recent publication a German researcher proposed classifying nitrite as a "prodrug" based on its many newly discovered physiological functions [52]. Clearly, nitrite is a metabolite and is naturally made in significant quantities. Exogenous nitrite ingestion is small by comparison, being at an average residual level of approximately 10 ppm in commercial cured processed meats [53–56]. Although it is not widely realized, potassium nitrate is used in many toothpaste formulations. Toothpaste designed for sensitive teeth is formulated with up to 5% potassium nitrate, (which is 5000 ppm) [57–63]. These products can be purchased at any drugstore.

We know that nitrite in food controls and stabilizes the oxidative state of lipids in meat products [4], thus preventing lipid oxidation. Carr and Frei [64] have previously shown that nitrite inhibits myeloperoxidase mediated LDL modification. Thus the underlying chemistry of nitrite in meats that has been exploited for centuries may then have similar effects in human physiology. In order to gain some insight into the role of nitrite in the context of a high cholesterol diet as would occur when consuming meat, the Bryan lab recently performed a series of experiments in mice. Hypercholesterolemia causes a pro-inflammatory phenotype in the microcirculation. This phenotype appears to result from a decline in NO bioavailability that results from a reduction in NO biosynthesis, inactivation of NO by superoxide ($O_2^{\bullet-}$), or both. Since nitrite has been shown to be potently cytoprotective and restore NO biochemical homeostasis, we investigated if supplemental nitrite could attenuate microvascular inflammation caused by a high cholesterol diet. C57Bl/6J mice were fed either a normal diet or a high cholesterol diet for 3 weeks to induce microvascular inflammation. The mice on the high cholesterol diet received either nitrite free drinking water or supplemental nitrite at 50 mg/L or 150 mg/L ad libitum in their drinking water. The results from this investigation reveal that mice fed a cholesterol-enriched diet exhibited significantly elevated leukocyte adhesion to, and emigration through the venular endothelium as well as impaired endothelium-dependent relaxation in arterioles. Administration of nitrite in the drinking water abrogated leukocyte adhesion and emigration to basal levels, and prevented the arteriolar dysfunction. This was associated with sparing of reduced tetrahydrobiopterin (BH_4) and decreased levels of C-reactive protein. These data reveal novel anti-inflammatory properties of nitrite and implicate the use of nitrite as a new natural therapy for microvascular inflammation and endothelial dysfunction associated with hypercholesterolemia [Stokes et al., *American Journal of Physiology* (in press)]. These data argue for a potent beneficial effect of nitrite in meats or any food products high in cholesterol.

Although the biomedical science community is aware of the emerging beneficial effects of nitrite, it is still regarded as an undesired food additive in cured and processed meats [65]. However studies reveal that dietary nitrite supplementation can restore NO biochemistry in eNOS$^{-/-}$ mice as well as prevent injury from ischemia-reperfusion insult [66–68], and most recent data reveal that nitrite attenuates inflammation and preserves endothelial function. Emerging evidence from animal models and human clinical studies indicate that, independent of its role as a source of NO in tissues by reduction, nitrite exerts unique intracellular signaling properties that mediate physiologic functions [69], and this is supported by the novel findings that tetrahydrobiopterin (BH_4) levels (critical cofactor for NOS enzymes to convert L-arginine to NO) are preserved by nitrite treatment. Because nitrite is a primary biologically active compound resulting from nitrate reduction in tissues, significant physiological benefits may be associated with the provision of nitrate from dietary sources. The United States Environmental Protection Agency put our limit at 1mg/L nitrate in drinking water. Despite the enormous effort over the past few decades to limit or even restrict dietary nitrite consumption due to the potential to form carcinogenic N-nitrosamines, to date there is no conclusive data to indicate that dietary sources of nitrite and nitrate may be unsafe, especially at doses naturally occurring in foods. Since the early 1980s there have been numerous reports on the association of N-nitrosamines and human cancers [14] but a causative link between nitrite exposure and cancer is still missing [70]. In fact, a two year study by the NIH on the carcinogenicity of nitrite conclusively found that there was no evidence of carcinogenic activity by sodium nitrite in male or female rats or mice [71]. Despite this, the negative connotations of nitrite and nitrate remain, and have led the government to regulate and restrict the levels in food and drinking water, particularly in cured and processed meats. However, this view of nitrite may be changing, as evidence is emerging for a protective role for nitrite against different cardiovascular-related disorders. One should not fear the nitrite contained in bacon or hot dogs. In fact, the nitrite in meats may provide vascular protection from the high fat and cholesterol content. It appears that we may have identified a critical component of our diet that many people are missing. In fact the one compound we have been taught to fear and avoid may be saving our life from inflammatory diseases. A 2005 symposium at the US National Institutes of Health highlighted advances in the understanding of nitrite biochemistry, physiology and therapeutics [72]. This is now a well attended conference held every two years highlighting new discoveries in the nitrite arena.

ABOUT THE AUTHORS

Randall D. Huffman, Ph.D.

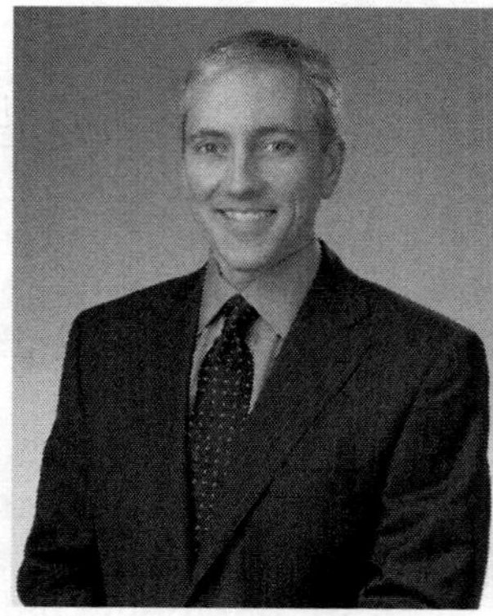

Randy Huffman is Chief Food Safety Officer of Maple Leaf Foods based at the company's corporate headquarters in Toronto, Ontario, Canada. In this capacity, Dr. Huffman has overall responsibility for leading Maple Leaf's food safety and quality programs across the Company. This involves identifying and assessing global best operating practices, technologies, ingredients and resources that support Maple Leaf's leadership in food safety and quality assurance. Maple Leaf Foods, with annual revenues in excess of $5 billion (CDN), is a leading consumer packaged food company which operates over 90 facilities across Canada and in the United States, United Kingdom, Asia and Mexico.

Dr. Huffman joined Maple Leaf Foods in January, 2009 after serving for 9 years as the Vice President and then President of the American Meat Institute (AMI) Foundation in Washington DC. In this capacity he was responsible for the day-to-day activities of the Foundation, including its research initiatives, industry best practices development and educational programming. The AMI Foundation's food safety research agenda assists AMI members and the industry at large in implementing solutions to food safety and meat quality challenges and serves as the liaison between AMI and various scientific organizations. The AMI Foundation sponsors research and educational programming on the major food safety hazards associated with meat processing. Among various responsibilities, Dr. Huffman has been a part of both the AMI Foundation-led Listeria Intervention and Control Task Force and the Beef Processing Best Practices Task Force that have developed and conducted multiple in-depth training workshops for industry and government.

Prior to joining the AMI Foundation, Dr. Huffman was director of technical services at Koch Industries, Inc., in Wichita, KS, where he managed food safety and product development issues at Koch Beef Company. Earlier in his career, he served as Vice President of Technical Services at Fairbank Farms a fresh meat processing firm based in Ashville, NY. Dr. Huffman received a B.S. in animal science from Auburn University in Auburn, AL; an M.S. and Ph.D. in animal sciences, with specialization in meat science from the University of Florida, Gainesville, FL.

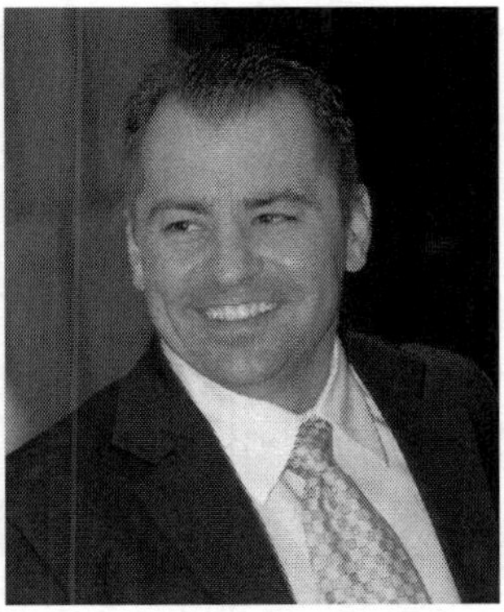

Nathan S. Bryan, Ph.D.

Dr. Bryan was born in Bryan Texas in November 1973. Nathan grew up in small town Texas. He spent his grade school years in Lexington (population 1000) and attended High School in Caldwell (population 3000). He earned his undergraduate Bachelor of Science degree in Biochemistry from the University of Texas at Austin and his doctoral degree from Louisiana State University School of Medicine in Shreveport where he was the recipient of the Dean's Award for Excellence in Research. He pursued his post-doctoral training as a Kirschstein Fellow at Boston University School of Medicine in the Whitaker Cardiovascular Institute. Dr. Bryan joined the Institute of Molecular Medicine, University of Texas Health Science Center in Houston, in June 2006 in the Center for Cell Signaling. He is also a faculty member of the Department of Integrative Biology and Pharmacology and Graduate School of Biomedical Sciences at the UT Houston Medical School. He is an active member of the Nitric Oxide Society, Society for Free Radical Biology and Medicine and the American Heart Association.

Dr. Bryan's research is dedicated to providing a better understanding of the interactions of nitric oxide (NO) and related metabolites with their different biological targets at the molecular and cellular level and the significance of these reactions for physiology and pathophysiology. Attempts are made to identify what particular changes in NO-related signaling pathways and reaction products occur in disease states such as endothelial dysfunction, ischemia/reperfusion, tissue/cardiac protection, diabetes, atherosclerosis and inflammation with the aim of testing their amenability as biomarkers for diagnosis and/or treatment of specific disease.

Current research is directed to understand the interactions of exogenous dietary nitrite/nitrate (NOx) on the endogenous NO/cGMP pathway and how perturbations in each system affect cardiovascular health. This involves mechanisms of nitrite transport and cellular uptake as well as mechanism of nitrite reduction back to NO and via direct NO-independent signaling actions of nitrite. Work in Dr. Bryan's lab involves molecular biology and analytical biochemistry utilizing gas phase chemiluminescence and HPLC in multiple organ systems and blood. Much of the work involves *in vivo* characterization of NO/nitrite metabolism using a number of transgenic and knockout animal models of disease. Dr. Bryan and colleagues recently discovered that nitrite is a biologically active molecule which was previously thought to be an inert breakdown product of NO production. These findings have unveiled many beneficial effects of nitrite in the treatment and prevention of human disease. These discoveries may provide the basis for new preventive or therapeutic strategies in diseases associated with NO insufficiency and new guidelines for optimal health. Since nitrite and nitrate are common constituents of many fruits and vegetables, changes in dietary habits may have profound effects on many diseases associated with NO insufficiency. NO insufficiency is a hallmark of a number of diseases including cardiovascular disease. The notion that nitrite can recapitulate NO biochemistry and serve as an alternative and compensatory mechanism of NO production is revolutionary. It may also serve as the endocrine mediator of NO signaling. Moreover, the direct signaling actions of nitrite may represent a novel NO independent pathway for nitrite. If our current understanding is true, then an optimal diet may then consist of a sufficient supply of nitrite and nitrate for health and disease prevention. Understanding this pathway will provide the basis for new preventive or therapeutic strategies in diseases associated with NO insufficiency and new guidelines for optimal health. To date Dr. Bryan has published over 20 peer reviewed papers that have been cited over 1000 times. He has been invited to speak at a number of national and international meetings.

Dr. Bryan currently resides in Houston with his wife Kristen and their two sons Grant and Lincoln. The Bryans spend their weekends at their ranch near Caldwell where they raise cattle and horses and enjoy the great outdoors. Nathan enjoys playing golf and calf roping and team roping on his ranch and in competition.

REFERENCES

1. Butler, A.R. and M. Feelisch, Therapeutic uses of inorganic nitrite and nitrate: from the past to the future. *Circulation,* 2008. 117(16): p. 2151–9.
2. Honikel, K., The use and control of nitrate and nitrite for the processing of meat products. *Meat Science,* 2008. 78: p. 68–76.
3. Binkerd, E.F. and O.E. Kolari, The history and use of nitrate and nitrite in the curing of meat. *Food Cosmet Toxicol,* 1975. 13: p. 665–661.
4. Shahidi, F. and C. Hong, Evaluation of malonaldehyde as a marker of oxidative rancidity in meat products. *J. Food Biochem,* 1991. 15: p. 97–105.
5. Haldane, J., The red color of salted meats. *J Hyg,* 1901. 1: p. 115–122.
6. Watts, B.M., A.M. Erdman, and J. Wentworth, Relation of free sulfhydryl groups to cured meat color. *J. Agric. Food Chem,* 1955. 3: p. 147.

7. Mirna, A. and K. Hofmann, *Uber den Verbleib von nitrit in fleischwaren. Die Fleischwirtschaft,* 1969. 10: p. 1361–1366.
8. Meat Inspections Regulations, in Code of Federal Regulations. 2008 Title 9 Section 434.21.
9. Magee, P.H. and J.M. Barnes, The production of malignant primary heptic tumors in the rat by feeding dimethylnitrosamine. *Br. J. Cancer,* 1956. 10: p. 114–122.
10. Druckrey, H. and R. Preussmann, Die Bilding carcinogener Nitrosamine am Beispiel des Tabakrauchs. *Naturewissenschaften,* 1962b. 49: p. 498–499.
11. Ender, F., et al., Isolation and identification of a hepatotoxic factor in herring meat produced from sodium nitrite preserved herring. *Naturwissenschaften,* 1964. 51: p. 637–638.
12. Sander, J. and F. Seif, Bakterielle Reduction von nitrat im magen des menschen als ursache einer Nitrosamin-Bildung. *Arzneimittel-Forsch,* 1969. 19: p. 1091–1093.
13. Bartsch, H. and R. Montesano, Relevance of nitrosamines to human cancer. *Carcinogenesis,* 1984. 5(11): p. 1381–1393.
14. Craddock, V.M., Nitrosamines and human cancer: proof of an association? *Nature,* 1983. 306: p. 638.
15. Ward, M.H., et al., Workgroup report: Drinking-water nitrate and health—recent findings and research needs. *Environ Health Perspect,* 2005. 113(11): p. 1607–14.
16. Reichert, E.T. and S.W. Mitchell, On the physiological action of potassium nitrite, with a note on the physiological action on man. *Am J Med Sci,* 1880. 159: p. 158–180.
17. Hunter, C.J., et al., Inhaled nebulized nitrite is a hypoxia-sensitive NO-dependent selective pulmonary vasodilator. *Nat Med,* 2004. 10: p. 1122–1127.
18. Kozlov, A.V., et al., Organ specific formation of nitrosyl complexes under intestinal ischemia-reperfusion in rats involves NOS-independent mechanism(s). *Shock,* 2001. 15: p. 366–371.
19. Chen, K.K. and C.L. Rose, Nitrite and thiosulfate therapy in cyanide poisoning. *J Am Med Assoc,* 1952. 149(2): p. 113–119.
20. Comly, H.H., Cyanosis in infants caused by nitrates in well water. *JAMA,* 1945. 129: p. 112–116.
21. Donohoe, W.E., Cyanosis in infants with drinking water as a cause. *Paediatrics,* 1949. 3: p. 308–311.
22. Lecks, H.I., Methemoglobinemia in infancy. *Am J Dis Child,* 1950. 79: p. 117–123.
23. Tannenbaum, S.R., et al., Nitrite and nitrate are formed by endogenous synthesis in the human intestine. *Science,* 1978. 200: p. 1487–1488.
24. Polenske, E., Uber den Verlust, welchen Rindfleisch and Nahrwert durch das Pokeln erleidet sowie uber die Veranderungen salpeterhaltiger Pokellaken. *Arbeiten aus dem kaiserlichen Gesendheitsamt,* 1891. 7: p. 471–474.
25. Haldane, J., The red color of salted meat. *Journal of Hygiene,* 1901. I: p. 115–122.
26. Moller, J.K. and L.H. Skibsted, Nitric oxide and myoglobins. *Chem Rev,* 2002. 102(4): p. 1167–78.
27. Fox, J.B.J. and S.A. Ackerman, Formation of nitric oxide myoglobin: Mechanisms of the reaction with various reductants. *Journal of Food Science,* 1968. 33: p. 364–370.
28. Duncan, C., et al., Protection against oral and gastrointestinal diseases: importance of dietary nitrate intake, oral nitrate reduction and enterosalivary nitrate circulation. *Comp Biochem Physiol A Physiol,* 1997. 118(4): p. 939–48.
29. Dykhuizen, R.S., et al., Antimicrobial effect of acidified nitrite on gut pathogens: importance of dietary nitrate in host defense. *Antimicrob Agents Chemother,* 1996. 40(6): p. 1422–5.

30. Dykhuizen, R.S., et al., Helicobacter pylori is killed by nitrite under acidic conditions. *Gut,* 1998. 42(3): p. 334–7.
31. Allaker, R.P., et al., Antimicrobial effect of acidified nitrite on periodontal bacteria. *Oral Microbiol Immunol,* 2001. 16(4): p. 253–6.
32. Weller, R., et al., Antimicrobial effect of acidified nitrite on dermatophyte fungi, Candida and bacterial skin pathogens. *J Appl Microbiol,* 2001. 90(4): p. 648–52.
33. Weller, R., et al., Nitric oxide release accounts for the reduced incidence of cutaneous infections in psoriasis. *J Am Acad Dermatol,* 1997. 36(2 Pt 1): p. 281–2.
34. Buchanan, R.L., M.H. Golden, and J.G. Phillips, Expanded models for the non-thermal inactivation of Listeria monocytogenes. *J Appl Microbiol,* 1997. 82(5): p. 567–77.
35. Duffy, L.L., P.B. Vanderlinde, and F.H. Grau, Growth of Listeria monocytogenes on vacuum-packed cooked meats: effects of pH, aw, nitrite and ascorbate. *Int J Food Microbiol,* 1994. 23(3–4): p. 377–90.
36. Gill, A.O. and R.A. Holley, Interactive inhibition of meat spoilage and pathogenic bacteria by lysozyme, nisin and EDTA in the presence of nitrite and sodium chloride at 24 degrees C. *Int J Food Microbiol,* 2003. 80(3): p. 251–9.
37. Legan, J.D., et al., Modeling the growth boundary of Listeria monocytogenes in ready-to-eat cooked meat products as a function of the product salt, moisture, potassium lactate, and sodium diacetate concentrations. *J Food Prot,* 2004. 67(10): p. 2195–204.
38. McClure, P.J., et al., Predictive modelling of growth of Listeria monocytogenes. The effects on growth of NaCl, pH, storage temperature and $NaNO_2$. *Int J Food Microbiol,* 1997. 34(3): p. 221–32.
39. Schlyter, J.H., et al., The effects of diacetate with nitrite, lactate, or pediocin on the viability of Listeria monocytogenes in turkey slurries. *Int J Food Microbiol,* 1993. 19(4): p. 271–81.
40. Seman, D.L., et al., Modeling the growth of Listeria monocytogenes in cured ready-to-eat processed meat products by manipulation of sodium chloride, sodium diacetate, potassium lactate, and product moisture content. *J Food Prot,* 2002. 65(4): p. 651–8.
41. Hecht, S.S., Approaches to cancer prevention based on an understanding of N-nitrosamine carcinogenesis. *Proc Soc Exp Biol Med,* 1997. 216(2): p. 181–91.
42. Mirvish, S.S., Inhibition by vitamins C and E of *in vivo* nitrosation and vitamin C occurrence in the stomach. *Eur J Cancer Prev,* 1996. 5 Suppl 1: p. 131–6.
43. Mirvish, S.S., Experimental evidence for inhibition of N-nitroso compound formation as a factor in the negative correlation between vitamin C consumption and the incidence of certain cancers. *Cancer Res,* 1994. 54(7 Suppl): p. 1948s–1951s.
44. Green, L.C., S.R. Tannenbaum, and P. Goldman, Nitrate synthesis in the germfree and conventional rat. *Science,* 1981. 212(4490): p. 56–8.
45. Green, L.C., et al., *Nitrate biosynthesis in man. Proc Natl Acad Sci U S A,* 1981. 78(12): p. 7764–8.
46. Tannenbaum, S.R., Nitrate and nitrite: origin in humans. *Science,* 1979. 205(4413): p. 1332, 1334–7.
47. Ignarro, L.J., et al., Endothelium-derived relaxing factor produced and released from artery and vein is nitric oxide. *Proc. Natl. Acad Sci.* USA, 1987. 84: p. 9265–9269.
48. Buga, G.M., et al., Endothelium-derived nitric oxide relaxes nonvascular smooth muscle. *Eur J Pharmacol,* 1989. 161(1): p. 61–72.
49. Deguchi, T. and M. Yoshioka, L-Arginine identified as an endogenous activator for soluble guanylate cyclase from neuroblastoma cells. *J Biol Chem,* 1982. 257(17): p. 10147–51.
50. Hibbs, J.B., Jr., R.R. Taintor, and Z. Vavrin, Macrophage cytotoxicity: role for L-arginine deiminase and imino nitrogen oxidation to nitrite. *Science,* 1987. 235(4787): p. 473–6.

51. Bryan, N.S., et al., Nitrite is a signaling molecule and regulator of gene expression in mammalian tissues. *Nat Chem Biol,* 2005. 1(5): p. 290–7.
52. Suschek, C.V., et al., Nitrite, a naturally occurring precursor of nitric oxide that acts like a 'prodrug'. *Biol Chem,* 2006. 387(5): p. 499–506.
53. Cassens, R.G., Residual nitrite in cured meat. *Food Technol,* 1997. 51: p. 53–55.
54. Cassens, R.G., Composition and safety of cured meats in the USA. *Food Chem,* 1997. 59: p. 561–566.
55. Kilic, B., R.G. Cassens, and L.L. Borchert, Influence of turkey meat on residual nitrite in cured meat products. *J Food Prot,* 2001. 64(2): p. 235–9.
56. Saccani, G., et al., Determination of nitrite, nitrate, and glucose-6-phosphate in muscle tissues and cured meat by IC/MS. *J AOAC Int,* 2006. 89(3): p. 712–9.
57. Cohen, S., et al., Anticalculus efficacy of a dentifrice containing potassium nitrate, soluble pyrophosphate, PVM/MA copolymer, and sodium fluoride in a silica base: a twelve-week clinical study. *J Clin Dent,* 1994. 5 Spec No: p. 93–6.
58. Manochehr-Pour, M., M. Bhat, and N. Bissada, Clinical evaluation of two potassium nitrate toothpastes for the treatment of dental hypersensitivity. *Periodontal Case Rep,* 1984. 6(1): p. 25–30.
59. Orchardson, R. and D.G. Gillam, The efficacy of potassium salts as agents for treating dentin hypersensitivity. *J Orofac Pain,* 2000. 14(1): p. 9–19.
60. Poulsen, S., et al., Potassium nitrate toothpaste for dentine hypersensitivity. *Cochrane Database Syst Rev,* 2001(2): p. CD001476.
61. Silverman, G., The sensitivity-reducing effect of brushing with a potassium nitrate-sodium monofluorophosphate dentifrice. *Compend Contin Educ Dent,* 1985. 6(2): p. 131–3, 136.
62. Tzanova, S., Z. Ivanova, and S. Velinova, Clinical evaluation of dentinal hypersensitivity treatment with 5% potassium nitrate dentifrice. *Folia Med* (Plovdiv), 2005. 47(2): p. 65–9.
63. Wara-aswapati, N., et al., The effect of a new toothpaste containing potassium nitrate and triclosan on gingival health, plaque formation and dentine hypersensitivity. *J Clin Periodontol,* 2005. 32(1): p. 53–8.
64. Carr, A.C. and B. Frei, The nitric oxide congener nitrite inhibits myeloperoxidase/H2O2/ Cl--mediated modification of low density lipoprotein. *J Biol Chem,* 2001. 276(3): p. 1822–8.
65. Research, W.C.R.F.A.I.f.C., *Food, Nutrition, Physical Activity, and the Prevention of Cancer: a Global Perspective.* 2007, AICR: Washington DC.
66. Bryan, N.S., et al., Dietary nitrite supplementation protects against myocardial ischemia-reperfusion injury. *Proc Natl Acad Sci U S A,* 2007. 104(48): p. 19144–9.
67. Bryan, N.S., et al., Dietary nitrite restores NO homeostasis and is cardioprotective in endothelial nitric oxide synthase-deficient mice. *Free Radic Biol Med,* 2008. 45(4): p. 468–74.
68. Elrod, J.W., et al., *Cardiac Derived Nitric Oxide Promotes Distant Organ Protection: Evidence for an Endocrine Role of Nitrite.* under review, 2007.
69. Bryan, N.S., Nitrite in nitric oxide biology: cause or consequence? A systems-based review. *Free Radic Biol Med,* 2006. 41(5): p. 691–701.
70. Ward, M.H., et al., Workgroup report: Drinking-water nitrate and health—recent findings and research needs. *Environ Health Perspect,* 2005. 113(11): p. 1607–14.
71. Program, N.T., On The Toxicology and Carcinogenesis Studues of Sodium Nitrite, U.S.D.o.H.a.H. Services, Editor. 2001, *National Institute of Health.* p. 1–276.
72. Gladwin, M.T., et al., The emerging biology of the nitrite anion. *Nat Chem Biol,* 2005. 1(6): p. 308–14.

CHAPTER 6

Physiological Effects and Mechanism of Action of Nitrite and Nitrate in Human Physiology

SRUTI SHIVA[1,2] and MARK T. GLADWIN[2,3]

[1]*Department of Pharmacology and Chemical Biology, University of Pittsburgh, Pittsburgh, PA 15260*

[2]*Hemostasis and Vascular Biology Research Institute, Department of Medicine, University of Pittsburgh, Pittsburgh, PA 15260*

[3]*Division of Pulmonary and Critical Care Medicine, Department of Medicine, University of Pittsburgh, Pittsburgh, PA 15260*

THE importance of the small anion nitrite (NO_2^-) in meat curing and as an antidote for cyanide poisoning has been recognized for centuries. However, its role as a physiological signaling molecule has been more elusive. This chapter will briefly describe the many emerging physiological effects of nitrite including the role of nitrite as a cell signaling molecule, focusing primarily on its vasodilatory activity during hypoxia and cytoprotective effects in the setting of ischemia/reperfusion.

THE FORMATION OF NITRITE *IN VIVO*

The concentration of nitrite *in vivo* appears to be highly regulated as the concentration of the anion in different compartments remains within a relatively narrow range. Plasma nitrite concentrations are maintained between 300 and 500 nM [1], while in tissue compartments nitrite concentration is much higher, in the 1–10 μM range [2]. Endogenous concentrations of nitrite are derived from two sources: oxidation of nitric oxide (NO) [3] and the dietary intake of nitrite and nitrate [4]. As described in Chapters 1 and 3, there are several mechanisms by which NO is generated in the body, including enzymatically by the NOS enzymes and non-enzymatically by acidic reduction of nitrite. Once NO is formed, it can be oxidized to nitrite or nitrate through its relatively slow reaction with oxygen. However, in most in vivo environments, this auto-oxidation reaction is not favored since NO reacts more rapidly with other targets, particularly heme based proteins. For example, in the blood, NO reacts with oxygenated hemoglobin at near diffusion limited rates ($k = 1 \times 10^7\ M^{-1}\ s^{-1}$) by a reaction that yields nitrate (NO_3^-) and methemoglobin [5]. Hence, kinetically, it is unexpected that any NO would be oxidized to nitrite in the blood. However, it has been shown that the addition of NO to blood does generate significant concentrations of plasma nitrite [3,6]. This paradoxical nitrite formation can be explained by the presence of an "NO oxidase", a protein that catalyzes the oxidation of NO to nitrite. It is now known that in the plasma, the multi-copper oxidase ceruloplasmin can act as a NO oxidase to generate nitrite (Figure 6.1). Consistent with this role for ceruloplasmin, mice deficient in ceruloplasmin have lower basal concentrations of plasma nitrite and less nitrite is formed in the plasma of these animals when NO is added *in vitro* [3].

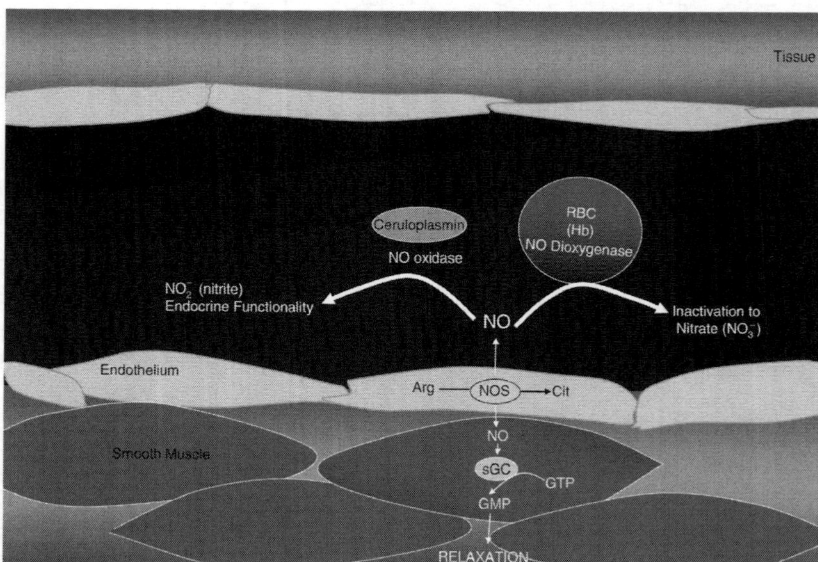

FIGURE 6.1 Ceruloplasmin is a NO oxidase. Nitric oxide is generated in the blood vessel by nitric oxide synthase (NOS). NO can mediate vasodilation by activating soluble guanylate cyclase in the smooth muscle cell or diffuse into the lumen of the vessel. In the lumen, NO reacts with hemoglobin in a dioxygenase reaction to form nitrate (NO_3^-) or is oxidized by ceruloplasmin to nitrite (NO_2^-), which can mediate vasodilation or cytoprotection after I/R.

The other source of nitrite *in vivo* is the dietary intake of both nitrite and nitrate. Nitrite itself has been used in curing meat (outlined in Chapter 5) and is present in leafy green vegetables. However, nitrate is much more abundant than nitrite in the diet. The concentration of nitrate is approximately 500 times that of nitrite in leafy green vegetables, and it is also present in beet roots as well as other components of the so-called Mediterranean diet [7]. Once nitrate enters the oral cavity, commensal bacteria in the posterior crypts of the tongue reduce the nitrate to nitrite. In addition, nitrate is concentrated and secreted into the saliva by the salivary glands, which allows for nitrate to come into close contact with and be reduced to nitrite by the oral flora. Consistent with this central role of the oral bacteria, Lundberg and colleagues have shown that the ingestion of nitrate leads to an increase in plasma nitrite levels, and these levels are decreased when an antiseptic mouthwash is used to remove the commensal bacteria [8].

NITRITE—FROM INERT METABOLITE TO PHYSIOLOGICAL VASODILATOR

Although it has been recognized for some time that nitrite is present *in vivo*, for decades this small anion was regarded as a physiologically inert metabolite of NO oxidation. One of the first formal tests of nitrite's vasoactivity was performed by Furchgott and colleagues in 1953, in which they demonstrated that high concentrations (100 μM–1 mM) of nitrite could mediate vasodilation when applied to isolated aortic rings *in vitro* [9]. However, since the concentration of nitrite in blood was found to be less than one micromolar [1], this precluded a role for nitrite as a physiological vasodilator [10]. In 2000, Gladwin and colleagues reported significant artery-to-vein gradients of nitrite in the human circulation and showed that nitrite consumption increased with exercise [11,12]. In addition, they demonstrated that inhaled NO gas mediated vasodilation, and this phenomenon was accompanied by a significant rise in plasma nitrite concentrations [11]. These seminal observations led to the re-evaluation of nitrite as a vasodilator. In 2003, Gladwin and colleagues tested whether nitrite could mediate vasodilation *in vivo* by infusing physiological concentrations of nitrite in the human brachial artery and simultaneously measuring forearm blood flow. In all cases, including when subjects were at rest, during exercise, or in the presence of the NOS inhibitor LNAME, nitrite significantly increased forearm blood flow [13]. Interestingly, vasodilation was associated with an increase in the formation of NO-modified hemoglobin [13], leading to the hypothesis that nitrite is reduced to NO and that hemoglobin may be responsible for the reduction of nitrite.

HEMOGLOBIN AS A REGULATOR OF HYPOXIC VASODILATION

The idea that hemoglobin could reduce nitrite to NO was supported by a previously described reaction between nitrite and deoxygenated hemoglobin [Equation (1)] by which deoxygenated hemoglobin (deoxyHb), in the presence of a proton, reduces nitrite to NO while being oxidized to methemoglobin (metHb) [14]:

$$\text{Nitrite} + \text{DeoxyHb}\ (Fe^{2+}) + H^{+} \rightarrow \text{NO} + \text{MetHb}\ (Fe^{3+}) + OH^{-} \qquad (1)$$

The bioactive NO generated from this reaction could then mediate vasodilation through the canonical NO-soluble guanylate cyclase-cGMP pathway. This idea was confirmed by a series of *in vitro* experiments in which various concentrations of nitrite were added to pre-constricted aortic rings. On its own, nitrite dilated the aortic rings at high micromolar concentrations, consistent with the early experiments of Furchgott and colleagues. However, in the presence of deoxygenated red blood cells, nanomolar concentrations of nitrite mediated significant vasodilation [13]. Indeed, consistent with the hypothesis of NO-mediated vasodilation, cyclic GMP was generated in the aortic rings in the presence of nitrite and deoxygenated red blood cells, and this effect was inhibited by the NO scavenger PTIO [13,15].

The nitrite reductase activity of hemoglobin is regulated by a number of factors including pH, oxygen concentration and the allosteric structural transition of the hemoglobin protein [16,17]. According to reaction (1) above, hemoglobin must be deoxygenated in order to reduce nitrite to NO, hence nitrite reduction is favored in hypoxic conditions. In addition, the reaction requires a proton to proceed, and hence as pH is lowered, the rate of hemoglobin-dependent nitrite reduction (and concomitant NO generation) increases [16,17].

Kinetic analysis of the hemoglobin nitrite reductase reaction also revealed that the nitrite reductase activity is regulated by the allosteric structural transition of the hemoglobin tetramer from the deoxy (T) to oxy (R) state [17]. These two allosteric conformations of hemoglobin possess different redox characteristics. Deoxy (T state) hemoglobin is not bound by oxygen and hence has free heme groups which are available to react with nitrite, while oxy (R state) hemoglobin has fewer sites for nitrite to bind, but possesses a lower reduction potential and hence is a better electron donor. As nitrite reacts with T state hemoglobin, the number of free heme sites (T state hemoglobin) decreases. However, as the reaction proceeds, R state hemoglobin is stabilized. These two opposing chemistries (the decrease in available binding sites and the increase in rate due to R state stabilization) reach an optimal balance at the P_{50} (the point at which half the ligands are saturated) of hemoglobin, which is the point of maximal nitrite reduction and NO generation [17] (Figure 6.2).

One major challenge facing the idea that NO generated from red blood cell deoxyhemoglobin-nitrite reaction can mediate vasodilation is that hemoglobin is a potent scavenger of NO and hence any NO generated would be scavenged before mediating vasodilation. It is now known that in addition to the chemistry described above, nitrite and deoxyhemoglobin can undergo a reductive anhydrase reaction which

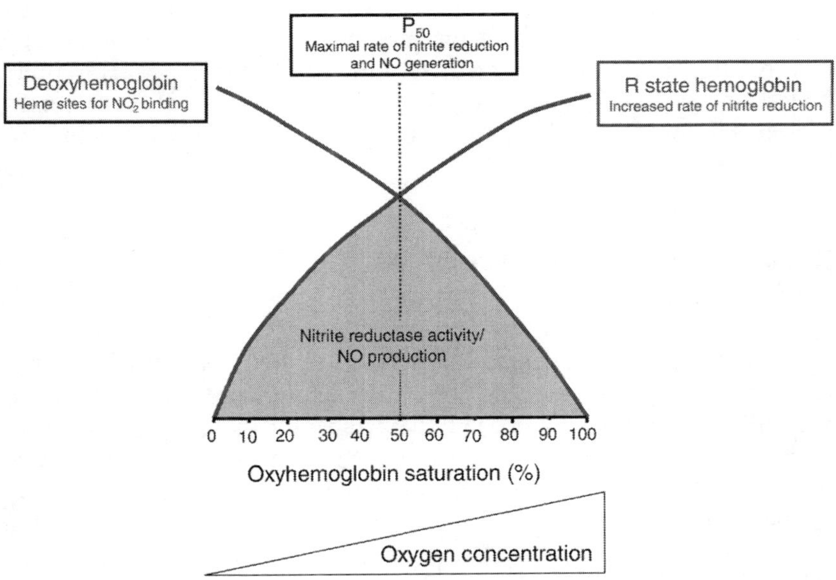

FIGURE 6.2 Allosteric regulation of nitrite reductase rate. The rate of hemoglobin-dependent nitrite reduction (black dashed line) is dependent on the number of available heme sites for reaction (blue line) and the amount of R state tetramers (red line). As oxygen saturation of hemoglobin increases, the number of available hemesites for nitrite binding decreases, decelerating the reaction. However, the R state tetramer is increasingly stabilized, which accelerates reaction rate. The maximal reaction rate occurs at an optimal balance of these two subprocesses, which occurs when 50% of the hemoglobin is saturated with oxygen. The partial pressure at which this occurs is the P_{50} of hemoglobin.

produces dinitrogen trioxide (N_2O_3), a unique species that is not scavenged by hemoglobin and can diffuse out of the red blood cell and homolyze into NO [18]. Briefly, one molecule of nitrite reacts with deoxyhemoglobin and generates NO and methemoglobin by the classical nitrite reductase reaction described in Equation (1). Another molecule of nitrite binds to methemoglobin, and this nitrite bound methemoglobin has an unusual electron configuration which appears to possess Fe^{2+}-$NO_2\cdot$ character Equation (2):

$$HbFe^{+3}\text{-}NO_2^- \text{ (metheme bound to nitrite)} \rightarrow Fe^{+2}\text{- } NO_2\cdot \quad \text{(Reaction 2)}$$

The $NO_2\cdot$ species can react rapidly with a molecule of NO to form dinitrogen trioxide (N_2O_3). By this reaction, hemoglobin essentially catalyzes the removal of a molecule of water from two molecules of nitrite to generate N_2O_3 [18]. This may allow the NO generated from nitrite to reach distal targets without being scavenged by hemoglobin. Furthermore, N_2O_3 is unique in that it reacts with free thiols and is a potent nitrosating agent, and hence lends another mechanism by which nitrite can modify proteins and mediate biological effects. This unique NO/N_2O_3 generating chemistry, which is maximized at the P_{50} of hemoglobin, has been hypothesized to be the mechanism responsible for hypoxic vasodilation [15,19–21].

NITRITE AS A MEDIATOR OF HYPOXIC VASODILATION

A maximal nitrite reductase activity at the hemoglobin P50 is biochemically consistent with the potential role of this reaction in hypoxic vasodilation. Hypoxic vasodilation is the physiological response to hypoxia by which oxygen delivery (via blood flow) is matched to tissue oxygen demand. This response requires the ability to detect changes in oxygen concentration or pH in the tissue, and to link this sensing to the generation of a vasodilator [22]. Although the exact mechanism of this response is unknown, the set point for humans at which this response occurs is between hemoglobin oxygen saturations of 40–60%, a value approximating the P_{50} of hemoglobin and the point of maximal nitrite reduction [23]. Studies investigating the gradients of hemoglobin oxygen saturation across the vasculature show that arteriolar oxygen concentration drops from A1 to A4 caliber arterioles. In skeletal muscle, this drop is substantial, resulting in hemoglobin saturation values of less than 40% (PO_2 of 20 mm Hg) in A4 level arterioles [24]. These data demonstrate that conditions ideal for maximal nitrite reductase activity occur within resistance vessels, consistent with a potential physiological role for nitrite-dependent hypoxic vasodilation. Indeed, evidence is accumulating that this chemistry may be responsible for hypoxic vasodilation. Consistent with this idea, Maher and colleagues demonstrated that in human subjects nitrite dilated the venous circulation in the forearm, and during experimental hypoxia (breathing of 11% oxygen), nitrite also dilated the arteriolar circulation [21].

OTHER NITRITE REDUCTASES

It is now recognized that the reduction of nitrite to bioavailable NO can be catalyzed by a number of proteins under appropriate conditions. Members of the heme globin family, other than hemoglobin, including myoglobin [25,26] and neuroglobin [27], have been shown to reduce nitrite by the same reaction as hemoglobin. Interestingly, these proteins possess a much lower reduction potential than T state hemoglobin, hence they reduce nitrite at a rate that is significantly greater than hemoglobin [26]. However, the P_{50} of these proteins is much lower (2.8 and 2.2 mm Hg for myoglobin and neuroglobin respectively) than that of hemoglobin. Thus, although they are much more efficient nitrite reductases, myoglobin and neuroglobin only become active at much lower oxygen tensions than hemoglobin.

In addition to the heme globin family, a number of other heme containing proteins have been shown to possess nitrite reductase chemistry, including xanthine oxidoreductase [28], cytochromes in the mitochondrial electron transport chain [29,30], endothelial NOS [31], and cytochrome P450 enzymes [32]. The differential distribution of these proteins in various biological compartments suggests that mechanisms of nitrite reduction may vary by tissue type. In addition, each of these reductases generate NO optimally at different pH and oxygen concentrations, ensuring that nitrite is reduced to NO along a broad range of physiological pH and oxygen concentrations.

NITRITE AS A CELL SIGNALING MOLECULE

The role of nitrite as a cell signaling molecule extends beyond mediating hypoxic vasodilation. In addition to stimulating soluble guanylate cyclase, NO generated from nitrite may form iron nitrosyl complexes with other proteins to mediate signaling. For example, nitrite reduction to NO binds $heme_{aa3}$ on cytochrome c oxidase to regulate mitochondrial respiration. Alternatively, nitrite may mediate S-nitrosation (the NO-dependent modification of thiols) to mediate signaling. While this may occur through the reductive anhydrase reaction (discussed above), nitrite-mediated N- and S-nitrosation has also been proposed to occur in the absence of NO formation. For example, Bryan *et al.* [33] recently reported that nitrite inhibits cytochrome P_{450} activity and affects the expression of two archetypical proteins, heat shock protein 70 and heme oxygenase-1. Nitrite mediated S-nitrosation will be discussed further in the context of ischemia/reperfusion injury below.

NITRITE MEDIATES CYTOPROTECTION DURING ISCHEMIA/REPERFUSION

Ischemia/reperfusion (I/R) injury, characterized by an inappropriate inflammatory response in the microcirculation, mitochondrial damage, and increased reactive oxygen species generation leading to oxidative modification of proteins and eventual cell death and tissue injury. Ischemia/reperfusion (I/R) is a component of many diseases and injury following I/R is a major cause of morbidity and mortality in the Western World [34]. In the right conditions, NO is known to be protective after I/R. However, NO cannot be enzymatically generated during ischemia since the NOS enzymes require oxygen as a substrate. The fact that nitrite is selectively reduced to NO in conditions of low oxygen and low pH led to the hypothesis that nitrite may be an important cytoprotective source of NO during tissue ischemia. Indeed, several studies have demonstrated that physiological concentrations of nitrite mediate potent cytoprotection in a number of animal models of ischemia/reperfusion (I/R) [35–44]. Webb and colleagues used an isolated perfused heart model of I/R to first demonstrate that micromolar concentrations of nitrite were cytoprotective, and that this cytoprotection was dependent on the reduction of nitrite to NO [43]. Duranski and colleagues were the first to demonstrate *in vivo* that nitrite could mediate cytoprotection [36]. They did this using murine models of hepatic ischemia/reperfusion and myocardial infarction, and in both models, nitrite mediated cytoprotection (measured as a decrease in circulating liver enzymes and a decrease in infarct size for each model respectively) in a dose dependent manner. Nitrite mediated protection in this model through NO signaling via soluble guanylate cyclase as administration of the NO inhibitor PTIO and the sGC inhibitor ODQ completely abolished protection. This cytoprotection was also eNOS and hemoxygenase-1 independent [36]. Nitrite is now known to be protective in a number of animal models of focal I/R in the heart, liver, brain, and kidney [35–44] (Table 6.1).

As a cytoprotective agent, nitrite demonstrates a great deal of versatility in terms of dose, as well as time and route of administration. Duranski and colleagues demonstrated that concentrations of nitrite within a large range (1.2–960 nmol) can reduce infarct size in a murine model of myocardial infarction. This dose response is biphasic, with the optimal dose at 48 nmols for a mouse [36]. Nitrite also mediates protection in a broad temporal window. Shiva and colleagues showed that a single dose of nitrite (48 nmol) given 24 hours before the ischemic episode is as protective in a murine model of hepatic I/R as when it is administered during ischemia [41]. Gonzalez and colleagues described a canine model of coronary artery occlusion in which the myocardium was made ischemic for 2 hours before reperfusion. In this model, a significant decrease in infarct size was observed whether nitrite was administered one hour or five minutes before reperfusion [37]. In addition, Bryan and colleagues have demonstrated that nitrite supplementation in the diet can attenuate injury in a murine model of myocardial I/R, while depletion of nitrite from the diet can exacerbate I/R-induced injury [35,45]. In the first demonstration that nitrite mediates cytoprotection in humans, study subjects drank nitrate rich beetroot juice to increase their plasma nitrite levels by 2-fold, and this increase was associated with prevention of I/R-induced endothelial damage in the forearm after an acute ischemic episode [44]. Nitrite also appears to be protective in a chronically ischemic setting, as Kumar and colleagues showed that nitrite can increase angiogenesis in a chronic murine model of hindlimb ischemia [46].

Importantly, the majority of studies demonstrating nitrite-dependent cytoprotection also show that this protection is dependent on the reduction of nitrite to NO, as the NO scavenger PTIO abolishes cytoprotection [36,43,46]. While acidic reduction of nitrite may be responsible for a small portion of nitrite-dependent NO generation in ischemic tissue, nitrite reductase proteins also play a role. Webb and colleagues reported that in the perfused Langendorff model of myocardial I/R, the xanthine oxidoreductase inhibitor, allopurinol, attenuated NO generation and nitrite dependent cytoprotection [43]. Rassaf and colleagues demonstrated using an *in vivo* murine model of myocardial infarction that myoglobin knockout mice are not protected by nitrite, suggesting that myoglobin is the predominant nitrite reductase during ischemia [39]. It is likely that different reductases play a role in different tissues, and that several proteins may synergize during ischemia to reduce nitrite to NO.

TABLE 6.1 Overview of Animal Models in which Nitrite Administration Reduced Ischemia Reperfusion Injury.

Species	I/R Model	Placebo	Nitrite Route	I/R Period	Measure of Outcome	Ref
			Heart			
Mouse	Left main coronary artery occlusion	Standard Chow	Supplemented in drinking water (50 mg/L for 7 d)	30-min ischemia 24-hr reperfusion	Infarct size	[35]
Mouse	Left main coronary artery occlusion	Nitrate or saline	2.4-1920 nmol i.v. injection 5 min before reperfusion	30-min ischemia 24-hr reperfusion	Infarct size	[36]
Mouse	Left main coronary artery occlusion	Saline	8 nmol i.p. Injection 24 h or 5 min before reperfusion	30-min ischemia 24-hr reperfusion	Infarct size	[41]
Rat	In vivo—Left anterior descending coronary artery occlusion	Nitrate or saline	In vivo - 0.04–10.0 mg/kg i.v. injection for 15 min before ischemia	In vivo-30 min ischemia	Infarct size	[47]
Rat	*In vitro*—isolated perfused heart (Langendorff)	Nitrate or saline	1.0–300.0 µmol/L infusion for 15 min before ischemia	30-min ischemia 180-min reperfusion	Left ventricular developed pressure (LVDP)	[47]
Rat	Isolated perfused heart	Saline	10 or100 uM for 15 min before I/R	30 min ischemia; 120 min reperfusion	Infarct size, LVDP; rate of change of pressure during diastole	[43]
Dog	In vivo—Left anterior descending coronary artery occlusion	Saline	0.20 µmol/min per kg 20 min infusion followed by 0.17 µmol/min/kg infusion for 40 min or 0.20 µmol/ min/kg infusion for 5 min during last 60 min or 5 min of ischemia	2-hr ischemia, 6 hr reperfusion	Infarct size, microvascular Perfusion, cardiomyocyte Apoptosis, left ventricular ejection fraction	[37]

(continued)

TABLE 6.1.(continued) Overview of Animal Models in which Nitrite Administration Reduced Ischemia Reperfusion Injury.

Species	I/R Model	Placebo	Nitrite Route	I/R Period	Measure of Outcome	Ref
			Liver			
Mouse	Hepatic artery/portal vein occlusion	Nitrate or saline	1.2–960 of nmol i.p. injection midway through ischemia 5	45-min ischemia 24-hr reperfusion	AST/ALT, Histopathology Hepatocellular necrosis and apoptosis	[36]
Mouse	Hepatic artery/portal vein occlusion	Saline	48 nmol of bolus i.p. Injection 24 h before ischemia or mid-way through ischemia or 200 μL of 100 mg/L oral gavage 24 h before ischemia onset	45-min ischemia 5-hr reperfusion	AST/ ALT	[41]
			Kidney			
Rat	Bilateral renal pedicle occlusion	Saline	0.12 nmol/g administered topically or i.v. 1 min before reperfusion	60-min ischemia 6-hr reperfusion	Serum creatinine, Creatinine clearance, Fractional excretion of sodium, AST, Renal injury (histology)	[42]
			Brain			
Rat	Middle cerebral artery occlusion	Nitrate	48-4800 nmol of i.v. infusion for 1 min at start of reperfusion	90 min ischemia 3-hr (LCBF) or 24-hr (infarct size) or 2-hr/1, 3, 7 d (neurologic testing) reperfusion	Infarct size, LCBF, neurologic scores	[40]

i.v. = intravenous, i.p. = intraperitoneal, ALT = alanine aminotransferase, AST= asparagine aminotransferase, MPO= myeloperoxidase, LCBF = left coronary blood flow. Modified from Sinha *et al.* [48] and reproduced with permission.

THE MECHANISM OF NITRITE-DEPENDENT CYTOPROTECTION

The pathology of I/R injury is complicated and stems from a number of processes. During ischemia, high energy phosphate stores are depleted and the ability to generate more ATP is dramatically decreased. While reperfusion is needed to supply the tissue with oxygen necessary for survival, reperfusion actually exacerbates injury and contributes to cell death. This is because the rapid re-introduction of oxygen is associated with a burst of reactive oxygen species generation which damages protein and lipids within the cell and accelerates cell death.

The mechanism of nitrite dependent cytoprotection is not completely understood, but potentially affects a number of processes. Nitrite regulates the expression of proteins important in the hypoxic response, including heat shock protein 70 and hemeoxygenase-1. Nitrite is also able to mediate post-translational modification of proteins [2,49], metal centers [16,17] and lipids [50]. Several of these modifications, including nitrosylation of heme and S-nitrosation of thiols, have been associated with nitrite-dependent cytoprotection in models of I/R [49]. While the identity of all these modified protein targets are not yet known, some targets have been identified.

Mitochondrial dysfunction is central in the progression of I/R injury and the mitochondria has been shown to be a target for nitrite within the cell. In cardiomyocytes, once nitrite is reduced by myoglobin, the resulting NO can inhibit mitochondrial respiration by binding complex IV of the respiratory chain [41]. This inhibition has been hypothesized to contribute to a phenomenon known as "cardiac hibernation", in which the energetic state of the heart is downregulated during ischemia to preserve energy [39,41]. Shiva and colleagues have shown that nitrite can also regulate pathological mitochondrial ROS generation at reperfusion. Upon reperfusion, mitochondria generate a burst of ROS which is thought to contribute to cell death [51–53]. Nitrite can modify critical thiol groups on mitochondrial complex I by S-nitrosation which inhibits the activity of the complex. By inhibiting this complex, the entry of electrons into the electron transport chain is decreased, and consequently, reactive oxygen species generation by the mitochondrion is also decreased, preventing oxidative protein and lipid damage, cytochrome c release, and eventual cell death.

CONCLUSIONS

In summary, the role for nitrite as a physiologically relevant signaling molecule is just being uncovered. Nitrite is formed from endogenous NO and is rapidly absorbed from the diet. The selective conversion of nitrite to NO at low pH and oxygen concentrations by a number of nitrite reductase proteins make it ideal for hypoxic cell signaling. Through its interaction with hemoglobin, nitrite is an ideal candidate to mediate hypoxic vasodilation. In addition, nitrite is a potent cytoprotective agent in the setting of ischemia/reperfusion. While there is much left to understand about the mechanisms of nitrite-mediated signaling, it is clear that nitrite is an important regulator of biological responses.

ABOUT THE AUTHORS

Sruti Shiva, Ph.D.

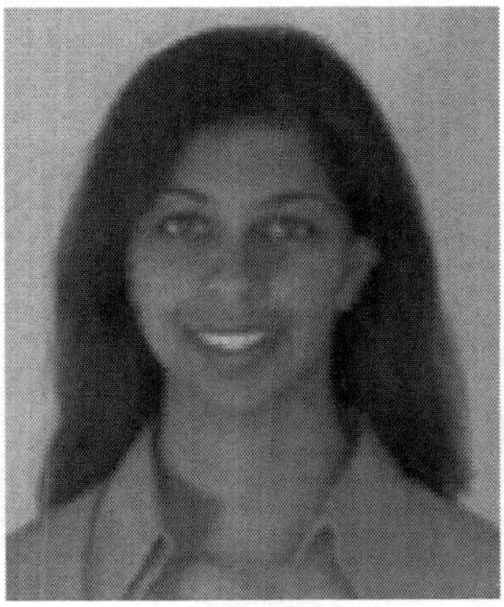

Sruti Shiva received her PhD from the University of Alabama at Birmingham in 2004. She then completed a four year post-doctoral fellowship under the mentorship of Mark Gladwin in the Pulmonary and Vascular Medicine Branch of NHLBI, NIH . Currently, Dr. Shiva is an Assistant Professor in the Department of Pharmacology and Chemical Biology and a member of the Hemostasis and Vascular Biology Research Institute at the University of Pittsburgh.

Dr. Shiva's research focuses on the regulation of mitochondrial function by nitric oxide, nitrite and other reactive nitrogen species, particularly in physiological conditions of hypoxia and pathological ischemia/reperfusion. She is an author on over 30 peer-reviewed articles and has been invited to speak at a number of national and international meetings.

Mark Gladwin, M.D.

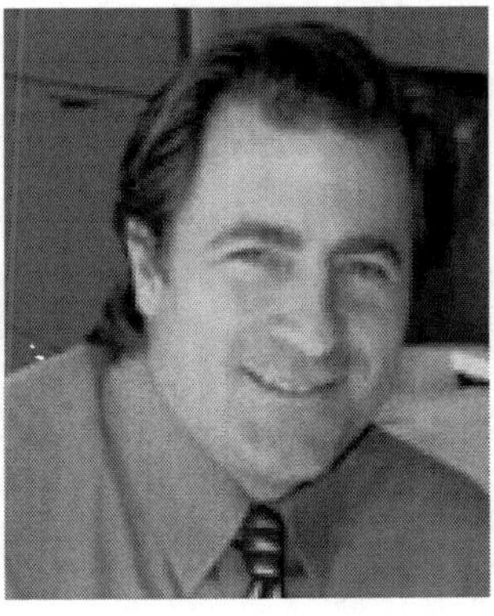

Mark Gladwin received his M.D. from the University of Miami Honors Program in Medical Education in 1991. After completing his internship and chief residency at the Oregon Health Sciences University in Portland, Ore., he joined the NIH in 1995 as a critical care fellow in the Clinical Center. After a one-year clinical fellowship in pulmonary medicine at the University of Washington in Seattle, he returned for a research fellowship at the Critical Care Medicine Department, CC, under the mentorship of James Shelhamer, Frederick Ognibene, Alan Schechter, and Richard Cannon. He then became the Chief of the Pulmonary and Vascular Medicine Branch within the NHLBI, NIH. In August of 2007, Dr. Gladwin became the Division Chief of the Pulmonary, Allergy and Critical Care Medicine Department at the University of Pittsburgh and is leading the newly formed Hemostasis and Vascular Biology Research Institute.

Since 1998, Dr. Gladwin's research activities have led to four major scientific discoveries. These discoveries have resulted in more than 150 published peer-reviewed manuscripts, 30 approved protocols, and more than 1000 patient protocol enrollments at the NIH Clinical Center. The four scientific discoveries include:

1. The discovery that the nitrite anion is a circulating storage pool for NO bioactivity (Gladwin, et al. PNAS 2002).
2. The discovery of a novel physiological function for hemoglobin as an electronically and allosterically regulated nitrite reductase (Cosby, et al. Nature Medicine 2003; Huang et al. JCI 2005). These studies reveal that nitrite is a potent vasodilator in humans, is bioactivated by reaction with deoxyhemoglobin to generate NO preferentially under hypoxic conditions and suggest that hemoglobin has an "enzymatic" property of a nitrite reductase that participates in hypoxic vasodilation. In related translational studies Dr. Gladwin has demonstrated that inhaled nitrite reverses hypoxic neonatal pulmonary hypertension in sheep (Hunter, et al. Nature Medicine 2004), and that infused nitrite solutions prevent post subarachnoid hemorrhage induced vasospasm in primates (Pluta et al. JAMA 2005) and prevent hepatic and cardiac ischemia-reperfusion injury and infarction in mice (Lefer et al. JCI 2005).
3. The characterization of a novel mechanism of disease, hemolysis-associated endothelial dysfunction (Reiter, et al. Nature 2003; Morris et al. JAMA 2005; Minneci et al. JCI 2005). This work has described a state of resistance to NO in patients with sickle cell disease caused by scavenging of nitric oxide by hemoglobin, released into plasma during hemolysis.
4. The mechanistic, clinical, and epidemiological description of a human disease syndrome, hemolysis-associated pulmonary hypertension (Gladwin, et al. NEJM 2004). He has found that pulmonary hypertension occurs in 30% of patients with sickle cell disease, is a major cause of mortality in this population (odds ratio 10:1), and is strongly associated with high hemolytic rate, iron overload and kidney disease.

REFERENCES

1. Dejam, A.; Hunter, C. J.; Pelletier, M. M.; Hsu, L. L.; Machado, R. F.; Shiva, S.; Power, G. G.; Kelm, M.; Gladwin, M. T.; Schechter, A. N. Erythrocytes are the major intravascular storage sites of nitrite in human blood. *Blood* 106:734–739; 2005.
2. Bryan, N. S.; Rassaf, T.; Maloney, R. E.; Rodriguez, C. M.; Saijo, F.; Rodriguez, J. R.; Feelisch, M. Cellular targets and mechanisms of nitros(yl)ation: an insight into their nature and kinetics *in vivo*. *Proc Natl Acad Sci U S A* 101:4308–4313; 2004.
3. Shiva, S.; Wang, X.; Ringwood, L. A.; Xu, X.; Yuditskaya, S.; Annavajjhala, V.; Miyajima, H.; Hogg, N.; Harris, Z. L.; Gladwin, M. T. Ceruloplasmin is a NO oxidase and nitrite synthase that determines endocrine NO homeostasis. *Nat Chem Biol* 2:486–493; 2006.
4. Lundberg, J. O.; Weitzberg, E.; Gladwin, M. T. The nitrate-nitrite-nitric oxide pathway in physiology and therapeutics. *Nat Rev Drug Discov* 7:156–167; 2008.
5. Olson, J. S.; Foley, E. W.; Rogge, C.; Tsai, A. L.; Doyle, M. P.; Lemon, D. D. No scavenging and the hypertensive effect of hemoglobin-based blood substitutes. *Free Radic Biol Med* 36:685–697; 2004.
6. Wang, X.; Tanus-Santos, J. E.; Reiter, C. D.; Dejam, A.; Shiva, S.; Smith, R. D.; Hogg, N.; Gladwin, M. T. Biological activity of nitric oxide in the plasmatic compartment. *Proc Natl Acad Sci U S A* 101:11477–11482; 2004.
7. Walker, R. Nitrates, nitrites and N-nitrosocompounds: a review of the occurrence in food and diet and the toxicological implications. *Food Addit Contam* 7:717–768; 1990.
8. Govoni, M.; Jansson, E. A.; Weitzberg, E.; Lundberg, J. O. The increase in plasma nitrite after a dietary nitrate load is markedly attenuated by an antibacterial mouthwash. *Nitric Oxide* 19:333–337; 2008.
9. Furchgott, R. F.; Bhadrakom, S. Reactions of strips of rabbit aorta to epinephrine, isopropylarterenol, sodium nitrite and other drugs. *J Pharmacol Exp Ther* 108:129–143; 1953.
10. Lauer, T.; Preik, M.; Rassaf, T.; Strauer, B. E.; Deussen, A.; Feelisch, M.; Kelm, M. Plasma nitrite rather than nitrate reflects regional endothelial nitric oxide synthase activity but lacks intrinsic vasodilator action. *Proc Natl Acad Sci U S A* 98:12814–12819; 2001.
11. Cannon, R. O., 3rd; Schechter, A. N.; Panza, J. A.; Ognibene, F. P.; Pease-Fye, M. E.; Waclawiw, M. A.; Shelhamer, J. H.; Gladwin, M. T. Effects of inhaled nitric oxide on regional blood flow are consistent with intravascular nitric oxide delivery. *J Clin Invest* 108:279–287; 2001.
12. Gladwin, M. T.; Shelhamer, J. H.; Schechter, A. N.; Pease-Fye, M. E.; Waclawiw, M. A.; Panza, J. A.; Ognibene, F. P.; Cannon, R. O., 3rd. Role of circulating nitrite and S-nitrosohemoglobin in the regulation of regional blood flow in humans. *Proc Natl Acad Sci U S A* 97:11482–11487; 2000.
13. Cosby, K.; Partovi, K. S.; Crawford, J. H.; Patel, R. P.; Reiter, C. D.; Martyr, S.; Yang, B. K.; Waclawiw, M. A.; Zalos, G.; Xu, X.; Huang, K. T.; Shields, H.; Kim-Shapiro, D. B.; Schechter, A. N.; Cannon, R. O., 3rd; Gladwin, M. T. Nitrite reduction to nitric oxide by deoxyhemoglobin vasodilates the human circulation. *Nat Med* 9:1498–1505; 2003.
14. Doyle, M. P.; Pickering, R. A.; DeWeert, T. M.; Hoekstra, J. W.; Pater, D. Kinetics and mechanism of the oxidation of human deoxyhemoglobin by nitrites. *J Biol Chem* 256:12393–12398; 1981.
15. Crawford, J. H.; Isbell, T. S.; Huang, Z.; Shiva, S.; Chacko, B. K.; Schechter, A. N.; Darley-Usmar, V. M.; Kerby, J. D.; Lang, J. D., Jr.; Kraus, D.; Ho, C.; Gladwin, M. T.; Patel, R. P. Hypoxia, red blood cells, and nitrite regulate NO-dependent hypoxic vasodilation. *Blood* 107:566–574; 2006.

16. Huang, K. T.; Keszler, A.; Patel, N.; Patel, R. P.; Gladwin, M. T.; Kim-Shapiro, D. B.; Hogg, N. The reaction between nitrite and deoxyhemoglobin. Reassessment of reaction kinetics and stoichiometry. *J Biol Chem* 280:31126–31131; 2005.

17. Huang, Z.; Shiva, S.; Kim-Shapiro, D. B.; Patel, R. P.; Ringwood, L. A.; Irby, C. E.; Huang, K. T.; Ho, C.; Hogg, N.; Schechter, A. N.; Gladwin, M. T. Enzymatic function of hemoglobin as a nitrite reductase that produces NO under allosteric control. *J Clin Invest* 115:2099–2107; 2005.

18. Basu, S.; Grubina, R.; Huang, J.; Conradie, J.; Huang, Z.; Jeffers, A.; Jiang, A.; He, X.; Azarov, I.; Seibert, R.; Mehta, A.; Patel, R.; King, S. B.; Hogg, N.; Ghosh, A.; Gladwin, M. T.; Kim-Shapiro, D. B. Catalytic generation of N2O3 by the concerted nitrite reductase and anhydrase activity of hemoglobin. *Nat Chem Biol* 3:785–794; 2007.

19. Gladwin, M. T. Hemoglobin as a nitrite reductase regulating red cell-dependent hypoxic vasodilation. *Am J Respir Cell Mol Biol* 32:363–366; 2005.

20. Gladwin, M. T.; Schechter, A. N.; Kim-Shapiro, D. B.; Patel, R. P.; Hogg, N.; Shiva, S.; Cannon, R. O., 3rd; Kelm, M.; Wink, D. A.; Espey, M. G.; Oldfield, E. H.; Pluta, R. M.; Freeman, B. A.; Lancaster, J. R., Jr.; Feelisch, M.; Lundberg, J. O. The emerging biology of the nitrite anion. *Nat Chem Biol* 1:308–314; 2005.

21. Maher, A. R.; Milsom, A. B.; Gunaruwan, P.; Abozguia, K.; Ahmed, I.; Weaver, R. A.; Thomas, P.; Ashrafian, H.; Born, G. V.; James, P. E.; Frenneaux, M. P. Hypoxic modulation of exogenous nitrite-induced vasodilation in humans. *Circulation* 117:670–677; 2008.

22. Tune, J. D.; Gorman, M. W.; Feigl, E. O. Matching coronary blood flow to myocardial oxygen consumption. *J Appl Physiol* 97:404–415; 2004.

23. Ross JM, F. H., Weldy J, Guyton AC. Autoregulation of blood flow by oxygen lack. Am J Physiol 202:21–24; 1963.

24. Tsai, A. G.; Johnson, P. C.; Intaglietta, M. Oxygen gradients in the microcirculation. *Physiol Rev* 83:933–963; 2003.

25. Rassaf, T.; Flogel, U.; Drexhage, C.; Hendgen-Cotta, U.; Kelm, M.; Schrader, J. Nitrite reductase function of deoxymyoglobin: oxygen sensor and regulator of cardiac energetics and function. *Circ Res* 100:1749–1754; 2007.

26. Shiva, S.; Huang, Z.; Grubina, R.; Sun, J.; Ringwood, L. A.; MacArthur, P. H.; Xu, X.; Murphy, E.; Darley-Usmar, V. M.; Gladwin, M. T. Deoxymyoglobin is a nitrite reductase that generates nitric oxide and regulates mitochondrial respiration. *Circ Res* 100:654–661; 2007.

27. Petersen, M. G.; Dewilde, S.; Fago, A. Reactions of ferrous neuroglobin and cytoglobin with nitrite under anaerobic conditions. *J Inorg Biochem* 102:1777–1782; 2008.

28. Xia, Y.; Zweier, J. L. Substrate control of free radical generation from xanthine oxidase in the postischemic heart. *J Biol Chem* 270:18797–18803; 1995.

29. Castello, P. R.; David, P. S.; McClure, T.; Crook, Z.; Poyton, R. O. Mitochondrial cytochrome oxidase produces nitric oxide under hypoxic conditions: implications for oxygen sensing and hypoxic signaling in eukaryotes. *Cell Metab* 3:277–287; 2006.

30. Kozlov, A. V.; Staniek, K.; Nohl, H. Nitrite reductase activity is a novel function of mammalian mitochondria. *FEBS Lett* 454:127–130; 1999.

31. Vanin, A. F.; Bevers, L. M.; Slama-Schwok, A.; van Faassen, E. E. Nitric oxide synthase reduces nitrite to NO under anoxia. *Cell Mol Life Sci.* 64:96–103; 2007.

32. Kozlov, A. V.; Dietrich, B.; Nohl, H. Various intracellular compartments cooperate in the release of nitric oxide from glycerol trinitrate in liver. *Br.J Pharmacol.* 139:989–997; 2003.

33. Bryan, N. S.; Fernandez, B. O.; Bauer, S. M.; Garcia-Saura, M. F.; Milsom, A. B.; Rassaf, T.; Maloney, R. E.; Bharti, A.; Rodriguez, J.; Feelisch, M. Nitrite is a signaling molecule and regulator of gene expression in mammalian tissues. *Nature chemical biology* 1:290–297; 2005.

34. Feelisch, M.; Fernandez, B. O.; Bryan, N. S.; Garcia-Saura, M. F.; Bauer, S.; Whitlock, D. R.; Ford, P. C.; Janero, D. R.; Rodriguez, J.; Ashrafian, H. Tissue Processing of Nitrite in Hypoxia: An Intricate Interplay of Nitric Oxide-Generating and -Scavenging Systems. *J Biol Chem* 283:33927–33934; 2008.

35. Bryan, N. S.; Calvert, J. W.; Elrod, J. W.; Gundewar, S.; Ji, S. Y.; Lefer, D. J. Dietary nitrite supplementation protects against myocardial ischemia-reperfusion injury. *Proc Natl Acad Sci U S A* 104:19144–19149; 2007.

36. Duranski, M. R.; Greer, J. J.; Dejam, A.; Jaganmohan, S.; Hogg, N.; Langston, W.; Patel, R. P.; Yet, S. F.; Wang, X.; Kevil, C. G.; Gladwin, M. T.; Lefer, D. J. Cytoprotective effects of nitrite during *in vivo* ischemia-reperfusion of the heart and liver. *J Clin Invest* 115:1232–1240; 2005.

37. Gonzalez, F. M.; Shiva, S.; Vincent, P. S.; Ringwood, L. A.; Hsu, L. Y.; Hon, Y. Y.; Aletras, A. H.; Cannon, R. O., 3rd; Gladwin, M. T.; Arai, A. E. Nitrite anion provides potent cytoprotective and antiapoptotic effects as adjunctive therapy to reperfusion for acute myocardial infarction. *Circulation* 117:2986–2994; 2008.

38. Hataishi, R.; Rodrigues, A. C.; Neilan, T. G.; Morgan, J. G.; Buys, E.; Shiva, S.; Tambouret, R.; Jassal, D. S.; Raher, M. J.; Furutani, E.; Ichinose, F.; Gladwin, M. T.; Rosenzweig, A.; Zapol, W. M.; Picard, M. H.; Bloch, K. D.; Scherrer-Crosbie, M. Inhaled nitric oxide decreases infarction size and improves left ventricular function in a murine model of myocardial ischemia-reperfusion injury. *Am J Physiol Heart Circ Physiol* 291:H379–384; 2006.

39. Hendgen-Cotta, U. B.; Merx, M. W.; Shiva, S.; Schmitz, J.; Becher, S.; Klare, J. P.; Steinhoff, H. J.; Goedecke, A.; Schrader, J.; Gladwin, M. T.; Kelm, M.; Rassaf, T. Nitrite reductase activity of myoglobin regulates respiration and cellular viability in myocardial ischemia-reperfusion injury. *Proc Natl Acad Sci U S A* 105:10256–10261; 2008.

40. Jung, K. H.; Chu, K.; Ko, S. Y.; Lee, S. T.; Sinn, D. I.; Park, D. K.; Kim, J. M.; Song, E. C.; Kim, M.; Roh, J. K. Early intravenous infusion of sodium nitrite protects brain against in vivo ischemia-reperfusion injury. *Stroke* 37:2744–2750; 2006.

41. Shiva, S.; Sack, M. N.; Greer, J. J.; Duranski, M.; Ringwood, L. A.; Burwell, L.; Wang, X.; MacArthur, P. H.; Shoja, A.; Raghavachari, N.; Calvert, J. W.; Brookes, P. S.; Lefer, D. J.; Gladwin, M. T. Nitrite augments tolerance to ischemia/reperfusion injury via the modulation of mitochondrial electron transfer. *J Exp Med* 204:2089–2102; 2007.

42. Tripatara, P.; Patel, N. S.; Webb, A.; Rathod, K.; Lecomte, F. M.; Mazzon, E.; Cuzzocrea, S.; Yaqoob, M. M.; Ahluwalia, A.; Thiemermann, C. Nitrite-derived nitric oxide protects the rat kidney against ischemia/reperfusion injury in vivo: role for xanthine oxidoreductase. *J Am Soc Nephrol* 18:570–580; 2007.

43. Webb, A.; Bond, R.; McLean, P.; Uppal, R.; Benjamin, N.; Ahluwalia, A. Reduction of nitrite to nitric oxide during ischemia protects against myocardial ischemia-reperfusion damage. *Proc Natl Acad Sci U S A* 101:13683–13688; 2004.

44. Webb, A. J.; Patel, N.; Loukogeorgakis, S.; Okorie, M.; Aboud, Z.; Misra, S.; Rashid, R.; Miall, P.; Deanfield, J.; Benjamin, N.; MacAllister, R.; Hobbs, A. J.; Ahluwalia, A. Acute blood pressure lowering, vasoprotective, and antiplatelet properties of dietary nitrate via bioconversion to nitrite. *Hypertension* 51:784–790; 2008.

45. Bryan, N. S.; Calvert, J. W.; Gundewar, S.; Lefer, D. J. Dietary nitrite restores NO homeostasis and is cardioprotective in endothelial nitric oxide synthase-deficient mice. *Free Radic Biol Med* 45:468–474; 2008.

46. Kumar, D.; Branch, B. G.; Pattillo, C. B.; Hood, J.; Thoma, S.; Simpson, S.; Illum, S.; Arora, N.; Chidlow, J. H., Jr.; Langston, W.; Teng, X.; Lefer, D. J.; Patel, R. P.; Kevil, C. G. Chronic

sodium nitrite therapy augments ischemia-induced angiogenesis and arteriogenesis. *Proc Natl Acad Sci U S A* 105:7540–7545; 2008.

47. Baker, J. E.; Su, J.; Fu, X.; Hsu, A.; Gross, G. J.; Tweddell, J. S.; Hogg, N. Nitrite confers protection against myocardial infarction: role of xanthine oxidoreductase, NADPH oxidase and K(ATP) channels. *J Mol Cell Cardiol* 43:437–444; 2007.
48. Sinha, S. S.; Shiva, S.; Gladwin, M. T. Myocardial protection by nitrite: evidence that this reperfusion therapeutic will not be lost in translation. *Trends Cardiovasc Med* 18:163–172; 2008.
49. Duranski, M. R.; Greer, J. J.; Dejam, A.; Sathya, J.; Hogg, N.; Langston, W.; Patel, R. P.; Yet, S. F.; Wang, X.; Kevil, C. G.; Gladwin, M. T.; Lefer, D. J. Cytoprotective effects of nitrite during in vivo ischemia-reperfusion of the heart and liver. *J Clin Invest;* 2005.
50. O'Donnell, V. B.; Eiserich, J. P.; Chumley, P. H.; Jablonsky, M. J.; Krishna, N. R.; Kirk, M.; Barnes, S.; Darley-Usmar, V. M.; Freeman, B. A. Nitration of unsaturated fatty acids by nitric oxide-derived reactive nitrogen species peroxynitrite, nitrous acid, nitrogen dioxide, and nitronium ion. *Chem Res Toxicol* 12:83–92; 1999.
51. Di Lisa, F. Mitochondrial contribution in the progression of cardiac ischemic injury. *IUBMB Life* 52:255–261; 2001.
52. Saikumar, P.; Dong, Z.; Weinberg, J. M.; Venkatachalam, M. A. Mechanisms of cell death in hypoxia/reoxygenation injury. *Oncogene* 17:3341–3349; 1998.
53. Sorescu, D.; Griendling, K. K. Reactive oxygen species, mitochondria, and NAD(P)H oxidases in the development and progression of heart failure. *Congest Heart Fail* 8:132–140; 2002.

CHAPTER 7

Polyphenols and Flavanols as Modulators of NO Activity

TIENUSH RASSAF and MALTE KELM

University Hospital Düsseldorf, Department of Internal Medicine, Division of Cardiology and Angiology—Düsseldorf, Germany

ENDOTHELIAL DYSFUNCTION is an early stage of cardiovascular disease and has been attributed to impaired endothelium-derived nitric oxide (NO) bioactivity and enhanced formation of oxygen-derived free radicals. Besides anthropological investigations, which suggested a protective role of flavanol-rich food in cardiovascular health, there is emerging evidence from recent interventional studies showing that flavanol-rich cocoa reverses endothelial dysfunction via modulation of the NO-pathway. Targeting endothelial dysfunction by means of nutritional rather than pharmacological intervention heralds a new strategy to halt progressive atherosclerotic disease and cardiovascular dysfunction. This chapter will discuss the action of polyphenols, particularly flavanols as modulators of NO activity and identify certain foods rich in polyphenols.

The endothelium regulates vascular tone, blood flow, antithrombotic, and antiadhesive properties of the vascular wall. Disturbances of these functions are termed endothelial dysfunction, which promotes the development of atherosclerosis leading to cardiovascular morbidity and mortality [1]. Endothelium-derived nitric oxide (NO) plays a major role in maintaining vascular homeostasis. Disturbance in the NO-pathway is a key element in the development of endothelial dysfunction. As one of the most important lifestyle factors, diet can strongly influence the incidence of cardiovascular diseases. In addition to the previously described benefits of dietary nitrite and nitrate, flavanol-rich food, such as wine, tea, various fruits, and cocoa, exert beneficial cardiovascular effects. Recent interventional studies with flavanol-containing cocoa have shown an improvement of endothelial function in healthy subjects and a reversion of endothelial dysfunction in smokers, in patients with coronary artery disease, and in diabetics [2–5]. These beneficial effects are mainly mediated via the NO-pathway. Dietary modulation of the NO-pathway and of endothelial dysfunction offers a novel approach in managing cardiovascular diseases.

ENDOTHELIAL FUNCTION AND NITRIC OXIDE

The endothelium is responsible for maintaining vascular tone, blood flow, blood fluidity, the clotting cascade and the fibrinolytic system. The endothelial L-arginine NO-pathway plays a major role in maintaining these functions and among various mediators released by the endothelium, nitric oxide plays an important role in regulating vascular tone and smooth muscle cell proliferation, blood cell adhesion, and lipid peroxidation. An interesting feature of the NO-synthases is that they not only generate NO but may also produce reactive oxygen species themselves. NOS are NADPH-consuming enzymes with electrons flowing from the reductase domain toward the heme-containing oxygenase domain. In the presence of oxygen a reactive superoxy ferrous-peroxy ferric complex is formed. If either the cofactor of NOS tetrahydrobiopterin or the substrate L-arginine are lacking, the superoxy ferrous-peroxy ferric complex dissociates to form superoxide anions or hydrogen peroxide. This state is called the uncoupled state of NOS. Due to the fact that NO can out-compete superoxide anions for superoxide dismutase, NO may thus react with superoxide anions to form peroxynitrite, which reacts relative slowly with most biological molecules, making peroxynitrite a selective oxidant. Disturbance in the NO-synthase (NOS)-dependent NO-pathway is a key element in the development of endothelial dysfunction, which results in the development of arteriosclerosis. The extent of endothelial dysfunction relates to the risk of patients for developing cardiovascular events such as myocardial infarction, stroke and claudication. Several risk factors including aging, hypertension, diabetes, hypercholesterolemia, smoking, obesity, chronic systemic inflammation, hyperhomocysteinemia, and a family history of premature atherosclerotic disease are all associated with an impairment of endothelial function. Recent studies have proven the prognostic value of endothelial dysfunction and primary- as well as secondary-preventive therapies, e.g. exercise, ACE inhibitors, and statins are believed to mediate their positive prognostic effect in large parts by improving endothelial function.

Adult endothelial progenitor cells (EPC) have been shown to effectively participate in endothelial homeostasis during injury and neo-vascularization. Experimental studies have shown that endothelium-derived NO modulates recruitment of EPC, which may contribute to impaired regeneration processes in e.g. patients with ischemic heart disease, who are characterized by a reduced NO bioavailability [6,7].

For a long time the signalling actions of NO in the vasculature have been thought to be short-lived as a result of the rapid reaction of NO with hemoglobin and the immense concentration of the latter in blood. Indeed, evidence suggests that free hemoglobin is an effective NO scavenger that can deplete NO bioavailability. Modelling analyses showed that if endothelium-produced NO reacted as rapidly with blood as it does with free hemoglobin, the NO concentration in vascular smooth muscle would be too low to activate soluble guanylate cyclase, the primary target of NO. Because 3–10 μM free hemoglobin can abolish NO-mediated vasodilation *in vitro*, it has been unclear for a long time how NO can exert its vasoregulatory function with 12–15 mM hemoglobin concentration in blood. However, in vivo, several compensation mechanisms exist allowing NO to be transported as NO itself, to react with plasma components to form nitrosospecies (RXNOs) [8,9], and to be oxidized to bioactive nitrite [10–12]. NO is not anymore the paracrine agent with only local effects, but, like a hormone, it disseminates throughout the body. Thus, a circulating NO-pool exists, opening new considerable pharmacological and therapeutical avenues in the diagnosis and therapy of cardiovascular diseases. It has recently been shown that the determination of changes in local plasma nitrite levels after five minutes of forearm-ischemia may offer a novel approach to determine endothelial function. Furthermore, changes in systemic plasma nitrite levels after ergometric exercise differentiates subjects with reduced from subject with regular vascular function [13,14]. Besides these rather novel biochemical attempts, several invasive and non-invasive approaches determining endothelium-dependent vasodilation have been employed to assess endothelial function. Especially the non-invasive examination of endothelium-dependent flow-mediated dilation (FMD) of the brachial artery using high resolution ultrasound has moved more and more into the focus. FMD represents the per cent diameter gain as calculated based on pre-ischemia and reactive hyperemia diameter measurements of the brachial artery. Ischemia is induced through vessel occlusion by means of inflating a blood pressure cuff around the forearm. The release of the cuff leads to an increased flow in the conduit brachial artery. The resulting sheer stress stimulates the endothelial NO-synthase and NO dilates the underlying vessel wall smooth muscle cells via the guanylate cyclase. FMD is in large parts mediated by NO synthesis and is used as a functional NO readout. The extent of endothelial function detected non-invasively in the brachial artery correlates with function in the coronary conduit arteries. As in the coronary circulation, endothelial function in the brachial artery is impaired in the setting of cardiovascular risk factors and responds to interventions known to reduce the risk of cardiovascular diseases [15]. This technique allows a safe application to diverse group of patients and repeated measurements can be made over time. The combination of the above mentioned biochemical approach together with the latter described technique to measure FMD offers an important diagnostic tool to sensitively assess vascular function [16].

DIETARY POLYPHENOLS AND HEALTH

Epidemiological studies have shown that cardiovascular and cerebrovascular ischemic events are decreased by moderate wine consumption [17–20]. Whereas the mechanism of this beneficial action is not fully established, several activities of wine, and especially of red wine, may be involved, such as the ability to raise high-density lipoprotein levels, to increase the antioxidant plasmatic potential, to improve endothelium-dependent vasodilation, and to inhibit platelet aggregation and leukocyte adhesion [21–23]. Studies in humans, as well as experiments on isolated tissues or organs, demonstrated that beneficial cardiovascular effects can be achieved also with de-alcoholized wine, suggesting that wine has beneficial effects partly dependent on components other than alcohol [21]. Grapes contain a variety of phenolic antioxidants, including quercetin, catechin, epicatechin, proanthocyanidins and resveratrol [24], mainly present in grape skin. The levels of the phenolic compounds in wines are highly variable, due to differences in fruit sources as well as in processing, ranging from ~200 mg of total phenols in a glass of red wine to 40 mg in a glass of white wine [25–28]. Red wine polyphenols have also been shown to increase the expression of endothelial nitric oxide (NO) synthase (eNOS) and consequently the release of NO by human umbilical vein endothelial cells *in vitro*; however, these actions were observed only with relatively high concentrations of polyphenols [29]. It has been proposed that resveratrol, a relevant wine constituent, is involved in vascular protection. Fresh grape skin contains 50–100 μg/g of resveratrol, whereas the concentration of resveratrol in wine ranges from ~0.1 to 14 mg/L for red wine and from 0.04 to 3.5 mg/L for white wine (with the highest concentrations reported in wines from pinot noir grapes) [25,26]. Indeed it has been shown that resveratrol itself stimulates NO production from human platelets [30].

WHAT ARE POLYPHENOLS?

Epidemiological studies have shown an inverse correlation between diets rich in polyphenols and reduced risk of cardiovascular disease (CVD) [31–33], cancer, and other chronic diseases [34,35]. Polyphenols are a group of chemical substances found in plants, characterized by the presence of more than one phenol unit or building block per molecule. Polyphenols are generally divided into hydrolyzable tannins (gallic acid esters of glucose and other sugars) and phenylpropanoids, such as lignins, flavonoids, and condensed tannins. Polyphenols are widely distributed in the Mediterranean diet, mainly in plant-derived foods and beverages, and include > 8000 phenolic structures. Notable sources of polyphenols include berries, tea, beer, grapes/wine, olive oil, chocolate/cocoa, coffee, walnuts, peanuts, pomegranates, yerba mate, and other fruits and vegetables. High levels of polyphenols can generally be found in the fruit skins. Daily consumption of polyphenols in the US ranges from 200 mg to 1 gram. Resveratrol is an exciting polyphenol which has been in the news a great deal for potential anti-cancer and anti-aging benefits. Green tea polyphenols and polyphenols from wine have attracted a great deal of media attention. While dietary anti-oxidants, such as vitamins E and C, have received considerable attention, relatively little is known about a similar anti-oxidant role for plant-derived polyphenols, such as the flavonoids and phenolic acids. Polyphenols occur in all plant foods and contribute to the beneficial health effects of vegetables and fruit. Their contribution to the antioxidant capacity of the human diet is much larger than that of vitamins. The total intake of polyphenols in a person's diet could amount to 1 gram a day, whereas combined intakes of beta-carotene, vitamin C, and vitamin E from food most often is about 100 mg a day. Phenolic acids account for about one third of the total intake of polyphenols in our diet, and flavonoids account for the remaining two thirds. There are several classes of polyphenols all of which may be structurally related (and may or may not be pigmented).

Phenolic acids are simple molecules such as caffeic acid, vanillin, and courmaric acid. Phenolic acids form a diverse group that includes the widely distributed hydroxybenzoic and hydroxycinnamic acids. Phenolic acid compounds seem to be universally distributed in plants. They have been the subject of a great number of chemical, biological, agricultural, and medical studies. Hydroxycinnamic acid compounds (p-coumaric, caffeic acid, ferulic acid) occur most frequently as simple esters with hydroxy carboxylic acids or glucose, while the hydroxybenzoic acid compounds (p-hydroxybenzoic, gallic acid, ellagic acid) are present mainly in the form of glucosides. Furthermore, phenolic acids may occur in food plants as esters or glycosides conjugated with other natural compounds such as flavonoids, alcohols, hydroxyfatty acids, sterols, and glucosides. Coffee is particularly rich in bound phenolic acids, such as caffeic acid, ferulic acid, and p-coumaric acid. Phenolic acids found in blueberries include gallic acid, p-hydroxybenzoic acid, coffeic acid, p-coumaric acid and vanillic acid.

Flavonoids are the main polyphenolic constituent, presenting with a common flavan core formed with 15 carbon atoms arranged in 3 rings (C_6-C_3-C_6) consisting of 2 aromatic ones linked through 3 carbons, usually forming an oxygenated heterocycle nucleus, the flavan nucleus. This is a very broad class of compounds that are defined by color (pigment). The term is derived from the Latin word “flavus,” which means yellow. For originally, and chemically speaking correctly so, flavonoid was the name for yellow plant pigments, like lemons, oranges and grapefruits. Flavonoids are widely distributed in nature, albeit not uniformly. As a result, specific groups of foods are often rich sources of one or more subclasses of these polyphenols. The polyphenolic structure of flavonoids and tannins renders them quite sensitive to oxidative enzymes and cooking conditions. Bioflavonoids are a subgroup of flavonoids that possess biological activity (“bio” is a Greek prefix that indicates a relationship to life). In some cases the differences between certain bioflavonoid members outnumber the similarities: some bioflavonoids are toxic, others are innocuous, some are inefficacious, others are useless, some are bioavailable, others are not. The different patterns of this nucleus permit the classification of flavonoids into several subgroups, i.e., flavanols (catechin, epicatechin), flavonols (quercetin, myricetin, kaempferol), anthocyanidins (cyanidin, delphinidin), flavones (apigenin, diosmin), and flavanones (naringenin, hesperetin). There is always a phenolic acid group attached to one of the benzene rings in flavonoids, therefore all flavonoids are also referred to as “polyphenols” or “phenols.” (“Poly” is from the Greek root which refers to “more than one” or “many” phenols.) Flavonols are found at high concentrations in onions, apples, red wine, broccoli, tea, and Ginkgo biloba. The most common in the American diet are Quercetin (70%), Kaempferol (16%), and Myricetin (6%). Grape seeds including have the monomeric flavan-3-ols catechin, epicatechin, gallocatechin, epigallocatechin, and epicatechin 3-O-gallate. Research shows that the cocoa bean is rich in specific antioxidants, with the basic structure of catechins and epicatechin, and especially the polymers procyanidins.

Anthocyanins are polyphenols that have red pigments. Anthocyanins and anthocyanidins are a large water-soluble pigment group found in a large number of fruits, vegetables and flowers. particularly grapes and berries. These pigments give plants their brilliant colors ranging from pink through scarlet, purple and blue. Bilberry and other berries have a high concentration of anthocyanins. Scientists have identified more than 500 different anthocyanins including cyanidin, pelargonidin, delphinidin, malvidin, and paeonidin. Anthocyanins are highly fragile and not interesting from a medical point of view unless they exist in an acidic environment, such as in red wine.

Proanthocyanidins are found in grapes, red wine, pine bark. Grape seed extract provides a concentrated source of polyphenols, many of which are proanthocyanidins. Red wine is rich in the complex polyphenols, the proanthocyanidins. Proanthocyanidins share common properties with other polyphenols, in particular their reducing capacity and ability to chelate metal ions.

Procyanidins (oligomeric catechins found at high concentrations in red wine, grapes and grape seeds, cocoa, cranberries, apples, and some supplements such as Pycnogenol) have pronounced effects on the vascular system. Apples contain many kinds of polyphenols, and the main components are oligomeric procyanidins. Applephenon is apple polyphenol extract produced commercially from unripe apples, and has been used as food additive in order to prevent oxidation of components in foods.

The most abundant polyphenols are the condensed tannins, found in virtually all families of plants, and comprising up to 50% of the dry weight of leaves. The convergent evolution of tannin-rich plant communities has occurred on nutrient-poor acidic soils throughout the world. Tannins were once believed to function as anti-herbivore defenses, but more and more ecologists now recognize them as important controllers of decomposition and nitrogen cycling processes. Tannins are found in red wine, tea, and nuts. They are large molecules. Many flavonoids in foods also occur as large molecules (tannins). These include condensed tannins (proanthocyanidins), derived tannins and hydrolysable tannins. There are many classes of polyphenols each found at different levels is certain foods.

FLAVANOLS AND NUTRITION

As discussed above, flavonoids represent a subclass of polyphenols, which are ubiquitous in human diet. They are synthesized as micronutrients in the secondary metabolism of plants, to protect against vermin or to serve as pigments. They are known to exert several health promoting effects. Among the six subclasses of flavonoids (Figure 7.1), flavanols attracted much attention due to their association with the reduced incidence of cardiovascular diseases. Important dietary sources of polyphenols also in Western societies are onions (flavonols); cocoa (proanthocyanidins); tea, apples, and red wine (flavonols and catechins); citrus fruit (flavanones); berries and cherries (anthocyanidins); and soy (isoflavones). Tea products account for a significant proportion of total polyphenol intake in different Western countries [36]. Thus, dietary recommendations are highly desirable. This requires in a first step the evaluation of food contents and the average consumption of those. However, although the containing amounts of substances are genetically determined, they are variations at different environmental conditions. Moreover, the methods described in the current literature to determine the contents in plant derived food and beverages vary and therefore lead to diverging results. The US Department of Agriculture has published a database with flavonoid contents of selected foods. Based on these data, the total actual daily intake of flavanols can be calculated [18]. However, besides the total daily intake, a limited bioavailability of flavanols has to be considered. Furthermore, it has to be considered that the nutritional habits differ between individuals, men and women, people in different

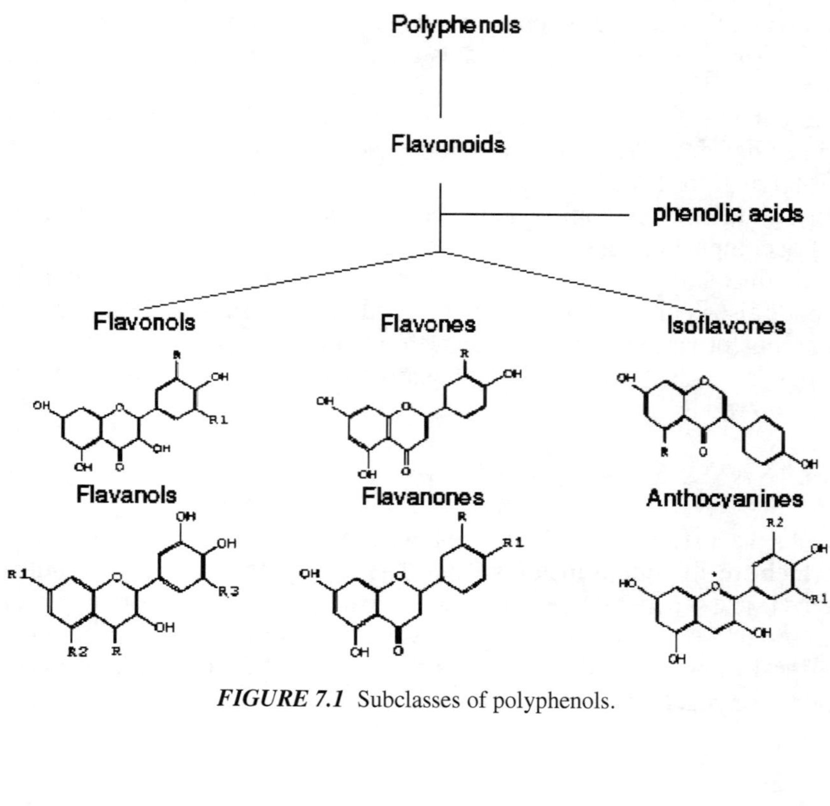

FIGURE 7.1 Subclasses of polyphenols.

stages of their lives, people from different countries, regions, religions, and ethnical groups.

FLAVANOLS AND CARDIOVASCULAR FUNCTION

Diets can strongly influence the incidence of cardiovascular diseases. Epidemiologic studies indicate an association between flavanol-rich diets and improved cardiovascular prognosis [19]. Flavanols, such as epicatechin and catechin, and their oligomers, the procyanidins, represent a major class of secondary, polyphenolic plant metabolites [5]. In this context, cocoa, some chocolates, red wine, and tea received much attention, because of their high content of flavanols. Several interventional studies have revealed acute and chronic increases in FMD after the ingestion of flavanol-rich foods/beverages such as red wine [20], purple grape juice [17], tea [37], cocoa [2,3,5,38,39], and chocolate [40]. Even in fully medicated type 2 diabetic patients beneficial health effects of flavanol-rich cocoa could be detected. Whereas the chronic consumption led to an increase in baseline FMD levels and additional "acute on chronic effect" was observed [3]. Furthermore, a chronic flavanol-rich cocoa consumption leads to an increase in urinary excretion of NO-metabolites [5]. Results that emanated from these studies corroborate the hypothesis that an increase in NO bioactivity represents the common underlying mechanistic principle for augmented vasodilation. Due to the fact that FMD is almost exclusively mediated by NO, increases in NO-synthase activity are principally paralleled by increases in plasma nitrite and/or RXNOs [41]. Thus, parallel measurements of FMD and circulating NO species represent a mechanistically strong experimental framework.

A recent experimental study in rats suggests that an epicatechin-rich diet exerts cytoprotective effects and thus protects from myocardial ischemia/reperfusion injury [42]. Future studies will have to follow in order to elucidate the underlying mechanisms and to proof a potential translation to human pathophysiology.

FLAVANOLS: MECHANISMS OF ACTION

Role of NADPH-Oxidase

As outlined before [43], several processes modulate the in vivo efficacy of flavanoids:

1. the rate and extent of absorption including the enterohepatic circulation,

2. the metabolic conversions in intestinal and liver cells/tissue,
3. the binding to serum proteins,
4. the plasma levels of aglycones and conjugates,
5. the accumulation in the vascular endothelium,
6. the urinary excretion, and
7. the molecular mode of actions.

Whereas it is well appreciated that flavanols exert positive effects on the NO-pathway, the exact mechanisms are still not known. The question raises whether flavanols improve bioavailability of NO in the vasculature via increasing production of endothelium-derived NO, or whether flavanols inhibit the breakdown of NO and thus increase its bioavailability. Recent data from *in vitro* cell experiments showed that treatment of endothelial cells with (-)-epicatechin elevated intracellular levels of NO and cyclic GMP [44]. Further investigations revealed that (-)-epicatechin inhibited NADPH oxidase, leading to a reduced production of superoxide anions, which are known to scavenge NO in a nearly diffusion-limited manner. The inhibition of the NADPH oxidase through flavanols thus increases NO without affecting NO-synthesis [44]. We have shown that a single dose of flavanol-rich cocoa acutely improves vascular function after 1–2 h following the time-course of (-)-epicatechin metabolites in plasma [3], an effect that may have been mediated via

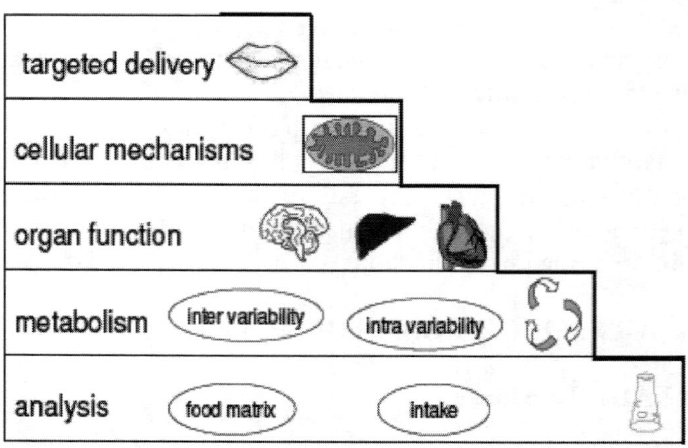

FIGURE 7.2 Steps in flavanol research. The basis for a targeted flavanol delivery includes the analysis of food contents, the characterization of the flavanol-metabolism, the consideration of individual variations, investigations of the organ functions, and analyses of the underlying cellular mechanisms. These aspects are necessary to design adequate food matrices.

TABLE 7.1 Human Interventional Studies with Flavanoid-rich Food (PAT = Peripheral Arterial Tone Technology measuring pulsatile blood volume changes; FMD = Flow-Mediated-Dilation for the determination of endothelial function; BP= Blood Pressure; QCA = Quantitative Coronary Analysis for the determination of diameters of coronary arteries).

Disease	Treatment	Outcome	Refs
Healthy volunteers	Cocoa drink	PAT ↑	Fisher *et al.* [38]
	Chocolate	FMD ↑	Grassi *et al.* [50]
	Chocolate	FMD ↑	Engler *et al.* [50]
	Chocolate	FMD ↑	Vlachopoulos *et al.* [51]
	Red wine	FMD ↑	Agewall *et al.* [20]
Cardiovascular risk factors	Cocoa drink	FMD ↑	Heiss *et al.* [2]
			Heiss *et al.* [4]
	Chocolate/ cocoa drink	BP ↓, FMD ↑	Faridi *et al.* [52]
Coronary artery disease	Black tea	FMD ↑	Duffy *et al.* [37]
	Grape juice	FMD ↑	Stein *et al.* [17]
Hypertension	Chocolate	BP ↓	Taubert *et al.* [53]
			Taubert *et al.* [54]
	Chocolate	BP ↓, FMD ↑	Grassi *et al.* [55]
Diabetes	Cocoa drink	FMD ↑	Balzer *et al.* [3]
Hypercholesterolemia	Black tea	FMD ↑	Hodgson *et al.* [56]
Heart transplant recepients	Chocolate	QCA ↑ Platelet adhesion ↓	Flammer *et al.* [57]

inhibition of NADPH oxidase. Chronic application of flavanols resulted into an increase in baseline levels of FMD [3]. It is assumed that this effect may—in addition to the inhibition of the NADPH oxidase—be mediated by an increase in endothelial NO-synthase expression in the vascular endothelium [43]. The chronic effect of flavanols differs from the acute effect by affecting gene expression patterns. It has to be considered that the above mentioned mechanisms on the influence of flavanols on NADPH oxidase have all solely been investigated in cell experiments. In vivo confirmation is still missing but crucial, as the results obtained from the cell experiments may differ from the in vivo situation.

Antioxidative Effects?

For a long time it has been proposed that flavanoids may be protective

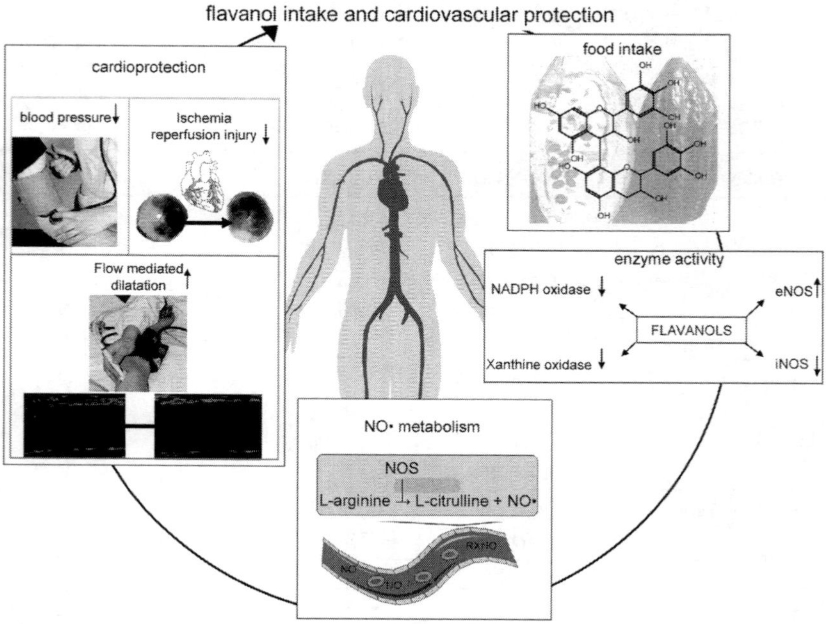

FIGURE 7.3 Flavanol intake and cardiovascular protection. Flavanols down-regulate NADPH-oxidase and xanthine-oxidase activity. This leads—together with the upregulation of the endothelial nitric oxide synthase (eNOS) activity—to an improvement of endothelial function (FMD), reduces blood pressure, and has cytoprotective effects in myocardial ischemia/reperfusion injury.

due to their antioxidative properties. *In vitro* studies supported this notion as flavanoids scavenge reactive oxygen radicals and nitrogen species. These results, however, have not been confirmed in vivo and studies on the role of flavanoids as antioxidants are not conclusive or are still missing [45,46]. In agreement with others [43] we thus suggest to see flavanoids as "antioxidants in a more broad sense" as they interfere with prooxidant processes or inhibit prooxidant enzymes as e.g. NADPH oxidases.

Facilitated Nitrite Reduction to NO

We know from previous chapters that nitrite can be a source of nitric oxide, particularly in highly acidic environments, such as the stomach. Dietary products can also contribute reductants that dramatically increase the production of NO from nitrite. Red wine has been attributed health promoting properties largely on basis of the reductive antioxidant properties of its polyphenolic fraction. Gago *et al.* [47] have recently shown *in vitro* that wine, wine anthocyanin fraction and wine catechol (caffeic acid) dose- and pH-dependently promote the formation of NO when mixed with nitrite. The production of NO promoted by wine from nitrite was substantiated *in vivo* in healthy volunteers by measuring NO in the air expelled from the stomach, following consumption of wine. Mechanistically, the reaction involves the univalent reduction of nitrite, as suggested by the formation of NO. Ascorbic and caffeic acids cooperate in the reduction of nitrite to NO. Moreover, reduction of nitrite is critically dependent on the phenolic structure and nitro-derivatives of phenols are also formed, as suggested by caffeic acid UV spectral modifications. The facilitated reduction of nitrite may reveal previously unrecognized physiologic effects of polyphenolic compounds found in many foods in connection with NO bioactivity. Therefore diets rich in polyphenols, nitrite and nitrate may provide the optimal combination for enhanced NO generation.

FLAVANOLS AND FUNCTIONAL FOOD

A very attractive research field is the development of functional food with a high flavanol content. Functional food can be defined as food with additional health benefits. Obviously, it can not replace a well-balanced diet and rather should be regarded to support a healthy way of living. Functional food which is offered as "whole food" and not in form of pills may provide several health promoting aspects. It differs from normal food by elimination or substitution of undesirable ingredients, enrichment or supplementation of useful ingredients, respectively. Flavanol-rich cocoa was already tested successfully on healthy male adults [5], smokers with endothelial dysfunction [4], patients with one cardiovascular risk factor [2], and diabetics [3]. Functional food containing flavanols could be obtained by an enrichment of the flavanol fraction in cocoa. A proposed production method uses blanch treated cocoa to diminish the loss of flavonoids during the processing of cocoa powder [48]. So may functional food containing flavanols provide a useful tool in the prevention of cardiovascular diseases? Studies on the administration of L-arginine to increase the synthesis of NO by endothelial NOS have taught us to temper our enthusiasm regarding the beneficial effects of functional food [49]. More experimental work will be required to confidently identify those individuals who would benefit from flavanol-containing functional food.

CONCLUSION

The emerging relevance of flavanols in the context of functional food opens new avenues for future preventive and therapeutic approaches. Experimental and interventional human studies suggest protective effects of flavanol-rich food (such as cocoa, chocolate, red-wine) in the cardiovascular system. Regarding these studies, it has to be considered that these foods and beverages contain complex mixtures of micro- and macronutrients. Hence, it should be differentiated between the research on isolated flavanols and research on flavanol containing food. Caution is advised in order to set the right signals for the public. The potential benefits of flavanols must not be misinterpreted as general benefits of chocolate. Chocolate or cocoa should rather be understood as a "carrier" of flavanols. In the future, recommended dietary intakes of flavanols will have to be established.

ABOUT THE AUTHORS

Tienush Rassaf, MD, PhD

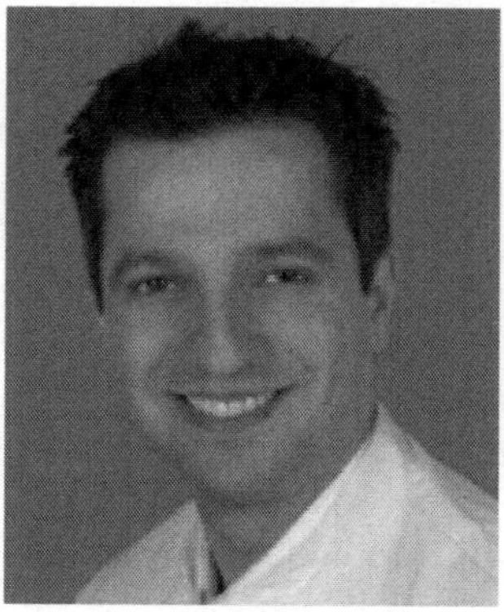

Dr. Rassaf is currently Associate Professor and Assistant Medical Director at the Department of Medicine, Division of Cardiology and Angiology at the University Hospital Dusseldorf, Germany. Dr. Rassaf is an interventional cardiologist and has been appointed director of the Heisenberg-Research program funded by the German Research Foundation at his Department. Dr. Rassaf studied medicine at the University of Dusseldorf, Germany and at the Texas Heart Institute, University of Texas. After receiving his PhD from the Heinrich-Heine-University in Dusseldorf, Dr. Rassaf had the following postdoctoral fellowships: from 2000–2001, he was at the Cardiovascular Research Laboratories at University Hospital Dusseldorf; from 2001–2002, he was at the Department of Molecular and Cellular Physiology at Louisiana State University Health Sciences Center; and from 2002–2003, he was at the Department of Cardiovascular Physiology, University of Dusseldorf, Germany. Dr. Rassaf passed his ECFMG license in 2005. Dr. Rassaf received his clinical training at the University of Dusseldorf and at the University of Aachen, Germany.

Dr. Rassaf is the recipient of 5 research scholarships and several scientific awards and has worked on several research grants. He is a member and reviewer in scientific communities and is a reviewer for various scientific journals. Dr. Rassaf's research has been continuously funded by the German Research Foundation and by the European Union.

Malte Kelm, MD, PhD

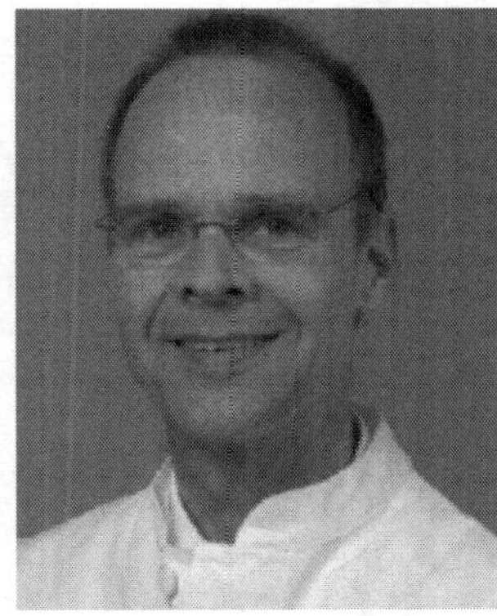

Dr. Kelm is currently Professor and Chairman of the Department of Cardiology and Angiology at the University Hospital Dusseldorf. From 1986–1987, Dr. Kelm completed an Internship at the Department of Neurology, University of Cologne and the Max-Plank Institute for Brain Research. From 1987–1989, he was a post-doctoral Fellow in the Department of Cardiovascular Physiology at the Heinrich-Heine-University, Dusseldorf and a Visiting Scientist at the Clinical Research Center, Section of Vascular Biology, London. From 1989–2005, Dr. Kelm worked in the Department of Medicine, Division for Cardiology, Pulmonary Diseases and Vascular Medicine, and Intensive Care Medicine at the Heinrich-Heine-University, Dusseldorf. From 1989–1995, Dr. Kelm was a Resident and Fellow in Internal Medicine, from 1995–1996 he was an Assistant Professor of Cardiology, Heinrich-Heine-University, Dusseldorf, and from 1996–1998, he was an Associate Professor of Cardiology. In 1998, Dr. Kelm became a Full Professor in Internal Medicine, Cardiology and Vascular Medicine (tenured position) at the Heinrich-Heine-University. In 2005 Dr. Kelm was appointed Head of the Medical Clinic, Department of Cardiology, Pulmonary Diseases, Vascular Medicine, and Intensive Care at the University Hospital Aachen. In April 2009, Dr. Kelm was appointed Head of the Department of Cardiology and Angiology at the University Hospital Dusseldorf.

REFERENCES

1. Loscalzo, J., Nitric oxide and vascular disease. *N Engl J Med,* 1995. 333(4): p. 251–3.
2. Heiss, C., et al., Vascular effects of cocoa rich in flavan-3-ols. *Jama,* 2003. 290(8): p. 1030–1.
3. Balzer, J., et al., Sustained benefits in vascular function through flavanol-containing cocoa in medicated diabetic patients a double-masked, randomized, controlled trial. *J Am Coll Cardiol,* 2008. 51(22): p. 2141–9.

4. Heiss, C., et al., Acute consumption of flavanol-rich cocoa and the reversal of endothelial dysfunction in smokers. *J Am Coll Cardiol*, 2005. 46(7): p. 1276–83.
5. Schroeter, H., et al., (-)-Epicatechin mediates beneficial effects of flavanol-rich cocoa on vascular function in humans. *Proc Natl Acad Sci U S A*, 2006. 103(4): p. 1024–9.
6. Gallagher, K.A., et al., Diabetic impairments in NO-mediated endothelial progenitor cell mobilization and homing are reversed by hyperoxia and SDF-1 alpha. *J Clin Invest,* 2007. 117(5): p. 1249–59.
7. Aicher, A., et al., Essential role of endothelial nitric oxide synthase for mobilization of stem and progenitor cells. *Nat Med*, 2003. 9(11): p. 1370–6.
8. Rassaf, T., et al., Plasma nitrosothiols contribute to the systemic vasodilator effects of intravenously applied NO: experimental and clinical Study on the fate of NO in human blood. *Circ Res*, 2002. 91(6): p. 470–7.
9. Rassaf, T., et al., Concomitant presence of N-nitroso and S-nitroso proteins in human plasma. *Free Radical Biology & Medicine,* 2002. 33(11): p. 1590–1596.
10. Rassaf, T., et al., NO adducts in mammalian red blood cells: too much or too little? *Nat Med*, 2003. 9(5): p. 481–2; author reply 482–3.
11. Schechter, A.N. and M.T. Gladwin, Hemoglobin and the paracrine and endocrine functions of nitric oxide. *N Engl J Med,* 2003. 348(15): p. 1483–5.
12. Cosby, K., et al., Nitrite reduction to nitric oxide by deoxyhemoglobin vasodilates the human circulation. *Nature Medicine,* 2003. 9: p. 1498–1505.
13. Rassaf, T., et al., Nitric oxide synthase-derived plasma nitrite predicts exercise capacity. *Br J Sports Med,* 2007. 41(10): p. 669–73; discussion 673.
14. Lauer, T., et al., Age-dependent endothelial dysfunction is associated with failure to increase plasma nitrite in response to exercise. *Basic Res Cardiol,* 2008. 103(3): p. 291–7.
15. Vita, J.A. and J.F. Keaney, Jr., Endothelial function: a barometer for cardiovascular risk? *Circulation,* 2002. 106(6): p. 640–2.
16. Rassaf, T., P. Kleinbongard, and M. Kelm, The L-arginine nitric oxide pathway: avenue for a multiple-level approach to assess vascular function. *Biol Chem,* 2006. 387(10–11): p. 1347–9.
17. Stein, J.H., et al., Purple grape juice improves endothelial function and reduces the susceptibility of LDL cholesterol to oxidation in patients with coronary artery disease. *Circulation,* 1999. 100(10): p. 1050–5.
18. Gu, L., et al., Concentrations of proanthocyanidins in common foods and estimations of normal consumption. *J Nutr,* 2004. 134(3): p. 613–7.
19. Arts, I.C. and P.C. Hollman, Polyphenols and disease risk in epidemiologic studies. *Am J Clin Nutr,* 2005. 81(1 Suppl): p. 317S–325S.
20. Agewall, S., et al., Does a glass of red wine improve endothelial function? *Eur Heart J,* 2000. 21(1): p. 74–8.
21. German, J.B. and R.L. Walzem, The health benefits of wine. *Annu Rev Nutr,* 2000. 20: p. 561–93.
22. Halpern, M.J., et al., Red-wine polyphenols and inhibition of platelet aggregation: possible mechanisms, and potential use in health promotion and disease prevention. *J Int Med Res,* 1998. 26(4): p. 171–80.
23. Ferrero, M.E., et al., Activity *in vitro* of resveratrol on granulocyte and monocyte adhesion to endothelium. *Am J Clin Nutr,* 1998. 68(6): p. 1208–14.
24. Nijveldt, R.J., et al., Flavonoids: a review of probable mechanisms of action and potential applications. *Am J Clin Nutr,* 2001. 74(4): p. 418–25.

25. Mark, L., et al., A validated HPLC method for the quantitative analysis of trans-resveratrol and trans-piceid in Hungarian wines. *J Chromatogr Sci,* 2005. 43(9): p. 445–9.
26. Pervaiz, S., Resveratrol: from grapevines to mammalian biology. *Faseb J,* 2003. 17(14): p. 1975–85.
27. Kopp, P., Resveratrol, a phytoestrogen found in red wine. A possible explanation for the conundrum of the 'French paradox'? *Eur J Endocrinol,* 1998. 138(6): p. 619–20.
28. Zern, T.L. and M.L. Fernandez, Cardioprotective effects of dietary polyphenols. *J Nutr,* 2005. 135(10): p. 2291–4.
29. Leikert, J.F., et al., Red wine polyphenols enhance endothelial nitric oxide synthase expression and subsequent nitric oxide release from endothelial cells. *Circulation,* 2002. 106(13): p. 1614–7.
30. Gresele, P., et al., Resveratrol, at concentrations attainable with moderate wine consumption, stimulates human platelet nitric oxide production. *J Nutr,* 2008. 138(9): p. 1602–8.
31. Stoclet, J.C., et al., Vascular protection by dietary polyphenols. *Eur J Pharmacol,* 2004. 500(1–3): p. 299–313.
32. Hertog, M.G., et al., Dietary antioxidant flavonoids and risk of coronary heart disease: the Zutphen Elderly Study. *Lancet,* 1993. 342(8878): p. 1007–11.
33. Geleijnse, J.M., et al., Inverse association of tea and flavonoid intakes with incident myocardial infarction: the Rotterdam Study. *Am J Clin Nutr,* 2002. 75(5): p. 880–6.
34. Hertog, M.G., et al., Flavonoid intake and long-term risk of coronary heart disease and cancer in the seven countries study. *Arch Intern Med,* 1995. 155(4): p. 381–6.
35. Scalbert, A., et al., Dietary polyphenols and the prevention of diseases. *Crit Rev Food Sci Nutr,* 2005. 45(4): p. 287–306.
36. Peters, U., C. Poole, and L. Arab, Does tea affect cardiovascular disease? A meta-analysis. *Am J Epidemiol,* 2001. 154(6): p. 495–503.
37. Duffy, S.J., et al., Short- and long-term black tea consumption reverses endothelial dysfunction in patients with coronary artery disease. *Circulation,* 2001. 104(2): p. 151–6.
38. Fisher, N.D., et al., Flavanol-rich cocoa induces nitric-oxide-dependent vasodilation in healthy humans. *J Hypertens,* 2003. 21(12): p. 2281–6.
39. Heiss, C., et al., Sustained increase in flow-mediated dilation after daily intake of high-flavanol cocoa drink over 1 week. *J Cardiovasc Pharmacol,* 2007. 49(2): p. 74–80.
40. Engler, M.B., et al., Flavonoid-rich dark chocolate improves endothelial function and increases plasma epicatechin concentrations in healthy adults. *J Am Coll Nutr,* 2004. 23(3): p. 197–204.
41. Rassaf, T., et al., Evidence for in vivo transport of bioactive nitric oxide in human plasma. *J Clin Invest,* 2002. 109(9): p. 1241–8.
42. Yamazaki, K.G., et al., Short- and long-term effects of (-)-epicatechin on myocardial ischemia-reperfusion injury. *Am J Physiol Heart Circ Physiol*, 2008. 295(2): p. H761–7.
43. Schewe, T., Y. Steffen, and H. Sies, How do dietary flavanols improve vascular function? A position paper. *Arch Biochem Biophys,* 2008. 476(2): p. 102–6.
44. Steffen, Y., T. Schewe, and H. Sies, (-)-Epicatechin elevates nitric oxide in endothelial cells via inhibition of NADPH oxidase. *Biochem Biophys Res Commun,* 2007. 359(3): p. 828–33.
45. Taubert, D., et al., Effects of low habitual cocoa intake on blood pressure and bioactive nitric oxide: a randomized controlled trial. *Jama*, 2007. 298(1): p. 49–60.
46. Mursu, J., et al., Dark chocolate consumption increases HDL cholesterol concentration and chocolate fatty acids may inhibit lipid peroxidation in healthy humans. *Free Radic Biol Med*, 2004. 37(9): p. 1351–9.

47. Gago, B., et al., Red wine-dependent reduction of nitrite to nitric oxide in the stomach. *Free Radic Biol Med*, 2007. 43(9): p. 1233–42.

48. Tomas-Barberan, F.A., et al., A new process to develop a cocoa powder with higher flavonoid monomer content and enhanced bioavailability in healthy humans. *J Agric Food Chem,* 2007. 55(10): p. 3926–35.

49. Blum, A., et al., Oral L-arginine in patients with coronary artery disease on medical management. *Circulation,* 2000. 101(18): p. 2160–4.

50. Grassi, D., et al., Short-term administration of dark chocolate is followed by a significant increase in insulin sensitivity and a decrease in blood pressure in healthy persons. *Am J Clin Nutr,* 2005. 81(3): p. 611–4.

51. Vlachopoulos, C., et al., Effect of dark chocolate on arterial function in healthy individuals. *Am J Hypertens,* 2005. 18(6): p. 785–91.

52. Faridi, Z., et al., Acute dark chocolate and cocoa ingestion and endothelial function: a randomized controlled crossover trial. *Am J Clin Nutr,* 2008. 88(1): p. 58–63.

53. Taubert, D., et al., Chocolate and blood pressure in elderly individuals with isolated systolic hypertension. *Jama*, 2003. 290(8): p. 1029–30.

54. Taubert, D., R. Roesen, and E. Schomig, Effect of cocoa and tea intake on blood pressure: a meta-analysis. *Arch Intern Med,* 2007. 167(7): p. 626–34.

55. Grassi, D., et al., Cocoa reduces blood pressure and insulin resistance and improves endothelium-dependent vasodilation in hypertensives. *Hypertension,* 2005. 46(2): p. 398–405.

56. Hodgson, J.M., et al., Regular ingestion of black tea improves brachial artery vasodilator function. *Clin Sci (Lond),* 2002. 102(2): p. 195–201.

57. Flammer, A.J., et al., Dark chocolate improves coronary vasomotion and reduces platelet reactivity. *Circulation,* 2007. 116(21): p. 2376–82.

CHAPTER 8

Nutritional Epidemiology

ANDREW L. MILKOWSKI AND JAMES R. COUGHLIN

TODAY, we are bombarded with media reports of studies relating diet to a number of chronic diseases, including coronary heart disease, cancer, type II diabetes and osteoporosis. For the past several decades, observational studies of diet and cancer have yielded many inconsistent results [1,2]. Given the limited variation in dietary intakes within many study populations and the seemingly weak diet–cancer associations that have been observed, results of such studies depend critically on an accurate assessment of the dietary exposure [3,4]. Measurement error in exposure can lead to serious errors in the reported relative risks of cancer for dietary intakes and can substantially reduce the statistical power to detect true existing relationships [3,4]. Extreme caution is required when interpreting associations, or the lack thereof, between dietary factors and disease.

Overall, the media does a fairly good job of reporting the limitations of the studies and the fact that the published results are merely expressions of risk probability. However, a recent, prominent *Perspective* article in the *New England Journal of Medicine* [5] noted that all too frequently, what is conveyed about health and disease by many journalists is wrong or misleading, especially when they ignore complexities or fail to provide context. When this happens, the authors believe that the public health messages they convey are inevitably distorted or inadequate. Therefore, the news media need to become more knowledgeable and to more fully embrace their role in delivering accurate, complete and balanced messages about health.

This is especially needed when the results being communicated to the public are diet-health associations, due mainly to the complexity of the diet compared to a drug/placebo clinical trial. There has been a dramatically increased interest in nutrition & health over the past decade. What we eat or don't eat is constantly being linked to various diseases, and there is a constant flow of anxiety-provoking media headlines on television, radio, print and more recently the Internet. "Carcinogen-of-the-month" reporting has become very alarming to consumers, and dietary epidemiological studies always seem to be contradicting each other, leading to much nutrition nonsense and food faddism. Because of these fears, consumers become sporadic or chronic avoiders of specific foods and ingredients, such as salt, fat, soft drinks, artificial sweeteners, carbohydrates in general, coffee/caffeine and meat.

In response to such reporting deficiencies, many individuals become either confused or alarmed about their own personal situation. There are also calls by numerous public health and consumer organizations to change our lifestyles as a matter of public policy.

Therefore, it is important for participants in the social debate to also understand the strengths and limits of epidemiological research. We will review the science of epidemiology, introduce the criteria for interpretation of the data and then discuss the published reports on diet and risk of disease. Since foods are heterogenous and complex in terms of their composition and contribution to the overall diet, ascribing an individual component of food as "good" or "bad" is fraught with difficulty. We will present a cursory review of current epidemiological data, but we will also focus primarily on the context of the nitrite and nitrate content of foods and what is reported about them, in order to present a balanced view of dietary sources of nitrite and nitrate and a potential risk-benefit analysis.

EPIDEMIOLOGY AS A SCIENTIFIC DISCIPLINE

Modern epidemiology is the branch of medicine that deals with the study of the causes, distribution and control of disease frequency in human populations. Historically, epidemiology began as the study of epidemics of infectious disease. Epidemiology essentially looks for patterns of disease (time, place, exposures, personal characteristics). The primary concern for exposure to dietary nitrite (and nitrate as a precursor to nitrite) is its propensity to form potentially carcinogenic N-nitrosamines and its consequent potential to cause human cancer. In terms of human cancer risk and diet, most of the publications, discussion and media attention have focused on data from epidemiological studies. Therefore, it is important to understand the different types of dietary epidemiological studies, while at the same time noting that epidemiological associations reported between dietary components, specific foods (or food groups) and chronic disease are rarely sufficient to establish cause and effect relationships. The results of epidemiological investigations must also be evaluated through other types of supportive studies (animal studies, metabolic studies, human clinical intervention trials, etc.) before persuasive causal relationships can be firmly established [6,7].

There are several types of epidemiological studies, each with their own strengths and weaknesses [7]. Ecologic/descriptive studies are the simplest and least persuasive type. They characterize differences between large and diverse populations by simple generalizations and can help formulate hypotheses; however, they cannot control for potential confounding factors. Case-control studies focus on individuals and provide stronger evidence for an association than ecologic studies. "Recalled" past diets of individuals diagnosed with a disease (cases) are compared to those of individuals without the disease (controls) in a retrospective case-control study. Many researchers rely on this type of study because of lower cost, smaller sample size and ability to study many potential factors. However, such retrospective studies are subject to recall bias and unavailable or incomplete data. There may also be questions regarding adequacy of the "control" group. Follow-up (prospective cohort) studies, on the other hand, are considered to provide the most definitive information and are the most persuasive study design. In these studies a cohort (group) of individuals, who do not yet have a specific disease, are selected and followed over a period of time while collecting specific information regarding diet and other factors related to the development of the disease. However, prospective studies are more costly and require more time and larger numbers of subjects. Following on the results of these types of epidemiological study, it is critical to conduct human, randomized clinical intervention studies in order to ultimately establish cause-effect relationships.

INTERPRETATION OF EPIDEMIOLOGICAL STUDIES DEMANDS CAUSATION CRITERIA

To evaluate research findings in any area of scientific investigation, certain scientific standards, established by experts in each field, need to be applied. This is especially true when trying to determine the health effects of the inclusion or exclusion or varying levels of components in the diets of humans. The eminent British biostatistician and epidemiologist A. Bradford Hill published a seminal paper in 1965 [8] offering a number of interpretation criteria that would be useful when interpreting the statistical results observed in epidemiological studies. The goal of these criteria was to guide epidemiologists in inferring causation (or establishing

TABLE 8.1 The Interpretation Criteria for Epidemiological Associations Presented by A. Bradford Hill in 1965.

1. Strength of Association	Magnitude of the effect
2. Temporality	Exposure must precede the disease
3. Consistency	Similar findings in many studies without contradictory results
4. Theoretical Plausibility	Biological/Physiological/Metabolic knowledge supports the findings
5. Coherence	No alternate hypotheses
6. Specificity	No confounding factors are found
7. Dose-response	Higher risk with higher exposure
8. Experimental Evidence	Animal and in-vitro experiments show the effect
9. Analogy	Similar findings in other situations can apply

"causal inference") from the associations observed in such studies. In effect, Bradford Hill tried to provide a framework to judge whether associations observed in a body of epidemiological work could be determined to be causal. Since the time of his publication, these criteria (which Bradford Hill urged others to call "viewpoints" and not true criteria) have become a de facto standard to evaluate the statistical associations found in epidemiological research.

Bradford Hill pointed out, however, that none of these nine viewpoints provide indisputable evidence for or against a cause and effect hypothesis. What he claimed they could do, with greater or less strength, was to help answer the fundamental question of whether there is any other way of explaining the set of observed facts, i.e., is there any other answer equally, or more likely than cause and effect? His criteria are still very relevant to the scientific and public discussion of diet and disease relationships. Bradford Hill's causation criteria are described below, with examples given to help illustrate each of the criteria.

1. *Strength of Association:* The stronger the relationship between the independent variable (the risk factor) and the dependent variable (the disease), the less likely it is that the relationship is due to an extraneous variable (a confounder). For example, the relative risk of smokers developing lung cancer is around 10 or above (i.e., a 10-fold higher risk than for non-smokers). The relative risks associated with consumption of grains containing mycotoxins and liver cancer is around 6. These are quite strong associations, and by contrast, modest relative risks on the order of 2 or less should be viewed with skepticism due to the likelihood of many potential confound-

ers. This was recognized in 1994 when the U.S. National Cancer Institute publicly indicated that relative risks values less than 2 were not strong enough to use for public policy pronouncements [9] (This document is available through the National Cancer Institute's CancerFax and CancerNet services, and in the News Section of the NCI's PDQ database. To get the document from CancerFax, dial (301) 402-5874 from the handset on your fax machine and follow the recorded instructions to receive the contents list: U.S. National Cancer Institute Press Release, Oct 16, 1994).

2. *Temporality:* The exposure must precede the disease by a reasonable amount of time, i.e., a cause must precede an effect in time. While this relationship seems obvious, there have been published findings that have occasionally violated this criterion. For example, cigarette smoking over a period of years is well established to increase lung cancer risk.
3. *Consistency:* Multiple observations of an association, with different people under different circumstances and with different measurement instruments, increase the credibility of a causal finding.

   Different methods (e.g., ecological, cohort and case-control studies) should produce the same conclusion. The relationship should also hold for different groups of people (in males and females, in different populations on different continents). This criterion is greatly debated, however, because consistency is often in the eye of the beholder. Some reviewers can conclude that six of ten studies with a statistically significant association represent a consistent finding, while others can see the same set of data as inconsistent.
4. *Theoretical Plausibility:* It is easier to accept an association as causal when there is a rational and theoretical basis for such a conclusion supported by known biological and other facts.

   While our knowledge of physiology today is vast, there is still much that is unknown about the complex interactions of ingested foods and food components and their metabolism and potential adverse effects.
5. *Coherence:* A cause-and-effect interpretation for an observed association is clearest when it does not conflict with what is known about the variables under study and when there are no plausible competing theories or rival hypotheses. In other words, the association must be coherent with other existing knowledge.

   The conclusion that smoking causes lung cancer, based on decades of epidemiologic, laboratory animal, pharmacokinetic, clinical and other biological data, showed that all available facts stuck together as a coherent whole.

6. *Specificity in the Causes:* In the ideal situation, the effect has only one cause. In other words, showing that a disease outcome is best predicted by one primary factor adds credibility to a causal claim. But this is often not the norm. High consumption of one food, food ingredient or nutrient can be covariate with low consumption of another food or ingredient, and it is often difficult to determine which of the two is more important.

   Other non-dietary confounders must also be considered. For example, chronic *Helicobacter pylori* infection is a strongly suspected risk factor for gastric cancer [10]. Nutritional epidemiological studies that fail to account for the incidence of this infection in the population studied should therefore be viewed with caution.

7. *Dose-Response Relationship:* There should be a direct biological gradient (or dose-response) between the risk factor (the independent variable) and people's status on the disease variable (the dependent variable).

   Many dietary epidemiological studies report a significant statistical trend for dose-response, but on closer examination, the data can be highly inconsistent. The data may only span a very narrow range of dietary intakes or in some cases such a wide range of intakes that upper intakes are representative of a grossly unbalanced diet. Calculated relative risks may sometimes decline to non-significant levels with higher intakes, or in some cases one quartile of intake may have a high enough calculated risk to skew the overall results. Such data patterns, when deviating from the linear dose-response, need to be considered as unlikely dose-response relationships and also be considered as part of the consistency criterion.

8. *Experimental Evidence:* Any related research (animal, *in vitro*, etc.) that is based on experiments and supports the conclusions of epidemiological studies will make a causal inference more plausible.

   This must be tempered with the understanding that animals are not people, and that results from lifetime, chronic feeding bioassays, where rodents are dosed at levels up to and sometimes exceeding maximum tolerated doses (MTDs), in such testing programs as the U.S. National Toxicology Program, may often be very useful but are not definitive by themselves.

9. *Analogy:* Sometimes a commonly accepted phenomenon in one area can be applied to another area.

   For instance, a newly discovered N-nitrosamine may be considered to be a carcinogen if it has structural similarities to other well-known carcinogenic N-nitrosamines. However, analogy is an obtuse criterion, and thus is considered to be a weaker form of evidence. This makes the application of the analogy consideration even more uncertain than the application of considerations on plausibility and coherence.

Bradford Hill developed his list of "criteria" that continues to be used today. When using them, it's important not to forget Hill's own advice: "None of these nine viewpoints can bring indisputable evidence for or against a cause and effect hypothesis. . . . What they can do, with greater or less strength, is to help answer the fundamental question—is there any other way of explaining the set of facts before us, is there any other answer equally, or more, likely than cause and effect?" Phillips and Goodman [11] have recently provided observations on the use of Hill's "causal criteria." They argued that the uncritical repetition of Hill's criteria is probably counterproductive in promoting sophisticated understanding of causal inference, but they set out a simplified list of the key considerations that can be found in Hill's address that they thought is worthy of repeating:

- "Statistical significance should not be mistaken for evidence of a substantial association.
- Association does not prove causation (other evidence must be considered).
- Precision should not be mistaken for validity (non-random errors exist).
- Evidence (or belief) that there is a causal relationship is not sufficient to suggest action should be taken.
- Uncertainty about whether there is a causal relationship (or even an association) is not sufficient to suggest action should not be taken."

The authors pointed out that while these points may seem obvious when stated so briefly and bluntly, causal inference and health policy decision-making would benefit tremendously if they were considered more carefully and more often.

The International Food Information Council Foundation has addressed the issue of "How to Understand and Interpret Food and

Health-Related Scientific Studies" [12]. They discuss the types of epidemiological research studies and what journalists, educators and health professionals should look for when critically reviewing scientific studies. When evaluating an epidemiological report, IFIC suggested that the following questions can be asked:

- Could the study be interpreted to say something else?
- Are there any methodological flaws in the study that should be considered when making conclusions?
- Are the study's results generalizable to other groups?
- How does the work fit with the body of research on the subject?
- What are the inherent limitations of this type of study and does the research design fit the stated purpose of the study?
- Has the author omitted important points in the background section which could have a meaningful effect on the study design or interpretation of the results?
- Are there any major design flaws in the study and are the data collection measures appropriate to answer the study questions?
- Were methodological limitations acknowledged and discussed and what influence might these have had on the results?
- What is the real and statistical significance of the results?
- To whom do the results apply and how do the results compare to those of other studies on the subject?
- Are the conclusions supported by the data?
- Are the conclusions of the study related to the stated purpose of the study? If not, does the study design and results support the secondary conclusions?

DIET AND CARDIOVASCULAR DISEASE

Now with these epidemiological criteria in mind, we will present the available data on certain foods and risk of specific diseases, namely cardiovascular disease (CVD) and cancer. Nothing is more important to our health than our diet, and there are well-established and recognized dietary patterns that confer health benefits. Numerous dietary epidemiological data have generally indicated an inverse relationship between dietary intake of fruits and vegetables and incidence of both CVD and cancer. The specific constituents of fruits and vegetables that afford protection from CVD have and continue to be widely researched and debated. Although there are many dietary components which may have protective effects, antioxidants appear to be one of the phytochemicals that play a significant role. One group of antioxidants present in fruits and vegetables is known as "polyphenols" or "polyphenolics" and is believed to neutralize free radicals formed in the body, thus minimizing or preventing damage to cell membranes and other cell structures. Many of these concepts were presented in chapter 4 and chapter 7. Although antioxidants are generally credited with improving states of oxidative stress, epidemiological studies which have evaluated the efficacy of supplementation with a high dose of an antioxidant alone, such as vitamin E, have shown no apparent improvement and in some cases a decrease in cardiovascular protection [13]. Yet, when these antioxidants are consumed through the diet in the form of fruits and vegetables, there is a significant degree of protection, best represented by the decrease in mortality rates from CVD of those consuming the popular Mediterranean diet [14]. Although Mediterranean diets vary by country, seasonal availability of ingredients and traditional cooking habits, they all tend to be rich in fruits, vegetables and monounsaturated fatty acids while low in saturated fat and meat. Epidemiological studies, such as the Seven Countries Study [15–21], have led to theories describing why and how the Mediterranean diet may promote a lower incidence of CVD, and antioxidants are emerging as a key component. However, since antioxidant supplementation alone does not confer the cardiovascular benefits, there must be more to explain the cardioprotection afforded by fruits and vegetables. The data and emerging story presented in this context provide a convincing argument for nitrite and nitrate as probable protective components. The Seven Countries Study constitutes the first nutritional epidemiological investigation that provided solid data for cardiovascular disease rates in different populations. In this study the results for all-cause death rates in Greece, Japan and Italy were quite favorable compared with the USA, Finland, the Netherlands, and the former Yugoslavia; the results also showed a lower incidence of CVD after a 5-year follow-up for the same countries that exhibited low mortality. The diet consumed by the Mediterranean cohorts studied was associated with a very low incidence of CVD and was called the *Mediterranean diet* by Keys [22]. Following the Seven Countries Study, the Mediterranean diet has oftentimes been singled out as a healthy diet. Additional studies later confirmed the association of the Mediterranean diet with decreased incidence and prevalence of chronic diseases, mainly CVD, in countries where it was consumed.

There are food peculiarities for the different populations in the Mediterranean basin. However, beyond the apparent differences, there are nutritional characteristics common to all or most of the diets in the Mediterranean region. The Mediterranean diet is characteristically low in saturated and high in monounsaturated fats (olive oil), low in animal protein, rich in carbohydrates, and rich in vegetables and leguminous fiber. People consuming a Mediterranean diet eat a relatively large amount of fish and white meat, abundant fruits and vegetables and a low amount of red meat, but they also drink moderate amounts of red wine [23]. We know from chapter 4 that fruits, vegetables, red wine and common foods of the Mediterranean diet are rich in nitrite and nitrate. The health benefits of Mediterranean diets have been attributed, at least in part, to the high consumption of antioxidants provided by fruit, vegetables and wine and to the type of fat, rich in monounsaturated and ω–3 fatty acids from vegetables and fish, and especially to a balanced ω–6/ω–3 fatty acid ratio, as is found in the traditional diet of Greece prior to 1960 [23]. Emerging data reveal that part of the health benefits may be mediated through their nitrite/nitrate content. Additionally, the Lyon Diet Heart Study was a randomized, single-blind, secondary prevention trial aimed at testing whether an experimental modified Cretan diet may reduce the risk of recurrence after a first myocardial infarction (MI). A significant reduction of the rates of cardiovascular complications was reported [24]. Adjusted risk ratios ranged from 0.28 to 0.53, with these reduced risk ratios indicating a protective effect of the diet on MI.

DIET AND CANCER

In contrast to the evidence on diet and CVD, epidemiological data on the consumption of meats and the risk of cancer sometimes reveal a slightly increased risk. It has been assumed for several decades that dietary factors are estimated to account for approximately one-third of all cancer deaths each year [25]. Since dietary factors, which can be numerous and complex, may yield both positive and negative risk associations, they are of great interest to the research community, public health agencies and to the public. Reports suggesting that red meat consumption may in some way affect the risk of cancer continue to be the subject of much research and media interest, and the scientific literature on this subject is quite extensive. In addition, the popular press coverage is intense, and sorting out all the data, interpretations and latest recommendations can be confusing.

The consumption of red meat and, in particular, processed or preserved or cured meats (i.e., meats treated with nitrite as a food additive, including ham, bacon, hot dogs, etc.), has been related to the incidence of colorectal cancer since 1975 in several epidemiological studies. A worldwide recommendation for moderation in the consumption of preserved meats, such as sausages, salami, bacon and ham, was launched by the World Health Organization in 2003 [26]. However, a 2008 international publication by the World Cancer Research Fund and the American Institute of Cancer Research (WCRF/AICR) has presented a recommendation to "avoid processed meats" [27], based on a meta-analysis of a limited number of selected cohort studies showing increased risk of colorectal cancer with increased intake of processed meats. The summary estimate of relative risk was determined to be 1.21 (95% confidence interval = 1.04–1.42) per 50 g intake/day and supported by case-control studies. A separate Swedish meta-analysis of 14 cohort studies reported a slightly lower summary hazard ratio estimate of 1.09 (95% confidence interval = 1.05–1.13) per 30 g intake/day [28]. However, this finding must be viewed with skepticism, considering that a relative risk ratio of 1.0 indicates no increase in risk and anything less than 2.0 should not be used for public policy recommendations, according to the U.S. National Cancer Institute [9].

According to the WCRF/AICR summary estimate of relative risk, a decrease of 50 g/day in processed meat consumption may then lower the total number of colorectal cancer cases by approximately 20%. However, a relative risk estimate of < 1.3 would normally receive little attention in the epidemiological community, but since exposure to processed meats is such a common event, then even a modest association, if proven to be causal, may have considerable public health consequences [29]. Curiously, the same literature review by the WCRF/AICR found a statistically significant 26% protective effect against rectal cancer for the highest meat consumption level, an important finding not referenced in the WCRF/AICR report or the press release that accompanied the report. There are also studies, however, showing no association between colorectal cancer and exposure to red or processed meats [30,31].

Red Meat and Cancer (NCBA) [32]: An earlier exhaustive review by Australian authors was entitled "Does Red Meat Cause Cancer?" [33]. This extensive review, with over 225 references, concluded that the associations of meat consumption and cancer risk were not consistent. They also concluded that any true effect of meat is likely to be small or even an artifact of a decreased consumption of fruit, vegetables and cereals by high meat consumers. This review discussed proposed mechanisms by which diet/meat might be associated with increased cancer risk. The two broad areas described were: high dietary fat intake, leading to bile acid secretion and conversion to potentially mutagenic compounds, oxidation of fats (especially unsaturated fats) and other unwanted effects exerted by specific dietary fats. The second area of potential concern related to the production of mutagens, such as heterocyclic amines (HA) and polyaromatic hydrocarbons (PAH) that are known to be produced in meat by specific cooking methods. These compounds (also found in cooked poultry and fish products) are not unique to red meat, and they can be dramatically controlled by alterations in cooking methods. The actual exposure level in humans, usually at very low parts per billion levels, is still unclear, as is the actual risk associated with such exposures. This Australian review also discussed the potential anticarcinogens that can be found in meat, including anti-oxidants, dipeptides and conjugated linoleic acid (CLA) and the possible role of methionine in gene regulation of cell proliferation.

Firm evidence of cancer causation in humans is lacking for dietary nitrite, nitrate and N-nitrosamines. A comprehensive review [34] could find no firm epidemiological evidence linking stomach, brain, esophageal and nasopharyngeal cancers to dietary intake of nitrate, nitrite or N-nitroso compounds. This conclusion was further supported by a study showing that cured meat consumption was not linked to adult or childhood brain cancer in the U.S. [35].

The epidemiological data on meats, particularly cured and processed meats, becomes important in terms of exposure because such products are known to contain nitrite and nitrate. There are many other confounding factors in meats (saturated fats for example), but the direct implications for nitrite and nitrate content are far from conclusive. Early reports implicated the nitrite and nitrate in processed meats as the culprit. Since the 1950's, when the potential to form carcinogenic N-nitrosamines from the reaction of nitrous acid with secondary amines was recognized, the use of nitrite salts as food preservatives has come under intense scrutiny. Numerous case-control studies have been conducted worldwide to determine if there is a link between gastric cancer and nitrate intake [34,36,37]. It is well known that elevated dietary nitrate intake leads to elevated salivary nitrate levels and, after reduction by oral bacteria, higher levels of ingested nitrite. Studies in Canada, Italy, Sweden and Germany involving thousands of study subjects have failed to show an association or have demonstrated an inverse association between estimated nitrate intake and gastric cancer, perhaps because much of the nitrate was from vegetables [37]. Occupational exposure to very high levels of nitrate occurs in nitrate fertilizer workers, who have elevated body burdens of nitrate and elevated salivary nitrate and nitrite levels, but no increase in gastric cancers has been observed [37]. Case-control studies attempting to link nitrate and nitrite consumption to brain, esophageal, and nasopharyngeal cancers have also been inconclusive [34]. In other studies published over two decades, the relationship between the consumption of cured meats during pregnancy and the risk of brain and other tumors in offspring was examined [36]. In this review of 14 epidemiological studies, 13 of which were case-control studies, Blot et al. [36] could not conclude that there was a relationship between cured meat consumption during pregnancy and brain or any other cancers. It may be that in the limited number of epidemiological studies linking nitrate, nitrite or cured meat to a specific cancer site, other as-yet uncharacterized dietary or environmental factors may be involved.

Thus, the concern for the use added nitrite in processed meats (added nitrate is only used in a very limited number of products outside the U.S.) has waxed and waned as numerous studies were published and as independent review and food regulatory panels have been convened to make determinations about nitrite for use as a food additive and public policy. In 2000, the results of a comprehensive battery of rodent carcinogenicity and mutagenicity studies by the U.S. National Toxicology Program, including a standard, two-year chronic cancer bioassay of sodium nitrite in rats and mice, were presented to the National Toxicology Program Technical Reports Review Subcommittee for evaluation. The final NTP Technical Report [38] indicated that the only adverse finding in both rats and mice was an "equivocal evidence" finding that sodium nitrite weakly increased the number of forestomach tumors in female mice. All other organ sites in both rats and mice showed no evidence of carcinogenicity. In short, any suspicion of sodium nitrite's carcinogenicity in rodents was not supported by this state-of-the-art cancer bioassay study. Shortly thereafter in 2000, nitrite was also reviewed and evaluated for potential listing as a developmental and reproductive toxicant under the Proposition 65 Statute in California. A review of 99 studies on sodium nitrite led the state's Developmental and Reproductive Toxicants Committee of eight independent scientists to conclude that sodium nitrite should not be listed as a developmental toxicant or as a male or female reproductive toxicant under California's Proposition 65 law. The literature and activities associated with the above events were reviewed and published by Archer [39].

The latest review of ingested nitrate and nitrite carcinogenicity was conducted in 2006 by an expert working group convened by the International Agency for Research on Cancer (IARC), a United Nations/World Health Organization organization headquartered in Lyon, France. IARC's mission is to coordinate and conduct research on the causes of human cancer, the mechanisms of carcinogenesis, and to develop scientific strategies for cancer control. The agency is involved in both epidemiological and laboratory research and disseminates scientific information through publications, meetings, courses, and fellowships. The IARC working group, whose report is not yet publicly available except in summary form IARC (2006). (http://monographs.iarc.fr/ENG/Meetings/94-nitratenitrite.pdf), made a decision to classify nitrate and nitrite for their potential as human carcinogens as follows:

Ingested nitrate or nitrite under conditions that result in endogenous nitrosation is probably carcinogenic to humans (Group 2A).

The expert group found that nitrate/nitrite were only weakly associated with human stomach cancer and no other cancers, and they also appeared to disregard or misinterpret the findings of the NTP cancer rodent bioassay, which showed that sodium nitrite was not carcinogenic in rats and mice. The above conclusion, which in a very narrow sense may be accurate, has in a broader biological sense questionable and minimal practical application. In simple terms, this overall evaluation means that the ingestion of food and water that contain nitrate or nitrite (e.g., spinach and other green leafy vegetables, root vegetables, bread, beer, cured meats), in combination with amines and amides commonly found in food, can react in the stomach to form N-nitrosamines and N-nitrosamides, which are known animal carcinogens already classified by IARC.

CONCLUSION

A long history of safe use as a food additive, minimal endogenous production of N-nitrosamines and natural metabolism of ingested nitrite all argue that nitrite as currently used is a safe food additive and even beneficial to human health. Dietary intake of nitrate is a well-known marker of a health-promoting fruit and vegetable diet. In addition, nitrite and nitrate per se, as individual chemical compounds, have never been shown to be carcinogens in animal or human studies. Nitrate itself is not capable of reacting with amines to form N-nitrosamines. One could ask the question, then, how simultaneous ingestion of nitrite/nitrate and nitrosatable amines/amides could be prevented or reduced by public policy considerations stemming from IARC's conclusion, when the majority of ingested (swallowed) nitrite is endogenously produced in saliva and when the major source of nitrate is the consumption of fruits and vegetables. Thus, to eat is to ingest nitrite, nitrate, amines and amides, regardless of the specific diet. Specifically, the ingestion of processed, cured meats would be no more or less risky given the low amount of residual nitrite in such products ready to consume (approximately 10 parts per million in individual servings, and sometimes undetectable).

There will very likely be considerable debate about the need for reviews by regulatory agencies and potential action on nitrite as a food additive as a result of the IARC classification. However, when considered in the context of evolving research about the biological function of all nitrogen oxides (including nitrite and nitrate) and their metabolism, any changes to current food regulations on nitrite are simply unwarranted, as are any regulatory implications for the unavoidable presence of nitrate in fruits and vegetables. The food additive use of nitrite represents only a small addition to the body burden of endogenously produced nitrogen oxides. It is hard to conceive that the ingestion of nitrite from cured meats or nitrate from fruits and vegetables could have any impact on potential adverse toxic outcomes. Due to the intense social and governmental desire to identify causes of CVD and cancer, we as a society have come to a point where some mechanistic/physiological observations and weak epidemiological associations can mislead us, even when the totality of evidence shows such findings to be biologically implausible. As more is understood about the human metabolic nitrogen oxide cycle, it will become apparent that nitrite is a safe and appropriate food additive providing many more benefits to society than risks, and that nitrate naturally occurring in fruits and vegetables and some drinking waters poses insignificant risks.

Overall, results from the epidemiological literature suggest that the association of meat consumption and cancer risk is very inconsistent. Examination of the literature yields evidence sometimes called "insufficient," "possible" or even "probable." However, this inconsistency has led to divided interpretations appearing in the literature. To date, we believe that the balance of the data has not provided "convincing" evidence of a consistent, specific link between red or processed meat consumption and any form of human cancer. This area of research will continue to be refined with additional studies, so that meaningful conclusions can be drawn from existing and new data, always keeping in mind Bradford Hill's causation criteria for evaluating the body of epidemiological evidence as well as a caution not to over interpret the mechanistic findings of animal studies. The consistency of the "inconsistency" in the data suggests that any real effect of meat intake is likely to be small, or perhaps even a result of an unbalanced consumption of other food groups among the higher meat consumers. While there is a need for the transfer of existing dietary information to consumers, such a transfer needs to carefully explain epidemiological risk levels and to also note inconsistencies in the data. For red meat, the importance of recommended cooking/preparation methods to minimize the already trace levels of known animal carcinogens (HAs and PAHs) needs to be stressed to consumers. And finally, the importance of dietary variety, balance and moderation should be stressed along with the importance of protective factors (including adequate consumption of fruits and vegetables) in the total diet, combined with a physically active lifestyle.

We should avoid getting caught up in fads to the point where we might ignore sound science and common sense. Dietary fads seem to have varying lifetimes, sometimes 3 months to even 3 years and, often in retrospect, some common sense critical thinking at the early stages of dietary research reporting could avoid a lot of poor dietary advice. We have seen a variety of diet vs. disease fads, some covering decades, such as the low-fat craze which according to some observers has led to significant increases in the incidence of both obesity and type II diabetes. Such fads can have large consequences in that they not only fail to improve public health, but actually result in unintended adverse effects. We believe that the weak and inconclusive data on nitrite and nitrate risks described here may be far outweighed by the health benefits of restoring nitric oxide homeostasis as described elsewhere in this book. The risk/benefit balance should be a strong consideration before there are any suggestions for new regulatory or public health guidelines for nitrite and nitrate exposures.

ABOUT THE AUTHORS

Andrew Milkowski, Ph.D.

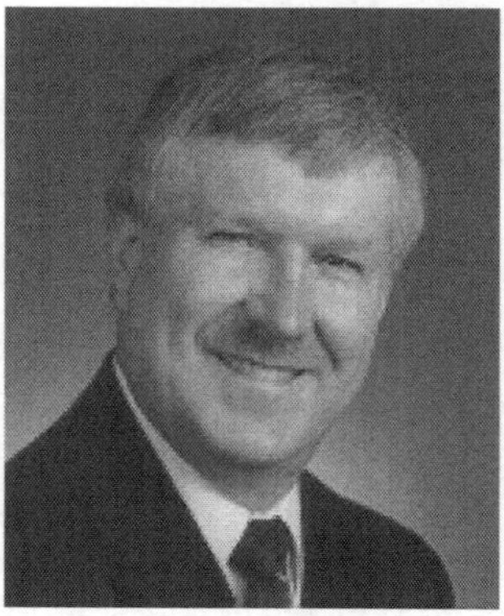

Andrew Milkowski serves as an Adjunct Professor in Muscle Biology Laboratory of the Department of Animal Sciences at the University of Wisconsin, Madison, WI (USA). He received his bachelor of science degree in chemistry from the University of Illinois Champaign-Urbana, and Ph.D. in in biochemistry from the University of Wisconsin, Madison.

Dr. Milkowski lectures in a variety of Animal Science courses and co-directs short courses in meat processing at the Muscle Biology Laboratory. He also is a member of the executive committee of the Food Research Institute and consults in many of the food safety related activities of the Institute.

Prior to joining the University of Wisconsin, Dr. Milkowski was a

Kraft Foods Fellow in the Oscar Mayer Division of Kraft Foods. There he was the leader for basic and applied research activities covering food chemistry, ingredient technology, sensory evaluation, product quality and food safety of processed meat products.

He is a member of the American Meat Science Association, Institute of Food Technologists, International Association for Food Protection and the American Chemical Society. He has been active with the American Meat Institute serving as chair of the nitrite subcommittee of the Scientific Affairs Committee.

Dr. Milkowski has received the American Meat Institute Industry Advancement Award and American Meat Science Association Meat Processing Award.

James R. Coughlin, Ph.D.

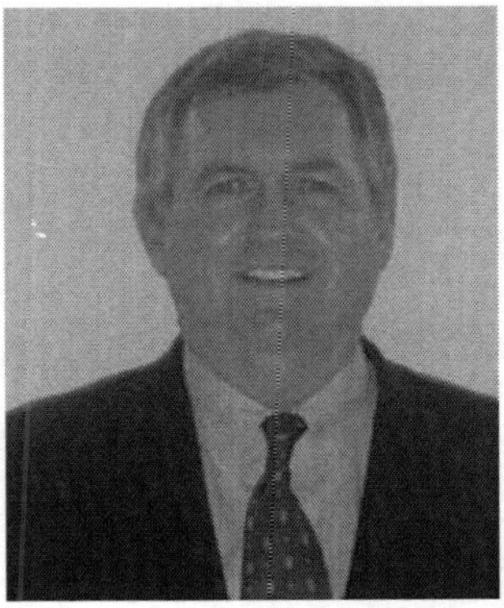

Dr. Coughlin is President of Coughlin & Associates, an independent consulting firm he established in 1992. He obtained his B.S. in Chemistry at Siena College, and his M.S. in Food Science and Technology and his Ph.D. in Agricultural and Environmental Chemistry at the University of California, Davis, where he also did a Postdoctoral Fellowship in Environmental Toxicology. He has over 30 years experience in food/nutrition science and regulatory affairs; food, chemical and environmental toxicology and safety; chemical risk assessment; GRAS safety evaluations; and scientific risk communication. He provides strategic toxicologic, nutritional, communications and regulatory counsel to many food, functional food, dietary supplement, chemical, mining and consumer products companies and their trade associations, law firms and public relations firms.

Before undertaking his current role, he spent two years as Food Chemical Safety Scientist at Armour Meats and ten years at General Foods and Kraft General Foods managing toxicology, safety and regulatory affairs, including several years as Director of International Scientific Relations at KGF. Health and regulatory issues surrounding coffee/caffeine, nitrite-cured processed meats, beverages, food additives/contaminants and environmental toxicants were among his areas of expertise. He served as President of the Association for Science and Information on Coffee (ASIC), the Paris-based scientific society dedicated to improving worldwide research on coffee growing, processing, biotechnology, quality, health and safety and is currently serving as a Member of the Board.

Dr. Coughlin has been involved in the assessment and management of California Proposition 65 requirements since the law's passage in 1986. He served for many years on the Editorial Advisory Board of *Prop 65 News* and currently serves on the *Prop. 65 Clearinghouse* Advisory Board. He has been elected three times as Chair of the Toxicology and Safety Evaluation Division of the Institute of Food Technologists and helped establish the IFT's International Division. He served for six years on the IFT Expert Panel assisting FDA in assessing food bioterrorism defense and is also serving as IFT's Codex Alimentarius Subject Expert on food contaminants. In addition, Dr. Coughlin served as Vice President of the International Society for Trace Element Research in Humans, an organization focused on both essential and toxic elements, with particular emphasis on guiding a decade-long research effort on boron's nutritional essentiality for humans and on the risk assessment of essential trace elements.

REFERENCES

1. Tarasuk, V.S. and A.S. Brooker, Interpreting epidemiologic studies of diet-disease relationships. *J Nutr,* 1997. 127(9): p. 1847–52.
2. Boyle, P., P. Boffetta, and P. Autier, Diet, nutrition and cancer: public, media and scientific confusion. *Ann Oncol,* 2008. 19(10): p. 1665–7.
3. Kipnis, V. and L.S. Freedman, Impact of exposure measurement error in nutritional epidemiology. *J Natl Cancer Inst,* 2008. 100(23): p. 1658–9.
4. Schatzkin, A. and V. Kipnis, Could exposure assessment problems give us wrong answers to nutrition and cancer questions? *J Natl Cancer Inst,* 2004. 96(21): p. 1564–5.
5. Dentzer, S., Communicating medical news—pitfalls of health care journalism. *N Engl J Med,* 2009. 360(1): p. 1–3.
6. van den Brandt, P., et al., The contribution of epidemiology. *Food Chem Toxicol,* 2002. 40(2–3): p. 387–424.
7. Langseth, L., Nutritional Epidemiology: Possibilities and Limitations, in *ILSI Europe Concise Monograph Series,* N.J. Jardine, Editor. 1996, International Life Sciences Institute: Brussels. p. 1–40.
8. Hill, A.B., The Environment and Disease: Association or Causation? *Proc R Soc Med,* 1965. 58: p. 295–300.
9. Anderson, L., *Abortion and Possible Risk for Breast Cancer: Analysis and Inconsistencies.* 1994, National Cancer Institute: Bethesda, MD.
10. Young, G.P. and B.H. Demediuk, The genetics, epidemiology, and early detection of gastrointestinal cancers. *Curr Opin Oncol,* 1992. 4(4): p. 728–35.
11. Phillips, C.V. and K.J. Goodman, The missed lessons of Sir Austin Bradford Hill. *Epidemiologic Perspective & Innovation,* 2004. 1: p. 1–5.

12. *How to Understand and Interpret Food and Health-Related Scientific Studies.* 2001, International Food Information Council Foundation: Washington DC. p. 1–11.
13. Yusuf, S., et al., Vitamin E supplementation and cardiovascular events in high-risk patients. The Heart Outcomes Prevention Evaluation Study Investigators. *N Engl J Med,* 2000. 342(3): p. 154–60.
14. Visioli, F., et al., Mediterranean food and health: building human evidence. *J Physiol Pharmacol,* 2005. 56 Suppl 1: p. 37–49.
15. Kimura, N. and A. Keys, Coronary heart disease in seven countries. X. Rural southern Japan. *Circulation,* 1970. 41(4 Suppl): p. I101–12.
16. Taylor, H.L., et al., Coronary heart disease in seven countries. IV. Five-year follow-up of employees of selected U.S. railroad companies. *Circulation,* 1970. 41(4 Suppl): p. I20–39.
17. Taylor, H.L., et al., Coronary heart disease in seven countries. XI. Five years of follow-up of railroad men in Italy. *Circulation,* 1970. 41(4 Suppl): p. I113–22.
18. Blackburn, H., H.L. Taylor, and A. Keys, Coronary heart disease in seven countries. XVI. The electrocardiogram in prediction of five-year coronary heart disease incidence among men aged forty through fifty-nine. *Circulation,* 1970. 41(4 Suppl): p. I154–61.
19. Buzina, R., et al., Coronary heart disease in seven countries. V. Five-year follow-up in Dalmatia and Slavonia. *Circulation,* 1970. 41(4 Suppl): p. I40–51.
20. Aravanis, C., et al., Coronary heart disease in seven countries. IX. The Greek islands of Crete and Corfu. *Circulation,* 1970. 41(4 Suppl): p. I88–100.
21. Fidanza, F., et al., Coronary heart disease in seven countries. VII. Five-year experience in rural Italy. *Circulation,* 1970. 41(4 Suppl): p. I63–75.
22. Keys, A., Mediterranean diet and public health: personal reflections. *Am J Clin Nutr,* 1995. 61(6 Suppl): p. 1321S–1323S.
23. Simopoulos, A.P., The Mediterranean diets: What is so special about the diet of Greece? The scientific evidence. *J Nutr,* 2001. 131(11 Suppl): p. 3065S–73S.
24. De Lorgeril, M., et al., Effect of a mediterranean type of diet on the rate of cardiovascular complications in patients with coronary artery disease. Insights into the cardioprotective effect of certain nutriments. *J Am Coll Cardiol,* 1996. 28(5): p. 1103–8.
25. Doll, R. and R. Petro, The causes of cancer: quantitative estimates of avoidable risks of cancer in the United States today. *Journal of National Cancer Institute,* 1981. 66: p. 1191–1308.
26. Diet, Nutrition and the Prevention of Chronic Disease. in *Diet Nutrition and the Prevention of Chronic Disease.* 2002. Geneva, Switzerland.
27. World Cancer Research Fund/American Institute for Cancer Research, in *Food, Nutrition, Physical Activity, and the Prevention of Cancer: A Global Perspective.* 2007, American Institute for Cancer Research: Washington D.C. p. 517.
28. Larsson, S.C. and A. Wolk, Meat consumption and risk of colorectal cancer: a meta-analysis of prospective studies. *Int J Cancer,* 2006. 119(11): p. 2657–64.
29. Demeyer, D., K. Honikel, and S. De Smet, The World Cancer Research Fund Report 2007: A challenge for the meat processing industry. *Meat Science,* 2008. 80: p. 953–959.
30. Kimura, Y., et al., Meat, fish and fat intake in relation to subsite-specific risk of colorectal cancer: The Fukuoka Colorectal Cancer Study. *Cancer Sci,* 2007. 98(4): p. 590–7.
31. Eunyoung, C. and S.A. Smith-Warner, Meat and fat intake and colorectal cancer risk: A pooled analysis of 14 prospective studies. *Proceedings of American Association Cancer Research,* 2004. 45.
32. Red Meat and Cancer: A Review of Current Epidemiological Findings. in *Chicago National Cattlemen's Beef Assoc.* 1997: National Cattlemen's Beef Association.

33. Baghurst, P., S. Record, and J. Syrette, Does red meat cause cancer? *Aust J Nutr Diet,* 1997. 54(4): p. S1–S44.

34. Eichholzer, M. and F. Gutzwiller, Dietary nitrates, nitrites, and N-nitroso compounds and cancer risk: a review of the epidemiologic evidence. *Nutr Rev,* 1998. 56(4 Pt 1): p. 95–105.

35. Murphy, R.S., C.J. Sadler, and W.J. Blot, Trends in cured meat consumption in relation to childhood and adult brain cancer in the United States. *Food Control,* 1998. 9(5): p. 299–305.

36. Blot, W.J., B.E. Henderson, and J.D. Boice, Jr., Childhood cancer in relation to cured meat intake: review of the epidemiological evidence. *Nutr Cancer,* 1999. 34(1): p. 111–8.

37. Moller, H. Adverse health effects of nitrate and its metabolites: epidemiological studies in humans. in *Health Aspects of nitrates and its metabolites* (particularly nitrite). 1995. Strasbourg Cedex, France: Council of Europe Press.

38. National Toxicology Program, in *NTP Technical Report on the toxicology and carcinogenesis studies of sodium nitrite* (CAS NO. 7632-00-0)IN F344/N rats and B6C3F1 mice(drinking water studies). 2001, NIH Publication No. 01-3954. p. 7–273.

39. Archer, D.L., Evidence that ingested nitrate and nitrite are beneficial to health. *J Food Prot,* 2002. 65(5): p. 872–5.

CHAPTER 9

Regulations Gone Awry: Addressing Public Health Concerns

NATHAN S. BRYAN and NORMAN G. HORD

Brown Foundation Institute of Molecular Medicine, The University of Texas Health Science Center, Houston, TX 77030

Department of Food Science and Human Nutrition, Michigan State University, East Lansing, MI

IT would not be appropriate to discuss all of the new emerging and exciting discoveries on nitric oxide, nitrite and nitrate without acknowledging the public perception of nitrite and nitrate in particular and the existing paradigm that has existed for decades. Nitrite became a research interest in the 1960s when it was discovered that nitrite in industry and in foods might increase the incidence of cancer by the formation of N-nitrosamines [1]. The paradigm on nitrite immediately developed into one in which nitrite and nitrate must be regulated and nitrite in any form was detrimental to health. In the late 1970s, despite all the fear and paranoia surrounding nitrite exposure, appreciation and understanding of nitrite and nitrate in the biomedical science community took a drastic turn. Studies on nitrogen balance in humans and analyses of fecal and ileostomy samples indicated that nitrite and nitrate are formed *de novo* in the intestine. These early findings by Tannenbaum *et al.* [2] significantly altered our conceptions of human exposure to exogenous nitrite and nitrate and represented the original observations that would eventually lead to the discovery of the L-arginine: NO pathway. However the paradigm did not spill over to the lay public and still today some 30 years later, public perception is that nitrite and nitrate are harmful food additives that should be avoided. We will address the scientific basis for health concerns of nitrite that have led to the public perception. As with any nutrient, nitrite is not completely innocuous and has toxic characteristics but we hope to dispel current myths and present the physiological context by which both nitrite and nitrate can be beneficial. As Paracelsus stated, "Poison is in everything, and no thing is without poison. The dosage makes it either a poison or a remedy". It is in that context that we hope to create a paradigm shift in nitrite and nitrate as natural indispensable nutrients that promote health and well-being.

POTENTIAL HEALTH RISKS OF EXCESSIVE NITRATE AND NITRITE EXPOSURE: REGULATION GONE AWRY

Analogous to all essential or indispensable nutrients, intake of excess nitrate and nitrite exposure is, in specific contexts, associated with increased risk of negative health outcomes. A set of Dietary Reference Intake (DRI) categories are set by the Food and Nutrition Board of the National Academy of Sciences for essential nutrients in order to clearly define, where possible, the contexts in which intakes are deficient, safe or potentially excessive. These DRI categories include the Recommended Dietary Allowance (RDA), Adequate Intake (AI), Tolerable Upper Level Intake (TUL) and Estimated Average Intake (EAI) [3]. The process of setting DRIs for nutrients considers a broad range of physiological factors, including nutritional status and potential toxicities. Rational methodologies such as these, including the consideration of normal dietary consumption patterns of nitrate- and nitrite-containing foods, have not been applied in setting exposure limits, or in considering the potential health benefits, for dietary nitrates and nitrites.

The fact that health risks due to excess nitrate and nitrite consumption appear only in specific subgroups of the population has not deterred regulators, toxicologists and epidemiologists and certain special interest groups from supporting generalized, non-specific regulations limiting or even eliminating nitrate and nitrite exposures. It is important to note that nitrate exposure limits are set on the basis of nitrate in drinking water, the route of exposure associated with nitrate toxicities, although accidental toxic exposures of nitrates and nitrites have occurred [4]. The permissible concentration of nitrate in drinking water is 50 mg nitrate per liter in the European Union (EU) and 44 mg per liter in the U.S. in accord with World Health Organization recommendations first established in 1970 and reaffirmed in 2004 [5]. The U.S. Environmental Protection Agency limits human exposure to inorganic nitrates to < 10 mg/L or 10 ppm nitrate nitrogen, and nitrites to 1 ppm nitrite nitrogen [6]. The Joint Food and Agricultural Organization/World Health Organization has set the Acceptable Daily Intake (ADI) for the nitrate ion is set at 3.7 mg/kg body weight and for the nitrite ion at 0.06 mg/kg body weight [7]. Likewise, EPA has set a Reference Dose (RfD) for nitrate of 1.6 mg nitrate nitrogen/kg bodyweight per day (equivalent to about 7.0 mg nitrate ion/kg body weight per day). Whereas the government has set regulations on the amount of nitrite and nitrate in our drinking water, there is no such oversight apparently on bottled mineral water or other commercially available drinks or juices. We found that bottled mineral water contains anywhere from 10–50 μmoles/liter or 1–4.5 mg/liter nitrate.

Due to their very high solubility, nitrates can enter groundwater. Elevated nitrate in groundwater is a concern for drinking water use because nitrate can interfere with blood-oxygen levels in infants and cause methemoglobinemia or blue-baby syndrome [8]. Where groundwater recharges stream flow, nitrate-enriched groundwater can contribute to eutrophication, a process leading to high algal, especially blue-green algal populations and the death of aquatic life due to excessive demand for oxygen. While not directly toxic to fish life like ammonia, nitrate can have indirect effects on fish if it contributes to this eutrophication. Nitrogen has contributed to severe eutrophication problems in some water bodies. As of 2006, the application of nitrogen fertilizer is being increasingly controlled in Britain and the United States. This is occurring along the same lines as control of phosphorus fertilizer, restriction of which is normally considered essential to the recovery of eutrophied waterbodies. Ammonia is highly toxic to fish and the water discharge level of ammonia from wastewater treatment plants must often be closely monitored. To prevent loss of fish, nitrification prior to discharge is often desirable. Land application can be an attractive alternative to the mechanical aeration needed for nitrification.

POTENTIAL CONTEXTS FOR NITRATE- AND NITRITE-ASSOCIATED TOXICITIES

Two types of exposure place susceptible individuals at high risk of adverse effects of excess nitrite exposure. First, infants less than six months of age may be exposed to excess nitrates in bacterially-contaminated well water that reduces nitrate to nitrite [9]. Infants consuming excess nitrite experience methemoglobinemia or "blue baby syndrome" due to nitrite-mediated oxidation of ferric (Fe^{2+}) iron in oxyhemoglobin that leads to hypoxia and cyanosis [10,11]. As such, an American Academy of Pediatrics consensus panel concluded that all prenatal and well-infant visits should include questions about the home water supply; if the water source is a private well, the water should be tested for nitrate [12]. The panel concluded that infants fed commercially prepared infant foods are generally not at risk of nitrate poisoning but that home-prepared infant foods from vegetables (e.g., spinach, beets, green beans, squash, carrots) should be avoided until infants are 3 months or older. Breastfed infants are not at risk of excessive nitrate exposure from mothers who ingest water with high nitrate content (up to 100 ppm nitrate nitrogen) as nitrate concentration does not increase significantly in the breast milk [12].

It is noteworthy that the few human nitrate and nitrite exposure studies, including children and adults, have not produced methemoglobinemia. Infants exposed to 175 to 700 mg nitrate per day did not experience methemoglobin levels above 7.5%, suggesting that nitrate alone is not causative for methemoglobinemia [13]. A more recent randomized 3-way crossover study exposed healthy volunteer adults to single doses of sodium nitrite that ranged from 150 to 190 mg per volunteer to 290 to 380 mg per volunteer [14]. Observed methemoglobin concentrations were 12.2% for volunteers receiving the higher dose of nitrite ion and 4.5% for those receiving the lower dose. Recent nitrite infusion studies of up to 110 μg/kg/minute for 5 minutes induced methemoglobin concentrations of only 3.2% [15]. These data have led scientists to propose alternative explanations for the observed methemoglobinemia in infants, including gastroenteritis and associated iNOS-mediated production of NO induced by bacteria-contaminated water [16,17]. These studies call into question the mechanistic basis for exposure regulations for nitrate and nitrite. At best, these findings highlight a serious, but context-specific, risks associated with nitrite overexposure in infants. Experts have questioned the veracity of the evidence supporting the hypothesis that nitrates and nitrites are toxic for healthy post-infant populations [7,10,18]. It appears that the biologically plausible hypothesis of nitrite toxicity (e.g., methemoglobinemia) has essentially transformed a plausible hypothesis into sacrosanct dogma [10] in spite of a lack of proof [16,17].

The second context in which nitrate and nitrite exposure has been associated with negative health effects is the consumption of red and processed meats [19]. Nitrites and nitrates added to meats serve as antioxidants, develop flavor and stabilize red color in meats but must be converted to nitrite to exert these actions. Sodium nitrite is employed as a colorant, flavor enhancer and antimicrobial agent in certain red and processed meats. Nitrate and nitrite use in meat products, including bacon, bologna, corned beef, hot dogs, luncheon meats, sausages, canned and cured meat and hams is subject to limits put forth in Food and Drug Administration (FDA) and U.S. Department of Agriculture (USDA) regulations. These regulations can be found in the Code of Federal Regulations (CFR) (21CFR 170.60, 172.170 and 172.175 for FDA and 9CFR 318.7 for USDA regulations, respectively). Nitrite is essential in the meat industry as it serves as a very effective anti-microbial to prevent growth of infectious or toxic bacteria [20]. In the US Code of Federal Regulation it states: "The food additive sodium nitrite may be safely used in or on specific foods as a preservative and color fixative with sodium nitrate, in meat curing preparations for the home curing of meat and meat products (including poultry and wild game), with directions for use which limit the amount of sodium nitrite to not more than 200 parts per million (mg/kg) in the finished meat product and the amount of sodium nitrate to not more than 500 parts per million in the finished meat product". Two hundred (200) parts per million or ppm converts to 200 mg/L in solution or 200 mg/kg in solid food products. As discussed and illustrated in Chapter 4, the nitrate content of many commercially available juice drinks and raw vegetables contain higher concentrations of nitrate than what the US code allows for in cured and processed meats.

Some studies report consumption of red and processed meats is associated with increased risk of certain types of cancer and chronic obstructive pulmonary disease [19,21–24]. Others on the contrary report that consumption of red or processed meat does not predict risk factors for coronary heart disease [25]. Based on the association with cancer risk, the American Institute for Cancer Research's Food, Nutrition, Physical Activity, and the Prevention of Cancer: a Global Perspective contains the following recommendation "Limit consumption of red meats (such as beef, pork and lamb) and avoid processed meats" [26]. Systematic review indicated that up to 18 ounces a week of red meat can be consumed without raising cancer risk. However, review panelists could not determine a safe consumption level for processed meat; cancer risk was shown to increase with any consumption of processed meats [26]. A discussion of this association in the context of nitrate and nitrite consumption and gastric physiology is warranted to illuminate the processes relevant to this association. Direct evidence for the participation of nitrate and nitrite in human carcinogenesis is lacking despite extensive epidemiologic and animal studies [16]. Rodent toxicological studies [27] and human epidemiological investigations have not shown an unequivocal relationship between nitrite exposure and the risk of cancer [28]. These data suggest that nitrite formation resulting from nitrate exposure from dietary sources pose no risk with regard to cancer. The association between nitrite consumption and gastrointestinal cancers was bolstered by findings that ingested nitrites may react with secondary amines or N-alkylamides to generate carcinogenic N-nitroso compounds

(NOCs) [28]. While NOCs have been shown in animal models to be carcinogenic [29] but proof in humans has been scant. The N-nitrosamides and N-nitrosoureas have been shown to be direct mutagens, while N-nitrosoamines do not act as direct mutagens but generally require activation by microsomal enzymes within the body, perhaps by microsomal enzymes [30]. The use of nitrites in bacon must be accompanied by the use of either sodium erythorbate or sodium ascorbate (vitamin C), antioxidants that inhibit the nitrosation effect of nitrites on secondary amines [31]. The use of these antioxidants, along with lower nitrate/nitrite levels in processed meats, has lowered residual nitrite levels in cured meat products in the U.S. by ~80% since the mid-1970s [32].

Although meat and meat products are important sources of saturated fat and sodium, they are also important sources of protein and iron. Meat is a diverse food group and the quantity of macro and micronutrients varies for different types of meat. There are a number of confounding ingredients and factors in meat. There are no data directly implicating nitrites or nitrates as health hazards, mainly because of the confounding issues of fat content or particular lifestyle habits of people who may preferentially consume meat. On the other hand, in the proper context and when consumed with certain other foodstuff, there is not enough data to exclude health risks, except perhaps for nitrate in vegetables since these have consistently been associated with reduced risks of multiple conditions. The high antioxidant content of vegetables combined with nitrite and nitrate likely contribute to its positive health effects whereas in meats containing nitrite and nitrate, there is less antioxidant capacity.

A recent study has yielded new insights into the ability of vitamin C to modulate the formation of carcinogenic NOCs under conditions simulating the proximal stomach during the digestion of foods like processed meats [33]. Nitrite in processed meats may be converted to nitrosating species and NOCs by acidification in the presence of thiocyanate at low gastric pH. The formation of NOCs was examined in these conditions in the presence and absence of vitamin C and lipid. In the absence of lipid, vitamin C prevented the formation of N-nitrosodiethylamine and N-nitrosopiperidine and decreased the formation of N-nitrosodimethylamine and N-nitrosomorpholine five-fold and one thousand-fold, respectively. In the presence of 10% lipid (a food matrix component for processed meats), the presence of vitamin C increased the formation of nitrosodimethylamine, nitrosodiethylamine, and N-nitrosopiperidine 8-, 60- and 140-fold, respectively. Thus, the presence of lipid converts vitamin C from inhibiting to promoting acid nitrosation. This effect is attributable to the ability of vitamin C to assist in the generation of NO in the aqueous phase which enables the regeneration of nitrosating species by reacting with oxygen in the lipid phase [33]. While these data require confirmation in animal models and humans, it provides a biologically plausible mechanism for the observed association between processed meat consumption and gastrointestinal cancer risk. Others have postulated that gastric formation of NOCs may be inhibited by nutrients and other components of vegetables and fruits [34]. Clearly, more research is needed to address the potential mechanisms by which certain NOCs are related to cancer risk.

DIETARY CONSUMPTION LEVELS OF NITRATES AND NITRITES RELATIVE TO THE WHO ADI

The WHO ADI level for nitrate (0–3.7 mg/kg) translates into an equivalent of 222 mg nitrate for a 60 kg adult. Our calculations from the previous chapter indicate that an individual following a DASH dietary pattern with high nitrate vegetable and fruit choices would exceed this ADI by 700%. In fact, as has been observed previously and confirmed here, a portion of spinach commonly consumed in one serving of salad can exceed the ADI for nitrate [35]. The fact typical consumption patterns of vegetables and fruit exceed regulatory limits for dietary nitrates calls into question the wisdom of the regulatory process. These data call into question the rationale for regulating the concentration of nitrates from food sources. To further illustrate the absurdity of current public perception and dogma, consuming a 50g hot dog equates to 0.026 mg of nitrite and 4.88 mg nitrate compared to eating a 125 g spinach salad which contains 0.023 mg nitrite and 881 mg nitrate based on the data presented in chapter 4. The unfair assertion that nitrite and nitrate in cured and processed meats should be avoided is therefore unjustified and unwarranted when a healthy spinach salad contains just as much nitrite and nitrate as the hot dog.

The DASH diet forms the basis for public dietary health recommendations in the U.S. (e.g., MyPyramid.gov) and is widely recommended by private health agencies like the American Heart Association [36]. Taken together, the data considered here supports conclusions of the European Food Safety Authority [7] benefits of vegetable and fruit consumption outweigh any perceived risk of developing cancer from the consumption of nitrate and nitrite in these foods. We have shown that the data on nitrate and nitrite content of vegetables and fruit bolsters the strength of the already solid evidence to recommend their consumption for health benefits. We also conclude that any health risks associated with cured and processed meats are not attributable to the nitrite and nitrate content.

Indeed, data from observational epidemiologic and human clinical studies support the hypothesis that nitrates and nitrites of plant origin play essential physiologic roles in supporting cardiovascular health and gastrointestinal immune function. We support the recent call for a multidisciplinary and systematic review of the biological consequences of dietary nitrate and nitrite consumption [16]. For the first time, evidence for the health benefits of plant sources of these compounds should be considered alongside the now suspect evidence for nitrate and nitrite toxicities [16]. In fact there are several clinical trials active for the use of nitrite to treat or cure certain cardiovascular complications (www.clinicaltrials.gov). To adapt a quote from epidemiologist John Potter, MD, who spoke of the cancer preventive efficacy of vegetables and fruit, "Vegetables and fruits contain the antiatherogenic cocktail to which we are adapted. We abandon it at our peril."

Despite historical use of nitrates as medicinal agents and demonstration of physiological roles for nitrate and nitrite in vascular and immune function, food sources of nitrates and nitrites as healthful dietary components have received little attention [37]. The questionable practice of causal inference with regard to the etiologic roles of dietary nitrates and nitrites in methemoglobinemia and cancer has exerted a detrimental effect on the health benefits of nitrate- and nitrite-containing foods. This has occurred in spite of the historically observed benefits of nitrate and nitrite in medical therapeutics [38] and the undisputed health benefits recently discovered [39–41]. A report from the National Research Council (*The Health Effects of Nitrate, Nitrite, and N-Nitroso Compounds,* NRC 1981) estimated based on food consumption tables that the average total nitrite and nitrate intake in the US was 0.77 mg and 76 mg respectively. An average daily intake of 0.77 mg of nitrite would equate to 11.1 μmoles per day and 76mg nitrate would equate to 894 μmoles per day or roughly 1 mmole NO_x per day from diet. Our body (70 kg person) produces 1.68 mmole NO per day (based on 1 μmole/kg/hr NO production). The amount of nitrite and nitrate consumed through our diet matches what our body makes from NO if we assume most of the endogenous NO goes to stepwise oxidation to nitrite and nitrate. Therefore our steady state levels of NO_x which are routinely used as clinical biomarkers of NO activity come almost 50% from diet. Moreover if nitrite were a carcinogen, we would be advised to avoid swallowing since saliva contains 50–100 μM nitrite which can increase to near millimolar levels [42] after a nitrate rich meal. Assuming 50 μM nitrite in saliva and daily production of up to 1.5 liters per day, the total nitrite exposure from swallowing saliva alone is 75 μmoles or 5.18 mg. The enterosalivary concentration and circulation of nitrate and ultimately nitrite provides an essential pathway for health and host defense [43]. Even more convincing, studies on high altitude natives of Tibet reveal that increasing nitrite and nitrate concentrations within the body is a natural physiological response that is devoid of harmful effects [44]. There should be a re-evaluation of current nitrite and nitrate consumption analysis based on 21st century dietary habits. The strategy of avoiding nitrite and nitrate rich foods imposed in the 1970s due to the propensity to form N-nitrosamines may prove to be unwarranted and even detrimental to cardiovascular health.

ABOUT THE AUTHORS

Nathan S. Bryan, Ph.D.

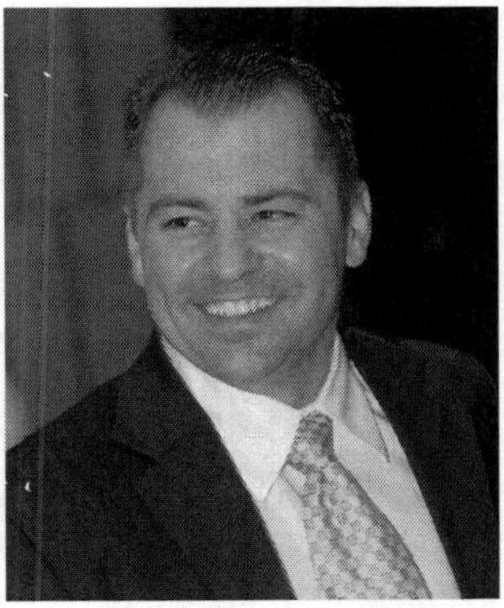

Dr. Bryan was born in Bryan Texas in November 1973. Nathan grew up in small town Texas. He spent his grade school years in Lexington (population 1000) and attended High School in Caldwell (population 3000). He earned his undergraduate Bachelor of Science degree in Biochemistry from the University of Texas at Austin and his doctoral degree from Louisiana State University School of Medicine in Shreveport where he was the recipient of the Dean's Award for Excellence in Research. He pursued his post-doctoral training as a Kirschstein Fellow at Boston University School of Medicine in the Whitaker Cardiovascular Institute. Dr. Bryan joined the Institute of Molecular Medicine, University of Texas Health Science Center in Houston, in June 2006 in the Center for Cell Signaling. He is also a faculty member of the Department of Integrative Biology and Pharmacology and Graduate School of Biomedical Sciences at the UT Houston Medical School. He is an active member of the Nitric Oxide Society, Society for Free Radical Biology and Medicine and the American Heart Association.

Dr. Bryan's research is dedicated to providing a better understanding of the interactions of nitric oxide (NO) and related metabolites with their different biological targets at the molecular and cellular level and the significance of these reactions for physiology and pathophysiology. Attempts are made to identify what particular changes in NO-related signaling pathways and reaction products occur in disease states such as endothelial dysfunction, ischemia/reperfusion, tissue/cardiac protection, diabetes, atherosclerosis and inflammation with the aim of testing their amenability as biomarkers for diagnosis and/or treatment of specific disease.

Current research is directed to understand the interactions of exogenous dietary nitrite/nitrate (NO_x) on the endogenous NO/cGMP pathway and how perturbations in each system affect cardiovascular health. This involves mechanisms of nitrite transport and cellular uptake as well as mechanism of nitrite reduction back to NO and via direct NO-independent signaling actions of nitrite. Work in Dr. Bryan's lab involves molecular biology and analytical biochemistry utilizing gas phase chemiluminescence and HPLC in multiple organ systems and blood. Much of the work involves in vivo characterization of NO/nitrite metabolism using a number of transgenic and knockout animal models of disease. Dr. Bryan and colleagues recently discovered that nitrite is a biologically active molecule which was previously thought to be an inert breakdown product of NO production. These findings have unveiled many beneficial effects of nitrite in the treatment and prevention of human disease. These discoveries may provide the basis for new preventive or therapeutic strategies in diseases associated with NO insufficiency and new guidelines for optimal health. Since nitrite and nitrate are common constituents of many fruits and vegetables, changes in dietary habits may have profound effects on many diseases associated with NO insufficiency. NO insufficiency is a hallmark of a number of diseases including cardiovascular disease. The notion that nitrite can recapitulate NO biochemistry and serve as an alternative and compensatory mechanism of NO production is revolutionary. It may also serve as the endocrine mediator of NO signaling. Moreover, the direct signaling actions of nitrite may represent a novel NO independent pathway for nitrite. If our current understanding is true, then an optimal diet may then consist of a sufficient supply of nitrite and nitrate for health and disease prevention. Understanding this pathway will provide the basis for new preventive or therapeutic strategies in diseases associated with NO insufficiency and new guidelines for optimal health. To date Dr. Bryan has published over 20 peer reviewed papers that have been cited over 1000 times. He has been invited to speak at a number of national and international meetings.

Dr. Bryan currently resides in Houston with his wife Kristen and their two sons Grant and Lincoln. The Bryans spend their weekends at their ranch near Caldwell where they raise cattle and horses and enjoy the great outdoors. Nathan enjoys playing golf and calf roping and team roping on his ranch and in competition.

Norman Hord, Ph.D., M.P.H., R.D.

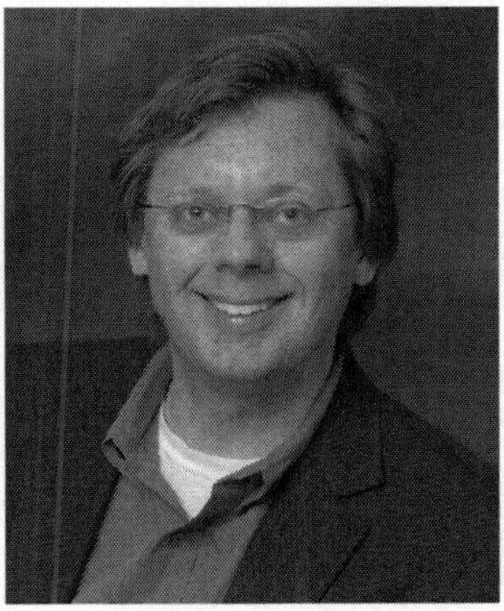

Norman Hord serves as an Associate Professor in Department of Food Science and Human Nutrition at Michigan State University (MSU), East Lansing, MI (USA). He received bachelor of science degree from Michigan State University, M.S. in nutrition from Clemson University, Ph.D. in nutrition from Purdue University, Master of Public Health degree from the Bloomberg School of Public Health from Johns Hopkins University and postdoctoral training as a Cancer Prevention Fellow at the National Cancer Institute. Dr. Hord is Chair of the Diet and Cancer Research Interest section of the American Society for Nutritional Sciences.

Dr. Hord supervises a research program that focuses on the role of dietary factors on phenotypes in colon epithelial cells related to colorectal cancer risk. His laboratory uses non-tumorigenic colon epithelial cell models to study dietary factor- and adipokine-induced cell behavior related to cancer risk. His laboratory is also characterizing the ability of probiotic bacteria to ameliorate the production of proinflammatory mediators caused by foodborne bacterial pathogens. Dr. Hord has received grant support from the USDA Higher Education Challenge Grant program, the National Cancer Institute (R03 grant program), the Kellogg Company, The J.F. Bell Institute for Health and Nutrition and various intramural funding sources. He has published research in nutrition, cancer research, cell biology and dietetics journals. He has served as a panel member of National Institutes of Health grant reviews, USDA NRI grant panel ad hoc reviewer and manuscript reviewer for cancer, cell biology, nutrition and dietetics journals.

Dr. Hord teaches courses in the undergraduate dietetics program and lectures in the Colleges of Human and Osteopathic Medicine as well as the Department of Epidemiology at MSU. He has served on the faculty of the Division of Cancer Prevention's Summer Curriculum in Cancer Prevention for the past ten years. He developed the MSU Dietetic Internship Program and currently serves as faculty coordinator for this program. This program recently received 10 year accreditation from The American Dietetic Association.

Dr. Hord advises forty undergraduate and two graduate students as well as two postdoctoral research associates. He serves on numerous theses and dissertation committees as well as on departmental, college and university committees.

REFERENCES

1. Ender, F.; Havre, C.; Helgebostad, A.; Kopping, N.; Masden, R.; Cehl, L. Isolation and identification of a hepatotoxic factor in herring meat produced from sodium nitrite preserved herring. *Naturwissenschaften* 51:637–638; 1964.
2. Tannenbaum, S. R.; Fett, D.; Young, V. R.; Land, P. D.; Bruce, W. R. Nitrite and nitrate are formed by endogenous synthesis in the human intestine. *Science* 200:1487–1488; 1978.
3. Otten JJ, H. J., Meyers, LD, Editors, *Dietary Reference Intakes: The Essential Guide to Nutrient Requirements.* National Academy Press, Food and Nutrition Board, Institute of Medicine, National Academy of Sciences; 2006.
4. Methemoglobinemia following unintentional ingestion of sodium nitrite—New York, 2002. Mmwr 51:639–642; 2002.
5. Organization, W. H. Recommendations; nitrate and nitrite. In: *Guidelines for Drinking Water Quality,* 3rd edition WHO, Geneva, Switzerland:417–420; 2004.
6. Agency, U. E. P. National Primary Drinking Water Regulations: Final Rule, 40. Fed Regist. CFR Parts 141–143:3526–3597; 1991.
7. Authority, E. F. S. Nitrate in vegetables: scientific opinion of the panel on contaminants in the food chain. *The EFSA Journal* 689:1–79; 2008.
8. Vitousek, P. M.; Aber, J.; Howarth, R. W.; Likens, G. E.; Matson, P. A.; Schindler, D. W.; Schlesinger, W. H.; Tilman, G. D. Human Alteration of the Global Nitrogen Cycle: Causes and Consequences. *Issues in Ecology* 1:1–17; 1997.
9. Johnson, C. J.; Kross, B. C. Continuing importance of nitrate contamination of groundwater and wells in rural areas. *American journal of industrial medicine* 18:449–456; 1990.
10. McKnight, G. M.; Duncan, C. W.; Leifert, C.; Golden, M. H. Dietary nitrate in man: friend or foe? *The British journal of nutrition* 81:349–358; 1999.
11. Fan, A. M.; Steinberg, V. E. Health implications of nitrate and nitrite in drinking water: an update on methemoglobinemia occurrence and reproductive and developmental toxicity. *Regul Toxicol Pharmacol* 23:35–43; 1996.
12. Greer, F. R.; Shannon, M. Infant methemoglobinemia: the role of dietary nitrate in food and water. *Pediatrics* 116:784–786; 2005.
13. Cornblath, M. a. H., AF. Methhemoglobinaemia in young infants. *J. Pediatr.* 33:421–425; 1948.
14. Kortboyer, J., Olling, M, and Zeilmaker, MJ *The oral bioavailability of sodium nitrite investigated in healthy adult volunteers.* National Institute of Public Health and the Environment Bilthoven, Netherlands; 1997.
15. Dejam, A.; Hunter, C. J.; Tremonti, C.; Pluta, R. M.; Hon, Y. Y.; Grimes, G.; Partovi, K.; Pelletier, M. M.; Oldfield, E. H.; Cannon, R. O., 3rd; Schechter, A. N.; Gladwin, M. T. Nitrite infusion in humans and nonhuman primates: endocrine effects, pharmacokinetics, and tolerance formation. *Circulation* 116:1821–1831; 2007.
16. Powlson, D. S.; Addiscott, T. M.; Benjamin, N.; Cassman, K. G.; de Kok, T. M.; van Grinsven, H.; L'Hirondel, J. L.; Avery, A. A.; van Kessel, C. When does nitrate become a risk for humans? *Journal of environmental quality* 37:291–295; 2008.
17. L'Hirondel J, L.; Avery, A. A.; Addiscott, T. Dietary nitrate: where is the risk? Environmental health perspectives 114:A458–459; author reply A459–461; 2006.
18. L'hirondel, J. L.-L. *Nitrate and man: Toxic, Harmless or Beneficial?* Wallingford, UK: CABI Publishing; 2001.

19. Norat, T.; Bingham, S.; Ferrari, P.; Slimani, N.; Jenab, M.; Mazuir, M.; Overvad, K.; Olsen, A.; Tjonneland, A.; Clavel, F.; Boutron-Ruault, M. C.; Kesse, E.; Boeing, H.; Bergmann, M. M.; Nieters, A.; Linseisen, J.; Trichopoulou, A.; Trichopoulos, D.; Tountas, Y.; Berrino, F.; Palli, D.; Panico, S.; Tumino, R.; Vineis, P.; Bueno-de-Mesquita, H. B.; Peeters, P. H.; Engeset, D.; Lund, E.; Skeie, G.; Ardanaz, E.; Gonzalez, C.; Navarro, C.; Quiros, J. R.; Sanchez, M. J.; Berglund, G.; Mattisson, I.; Hallmans, G.; Palmqvist, R.; Day, N. E.; Khaw, K. T.; Key, T. J.; San Joaquin, M.; Hemon, B.; Saracci, R.; Kaaks, R.; Riboli, E. Meat, fish, and colorectal cancer risk: the European Prospective Investigation into cancer and nutrition. *Journal of the National Cancer Institute* 97:906–916; 2005.

20. Skovgaard, N. Microbiological aspects and technological need: technological needs for nitrates and nitrites. *Food additives and contaminants* 9:391–397; 1992.

21. Jiang, R.; Camargo, C. A., Jr.; Varraso, R.; Paik, D. C.; Willett, W. C.; Barr, R. G. Consumption of cured meats and prospective risk of chronic obstructive pulmonary disease in women. The *American journal of clinical nutrition* 87:1002–1008; 2008.

22. Jiang, R.; Paik, D. C.; Hankinson, J. L.; Barr, R. G. Cured meat consumption, lung function, and chronic obstructive pulmonary disease among United States adults. *American journal of respiratory and critical care medicine* 175:798–804; 2007.

23. Varraso, R.; Jiang, R.; Barr, R. G.; Willett, W. C.; Camargo, C. A., Jr. Prospective study of cured meats consumption and risk of chronic obstructive pulmonary disease in men. *American journal of epidemiology* 166:1438–1445; 2007.

24. Santarelli, R. L.; Pierre, F.; Corpet, D. E. Processed meat and colorectal cancer: a review of epidemiologic and experimental evidence. *Nutrition and cancer* 60:131–144; 2008.

25. Wagemakers, J. J.; Prynne, C. J.; Stephen, A. M.; Wadsworth, M. E. Consumption of red or processed meat does not predict risk factors for coronary heart disease; results from a cohort of British adults in 1989 and 1999. *European journal of clinical nutrition;* 2007.

26. Research, W. C. R. F. A. I. f. C. Food, Nutrition, Physical Activity, and the Prevention of Cancer: a Global Perspective. *Second Expert Report;* 2007.

27. Toxicology and carcinogenesis studies of sodium nitrite in F344/N rats and B6C3F1 mice (drinking water studies). *Natl Toxicology Program Tech Rep Ser,* 2001: 7–273.

28. Mensinga, T. T.; Speijers, G. J.; Meulenbelt, J. Health implications of exposure to environmental nitrogenous compounds. *Toxicological reviews* 22:41–51; 2003.

29. Adamson, R. H. Induction of hepatocellular carcinoma in nonhuman primates by chemical carcinogens. *Cancer detection and prevention* 14:215–219; 1989.

30. Anonymous. *Nitrates and nitrites in food and water.* Cambridge, England: Woodhead Publishing Limited;1996.

31. Rao, G. S.; Osborn, J. C.; Adatia, M. R. Drug-nitrite interactions in human saliva: effects of food constituents on carcinogenic N-nitrosamine formation. *Journal of dental research* 61:768–771; 1982.

3.] Cassens, R. G. Residual nitrite in cured meat. *Food Technology* 51:53–55; 1997.

33. Combet, E.; Paterson, S.; Iijima, K.; Winter, J.; Mullen, W.; Crozier, A.; Preston, T.; McColl, K. E. Fat transforms ascorbic acid from inhibiting to promoting acid-catalysed N-nitrosation. *Gut* 56:1678–1684; 2007.

34. de Kok, T. M.; Engels, L. G.; Moonen, E. J.; Kleinjans, J. C. Inflammatory bowel disease stimulates formation of carcinogenic N-nitroso compounds. *Gut* 54:731; 2005.

35. Lundberg, J. O.; Govoni, M. Inorganic nitrate is a possible source for systemic generation of nitric oxide. *Free radical biology & medicine* 37:395–400; 2004.

36. Appel, L. J.; Brands, M. W.; Daniels, S. R.; Karanja, N.; Elmer, P. J.; Sacks, F. M. Dietary ap-

proaches to prevent and treat hypertension: a scientific statement from the American Heart Association. *Hypertension* 47:296–308; 2006.

37. Lundberg, J. O.; Feelisch, M.; Bjorne, H.; Jansson, E. A.; Weitzberg, E. Cardioprotective effects of vegetables: is nitrate the answer? *Nitric Oxide* 15:359–362; 2006.
38. Butler, A. R.; Feelisch, M. Therapeutic uses of inorganic nitrite and nitrate: from the past to the future. *Circulation* 117:2151–2159; 2008.
39. Bryan, N. S.; Calvert, J. W.; Elrod, J. W.; Gundewar, S.; Ji, S. Y.; Lefer, D. J. Dietary nitrite supplementation protects against myocardial ischemia-reperfusion injury. *Proceedings of the National Academy of Sciences of the United States of America* 104:19144–19149; 2007.
40. Bryan, N. S.; Calvert, J. W.; Gundewar, S.; Lefer, D. J. Dietary nitrite restores NO homeostasis and is cardioprotective in endothelial nitric oxide synthase-deficient mice. *Free Radic Biol Med* 45:468–474; 2008.
41. Webb, A. J.; Patel, N.; Loukogeorgakis, S.; Okorie, M.; Aboud, Z.; Misra, S.; Rashid, R.; Miall, P.; Deanfield, J.; Benjamin, N.; MacAllister, R.; Hobbs, A. J.; Ahluwalia, A. Acute blood pressure lowering, vasoprotective, and antiplatelet properties of dietary nitrate via bioconversion to nitrite. *Hypertension* 51:784–790; 2008.
42. McKnight, G. M.; Smith, L. M.; Drummond, R. S.; Duncan, C. W.; Golden, M.; Benjamin, N. Chemical synthesis of nitric oxide in the stomach from dietary nitrate in humans. *Gut* 40:211–214; 1997.
43. Petersson, J.; Phillipson, M.; Jansson, E. A.; Patzak, A.; Lundberg, J. O.; Holm, L. Dietary nitrate increases gastric mucosal blood flow and mucosal defense. *Am J Physiol Gastrointest Liver Physiol* 292:G718–724; 2007.
44. Erzurum, S. C.; Ghosh, S.; Janocha, A. J.; Xu, W.; Bauer, S.; Bryan, N. S.; Tejero, J.; Hemann, C.; Hille, R.; Stuehr, D. J.; Feelisch, M.; Beall, C. M. Higher blood flow and circulating NO products offset high-altitude hypoxia among Tibetans. *Proceedings of the National Academy of Sciences of the United States of America* 104:17593–17598; 2007.

CHAPTER 10

Diet and Endothelium: Two Systems, Redundant Functions

NATHAN S. BRYAN and NORMAN G. HORD

Brown Foundation Institute of Molecular Medicine, The University of Texas Health Science Center, Houston, TX 77030

Department of Food Science and Human Nutrition, Michigan State University, East Lansing, MI

THE preceding chapters have discussed the critical importance of nitric oxide and described natural dietary means to enhance NO availability either by providing antioxidants to prevent its rapid degradation, by enhancing its production from L-arginine by the NOS enzymes or through the reduction of nitrate and nitrite back to NO or through formation and maintenance of nitrosothiols. The number of diseases and conditions associated with NO insufficiency are well described and the list continues to grow. Up to this point, the strategies employed to restore NO homeostasis were concentrated solely on priming the NOS system to convert more L-arginine to NO. While the concept to enhance and restore NO production is appreciated and well-recognized, the strategy of feeding L-arginine may not be sufficient especially for those that are NO insufficient and would benefit most. These strategies have not been remarkably successful due to the complex spatial and temporal regulation of substrate availability, sub-cellular compartmentalization, sufficient supply of available co-factors and prosthetics groups and the redox environment in which the NO is produced. Conditions of endothelial dysfunction are characterized by enhanced oxidative stress. Even if such strategies are successful at converting more L-arginine to NO, it is likely to be quickly inactivated before it can reach its physiological target. The concepts and principles introduced in the preceding chapters provide an alternative and viable approach and strategy to restore NO biochemistry that may be best fit for such an environment when NOS is inactive. This chapter will focus on the intricate balance between our diet and endothelial production of NO and how one may compensate for the other.

To put this in focus, we will review some of the information presented earlier. Nitric oxide synthase (NOS) enzymes produce ·NO by catalyzing a five electron oxidation of a guanidino nitrogen of L-arginine (L-Arg). Oxidation of L-Arg to L-citrulline occurs via two successive monooxygenation reactions producing N^{ω}hydroxy L-arginine as an intermediate. Two moles of O_2 and 1.5 moles of NADPH are consumed per mole of ·NO formed [1]. NOS enzymes are the only enzymes known to simultaneously require five bound co-factors/prosthetic groups: FAD, FMN, heme, tetrahydrobiopterin (BH_4) and Ca^{2+}-calmodulin (CaM). CaM also facilitates NADPH dependent reduction of cytochrome *c* and ferricyanide in BH_4 and heme depleted nNOS. If any of the co-factors become limiting, then NO production from NOS shuts down, and in many cases NOS then produces superoxide instead. This is indeed a very complex and coordinated effort to enzymatically produce NO which normally proceeds very efficiently. However, in disease characterized by oxidative stress where cofactors become oxidized, NOS uncoupling, or conditions of hypoxia where oxygen is limiting, this process can no longer maintain NO production. Therefore there has to be an alternate route to NO production. It is highly unlikely that Nature devised such a sophisticated mechanism of NO production as a sole source of a critical molecule. The data presented throughout this book provides a compelling and convincing argument that dietary nitrite and nitrate act as a backup system to the L-arginine:NO pathway. Part of this may occur through nitrite reduction facilitated by polyphenols or antioxidants or during low oxygen availability in the acidic environment of the stomach. Restoring NO homeostasis may occur primarily through the maintenance of nitrosylation in tissues by utilizing nitrite as a substrate.

Nitrite reduction to NO can occur in a much simpler mechanism than the 5-electron oxidation of L-arginine. The 1-electron reduction of nitrite can occur by ferrous heme proteins (or any redox active metal) and an electron donor through the following reaction:

$$NO_2^- + Fe^{(II)} + H^+ \leftrightarrow NO + Fe^{(III)} + OH^-$$

This reaction is accelerated by acidity or reducing agents. We know from previous chapters than since the pKa of nitrite is 3.4, at acid pH, nitrous acid can be produced which then dissociates to form NO. This is the same biologically active NO as that produced by NOS just instead of using L-arg as the substrate, nitrite is used. Blood and tissue nitrite reduction is an extremely inefficient process [2]. Therefore for this to occur, the tissues or biological compartment must have a sufficient pool of nitrite stored. Since plasma nitrite is a direct measure of NOS activity, a compromised NOS system can also affect downstream nitrite production and metabolism. This can perhaps exacerbate any condition associated with decreased NO bioavailability. Nitrite or nitrate supplementation through dietary means may therefore act as a protective measure to compensate for insufficient NOS activity under conditions of hypoxia or in critically ill patients unable to swallow [3]. It is very likely that exogenous nitrite contributes to whole body NO production and homeostasis. Considerable published support for this theory derives from the following facts: NO produced from nitrite in the upper intestine is up to 10,000 times the concentrations that occur in tissues from enzymatic synthesis [4], nitrite can act as a circulating NO donor [5] and nitrite can itself perform many actions previously attributable to NO [6] without the intermediacy of NO [7].

Emerging physiological evidence from the Bryan research lab reveals that nitrite may be acting more than a NOS-independent source of NO. Clearly, much more has to be learned before an informed judgment can be made as to the physiological role of individual regulatory pathways that are modulated or triggered by nitrite. Nevertheless, one clear picture emerging from these results is that changes in nitrite availability into either direction may have a direct effect on endogenous NO production and elicit measurable changes in the activity and expression of multiple proteins and enzyme products as well as outcome from physiological insults.

Although it may be argued that nitrite is simply a storage pool that can be reduced to NO under appropriate conditions, we consider this not the primary role for nitrite in physiology, i.e. normoxic and neutral pH, conditions under which nitrite is stable and tightly regulated. Alternatively, nitrite acts as an important molecule in its own right but which has regulatory effects on the NO pathway. It may be that both hypoxic reduction of nitrite to NO and normoxic metabolism of nitrite represent an advantageous oxygen sensing system which is a vestige of denitrifying microorganisms that existed long before the advent of aerobic respiration and the emergence of an NO synthase system [8]. The fact that both systems still exist today highlight the importance of nitrite in all cellular processes throughout the entire physiological oxygen gradient [6].

An explosion of new discoveries in the field of nitrate and nitrite biology has provided mechanistic insights into the potential new physiologic roles of dietary nitrate and nitrite and their potential health benefits [9–11]. A brief review of the biology of NO production in the vasculature and NO-requiring tissues will provide the appropriate context for understanding the importance of dietary nitrate and nitrite. These pathways have been discussed in the preceding chapters. There is consensus that dietary nitrates are essentially inert and acquire biological activity only after reduction to nitrite. As such, nitrate serves as a source, via successive reduction, for the production of nitrite and NO as well as other metabolic products. The late Speaker of the U.S. House of Representatives, Rep. Thomas "Tip" O'Neil, famously stated "All politics are local". There is no more apropos analogy in biology than the regulation of the availability of nitrogen oxides—by localization, oxygen tension, pH, inflammatory microenvironment, local redox milieu, organ and tissue specificity—that determines how much nitrate, nitrite, nitric oxide and other NOx species a tissue will be exposed to.

Normal functioning of human vasculature requires both the presence of nitrite and NO along with the necessity to respond to these important signaling molecules [10,12]. The generation of approximately 70% of systemic NO is accomplished by endothelial nitric oxide synthase (eNOS), one of three members of the NOS family of enzymes, in the vascular endothelium [13]. These enzymes synthesize NO from the amino acid L-arginine and molecular oxygen to accomplish vasodilation, blood pressure regulation, and the prevention of the atherogenic phenotype (i.e., endothelial inflammatory cell recruitment and platelet aggregation) [10]. The major pathway for NO metabolism is the stepwise oxidation to nitrite and nitrate [14]. As a result, the normal production of nitrite, NO and NO_x, and ability of the endothelium to respond to these species, may prevent various types of cardiovascular disease including hypertension, atherosclerosis as well as subsequent clinical sequelae such as heart attack and stroke [11].

Many of the biological effects of NO are caused by the initiation of cyclic GMP-mediated intracellular signals in the endothelium and surrounding cells. Two other members of the NOS family serve neuronal function (nNOS) and inflammatory immune function (inducible NOS or iNOS) [15]. In neuronal tissue, nNOS provides NO for normal neuron function. The function of iNOS is an essential signaling mechanism in the innate immune response [16]. In tissues experiencing chronic inflammation, such as inflammatory bowel disease or ulcerative colitis, iNOS can generate high concentrations of NO that promote carcinogenesis by inhibiting apoptosis, enhancing prostaglandin formation and promoting angiogenesis in the early stage of carcinogenesis [17–19]. In atherosclerosis, hypoxic conditions can limit eNOS-derived NO production; nitrite can directly induce vasodilation in hypoxic endothelium [20]. Indeed, the Bryan lab has demonstrated that dietary nitrite can restore vascular tone after ischemia/reperfusion and substitutes for loss of eNOS-derived NO in both healthy and eNOS-deficient mice [21,22].

Unlike the provision of eNOS-derived NO to the endothelium to maintain vasomotor tone, most tissues use nitrite as a source of NO production [23] and to mainstain nitroso-redox homeostasis [24]. There are two systems of reducing nitrate to nitrite in mammals. The first system identified to accomplish this was the action of commensal, Gram negative bacteria on the tongue to reduce salivary nitrate [25]. Concentration of plasma nitrate in saliva occurs as part of enterosalivary circulation of dietary nitrate [26]. Approximately 25% of ingested nitrate is secreted in saliva, where some 20% (or approximately 5–8% of the nitrate intake) is converted to nitrite by commensal bacteria on the tongue [27]. Saliva contains 50–100 μM nitrite which can increase to near millimolar levels [28] after a nitrate rich meal. The nitrite supplied to the gastrointestinal tract serves to enhance gastric mucin production [29] and serve as a substrate for generation of nitrogen oxides for antimicrobial actions and support of gastric homeostasis [30]. Recently, NO synthesis in healthy tissues has been shown to occur independent of the L-arginine-NOS pathway. Because inorganic nitrate is considered a biologically inert compound, the reduction of nitrate to nitrite must be accomplished by either bacterial nitrate reductases or several different mammalian enzymes and metalloproteins that possess nitrate reductase activity, including xanthine oxidoreductase (XOR), aldehyde oxidase (AO), heme proteins and mitochondria [31–33]. NO synthesis in tissues, therefore, can occur by reduction of nitrate to nitrite and nitrite can be subsequently reduced to NO. Nitrite reduction to NO can be carried out by numerous metalloproteins, enzymes, and compounds with redox potential including hemoglobin [34], deoxyhemoglobin [35], deoxymyoglobin [36], XOR [37], vitamin C [38] and polyphenols [39]. As noted above, nitrite reduction to NO is greatly enhanced during the stress of hypoxemia and ischemia [40]. These redundant physiologic systems for the provision of NO under normoxic or hypoxic conditions indicate that nitrite may serve as systemic reservoir for NO production.

Emerging evidence from animal models and human clinical studies indicate that nitrite exerts unique intracellular signaling properties that mediate physiologic functions independent of its role as a source of NO in tissues by reduction [11]. Nitrite infusion in humans induces rapid vasodilation, reduces blood pressure acutely, serves as an endocrine reservoir of nitric oxide and, unlike organic nitrates, does not induce tolerance [41]. Nitrite has also been shown to play a role in mitochondrial respiration [42], cardiac function [36], activation the alpha form of the estrogen receptor [43] and exertion of antiapoptotic effects [44]. Because nitrite is a primary biologically active compound resulting from nitrate reduction in tissues, significant physiological benefits may be associated with the provision of nitrate from dietary sources.

REGULATION OF THE NITRITE ECONOMY: ROLE OF DIET, TISSUE NITRATE REDUCTASES AND DISEASE STATES

The stepwise reduction of nitrate to nitrite to NO is, by necessity, an inefficient process by which each step yields a 3 log lower concentration of product than substrate [31]. Therefore, a 10 mg/kg infusion of nitrate given over 5 minutes yields a plasma concentration of nitrite of ~1 μM and results in ostensibly NO-mediated vasodilation after experimentally-induced ischemia [31]. Table 10.1 contains the typical plasma concentrations, half-lives and sources of nitrate, nitrite and NO. The one to five minute half-life of nitrite is intermediate between that of nitrate (5–8 hours) and nitric oxide (milliseconds) [45]. Notably, the short half-life of NO results from efficient oxidation of NO to nitrite and other nitrogen oxides compounds by enzymes (so-called "NO oxidases") that utilize transition metals in their active sites, such as copper-containing ceruloplasmin [46] (Cu), myeloperoxidase (which uses heme (Fe) as a cofactor) and even endothelial NOS [47]. Oxidation of nitric oxide to nitrite and nitrite to nitrate contributes to the pool of NO_x compounds that serve as signaling molecules systemically or as a local substrate for NO production. In situations such as iNOS-mediated inflammatory processes in ulcerative colitis, the large concentrations of NO produced can lead to high concentrations of secondary reaction products of NO notably nitrotyrosine and induce a state of nitrosative stress. Figure 10.1 il-

TABLE 10.1 Plasma Levels, Half-life and Sources of NO_x Species (nitrate, nitrite and nitric oxide or NO) [49].

NO_x Species	Fasting Plasma Levels (nmol/l)	Half-life ($t_{1/2}$)	Exogenous or Endogenous Source
Nitrate	20–50,000	5–8 hours	Diet or endogenous oxidation of nitrite
Nitrite	100–500	1–5 minutes	Endogenous nitrate, diet, oxidation of nitrite
NO	< 1	1–2 milliseconds	Endogenous nitrite

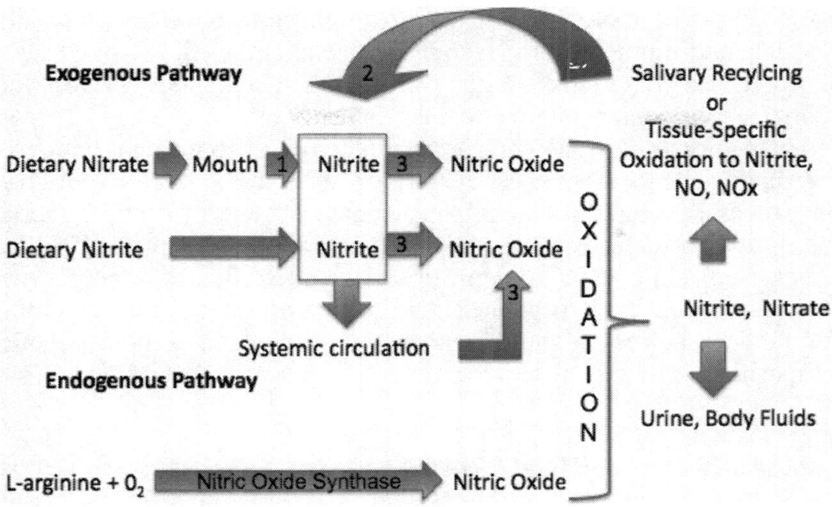

FIGURE 10.1 A schematic diagram of the physiological disposition of nitrate, nitrite and nitric oxide (NO) from exogenous (dietary) and endogenous sources. The action of mammalian bacterial nitrate reductases are noted by the number 1, bacterial nitrate reductases by number 2; nitrite reductase activity is noted by the number 3.

lustrates the elegant physiologically redundant mechanisms by which nitrite and nitrate are produced and reformed by oxidation of NO to ensure an abundant supply for the myriad processes that require them for adequate functioning. Dietary sources of nitrate and nitrite may bolster the reserve of these compounds for optimal functioning through periods of physiological stress and disease [11,21,22,48].

SOURCES OF ENDOGENOUS AND DIET-DERIVED NO GENERATION

In addition to the provision of nitrate and nitrite by diet or via the oxidation of NO or nitrite, vascular and gastrointestinal NO production can be enhanced through various means based on lifestyle and food choices. Physical activity, commensal bacteria and dietary factors can influence NO production. Exercise enhances NO production in healthy vascular endothelium [50] and post-exercise plasma nitrite levels have been proposed as an index of exercise capacity [51]. In fact, aging is associated with an impaired capacity of the vasculature to increase plasma nitrite during exercise [52]. Strikingly, it has been found that dietary nitrate supplementation, at concentrations achievable by vegetable consumption, results in more efficient energy production without increasing lactate concentrations during submaximal exercise [48].

Foods can increase generation of NO in the gastrointestinal tract via polyphenolic content of, for example, apples or red wine [53,54]. Pomegranate juice as been shown to protect nitric oxide from oxidation while enhancing its biological activity [55]. The metabolic activity of commensal bacteria in the gastrointestinal tract and probiotic bacteria also provide NO from nitrite, and to a lesser extent, from nitrate [56,57]. These data add layers of complexity to the estimation of nitrate/nitrite exposure levels in vivo and the determination of whether specific foods or lifestyle choices can significantly affect the production and metabolic disposition of dietary and endogenous NO_x species.

QUANTIFYING THE NITRITE ECONOMY

Given the complex interactions between endogenous nitrite, nitrate and that of dietary origin, the endogenous production of nitrate and nitrite from NO and other nitrogen oxides (NO_x) (Figure 10.1), the effect of physiological conditions like atherosclerosis and inflammatory disease, dietary sources of NO_x, physical activity, nitrate and nitrite balance studies are not, at present, feasible. Therefore, a simple characterization of an optimal concentration of dietary nitrate and nitrite based on an overall picture of the nitrate and nitrite economy is not possible. However, we can make two generalizations that summarize our current knowledge. First, the majority of nitrite utilization and NO production occur in healthy individuals in two compartments: vascular and somatic tissues. Normal vascular function requires NO production from the L-arginine-NOS pathway; in ischemic conditions, nitrite can substitute for L-arginine-NOS-derived NO [21,22,58]. Most healthy somatic tissues possess mammalian enzymes that exert nitrate reductase activity (the tongue utilizes nitrate reductases of commensal bacteria) to generate biologically active nitrite to maintain GI and cardiovascular health. In inflammatory conditions, iNOS in epithelial and immune cells can produce NO as part of the innate immune response. In cardiovascular disease states characterized by hypoxia and/or ischemia/reperfusion injury, eNOS-supplied NO may be limiting and nitrite can be utilized to support vascular function under these conditions. These generalizations support conjecture for a second generalization: dietary consumption of foods high in nitrate and nitrite may supply nitrite in situations where substrates for endogenous NO_x production are limiting, as in cardiovascular conditions, to support cardiovascular and gastrointestinal function

[11]. As such, when dietary intake of nitrate and nitrite intake is low and no additional endogenous "sources" of NO_x (e.g., gastrointestinal infections involving iNOS activation), the endogenous production of nitrate, via oxidation of NO and nitrite, provides more substrate for NO_x production than dietary sources. Long-term consumption of diets containing high levels of nitrate and nitrite may have important implications for providing health benefits by ensuring high concentrations of NOx as a "reserve" for tissue defense and homeostasis in stress and disease [11].

We propose a scenario depicted in the schematic below, whereby dietary sources of both L-arginine and nitrite work in unison to maintain normal NO homeostasis. Conditions of sufficient nitrite and NO production from NOS or by dietary consumption are hallmarks of health and vitality. During periods of fasting or low nitrite intake NOS becomes more active to maintain NO production as well as a sufficient pool of nitrite, provided ample L-arginine and reduced cofactors are available and a functional NOS. Under conditions when NOS is insufficient due to de-

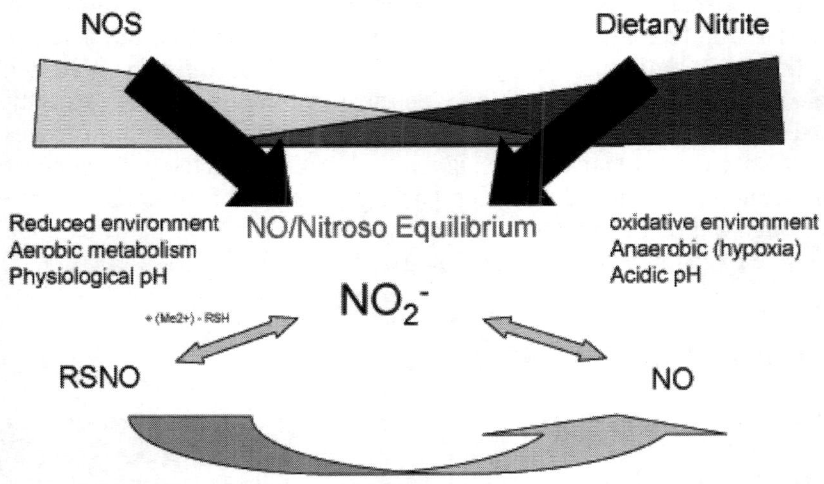

FIGURE 10.2 Both NOS and dietary sources provide NO and NO_x for optimal NO/nitroso homeostasis. Under normal physiological conditions, reduced cellular environment and normal pH, NOS likely provides sufficient NO for homeostasis. These same conditions render nitrite extremely reactive with thiols to form nitrosothiols. On the contrary, under conditions when NOS is dysfunctional dietary sources of nitrite and nitrate can maintain NO-nitroso redox status and rescue the phenotype. These conditions favor the reduction of nitrite to NO. There is a concerted effort through dietary NO_x and NOS to maintain both nitrite and NO bioavailability and thus steady state tissue nitroso/nitrosyl. One may compensate for the other provided both pathways are active with ample substrate.

pletion of L-arginine or oxidation of co-factors combined with a poor diet low in NO_x such as in atherosclerosis, neither system can maintain homeostasis and disease ensues. Therefore nitrite becomes an important regulatory molecule in physiology and may serve as potential therapy under conditions of insufficient NO as a result of impaired NOS activity. Supplemental nitrite can increase steady state plasma and tissue nitrite/RSNO. Increases in nitrite bioavailability can inhibit MPO mediated LDL modification, protect thiols from oxidation and provide an alternate source of NO thereby protecting from the development of cardiovascular disease including the onset and progression of atherosclerosis.

Nature has a way of ensuring that important molecules and signal transduction pathways are maintained in the face of extraordinary circumstance. This is the basis for the number of redundant systems in physiology. The concept described above is no different. We can now appreciate that the conversion of L-arginine to NO is complex and requires a number of substrates and co-factors to be available at any given time. The fact that NOS enzymes can produce NO in such a fashion is impressive and remarkable. Inherent to this complex design is the susceptibility to dysregulation and dysfunction if any of the required participants are not available at a time of need. The absolute import of NO in virtually every cell and organ system is well documented. Therefore we propose that Nature would not have designed such pathway as the only means to generate NO or transduce NO signaling. The use of nitrite and nitrate through our diet provides the rescue system for the NOS pathway and a source of redundancy for NO biology.

ABOUT THE AUTHORS

Nathan S. Bryan, Ph.D.

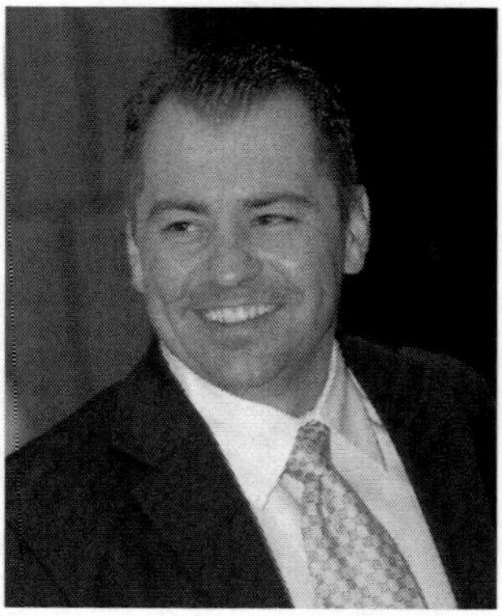

Dr. Bryan was born in Bryan Texas in November 1973. Nathan grew up in small town Texas. He spent his grade school years in Lexington (population 1000) and attended High School in Caldwell (population 3000). He earned his undergraduate Bachelor of Science degree in Biochemistry from the University of Texas at Austin and his doctoral degree from Louisiana State University School of Medicine in

Shreveport where he was the recipient of the Dean's Award for Excellence in Research. He pursued his post-doctoral training as a Kirschstein Fellow at Boston University School of Medicine in the Whitaker Cardiovascular Institute. Dr. Bryan joined the Institute of Molecular Medicine, University of Texas Health Science Center in Houston, in June 2006 in the Center for Cell Signaling. He is also a faculty member of the Department of Integrative Biology and Pharmacology and Graduate School of Biomedical Sciences at the UT Houston Medical School. He is an active member of the Nitric Oxide Society, Society for Free Radical Biology and Medicine and the American Heart Association.

Dr. Bryan's research is dedicated to providing a better understanding of the interactions of nitric oxide (NO) and related metabolites with their different biological targets at the molecular and cellular level and the significance of these reactions for physiology and pathophysiology. Attempts are made to identify what particular changes in NO-related signaling pathways and reaction products occur in disease states such as endothelial dysfunction, ischemia/reperfusion, tissue/cardiac protection, diabetes, atherosclerosis and inflammation with the aim of testing their amenability as biomarkers for diagnosis and/or treatment of specific disease.

Current research is directed to understand the interactions of exogenous dietary nitrite/nitrate (NO_x) on the endogenous NO/cGMP pathway and how perturbations in each system affect cardiovascular health. This involves mechanisms of nitrite transport and cellular uptake as well as mechanism of nitrite reduction back to NO and via direct NO-independent signaling actions of nitrite. Work in Dr. Bryan's lab involves molecular biology and analytical biochemistry utilizing gas phase chemiluminescence and HPLC in multiple organ systems and blood. Much of the work involves in vivo characterization of NO/nitrite metabolism using a number of transgenic and knockout animal models of disease. Dr. Bryan and colleagues recently discovered that nitrite is a biologically active molecule which was previously thought to be an inert breakdown product of NO production. These findings have unveiled many beneficial effects of nitrite in the treatment and prevention of human disease. These discoveries may provide the basis for new preventive or therapeutic strategies in diseases associated with NO insufficiency and new guidelines for optimal health. Since nitrite and nitrate are common constituents of many fruits and vegetables, changes in dietary habits may have profound effects on many diseases associated with NO insufficiency. NO insufficiency is a hallmark of a number of diseases including cardiovascular disease. The notion that nitrite can recapitulate NO biochemistry and serve as an alternative and compensatory mechanism of

NO production is revolutionary. It may also serve as the endocrine mediator of NO signaling. Moreover, the direct signaling actions of nitrite may represent a novel NO independent pathway for nitrite. If our current understanding is true, then an optimal diet may then consist of a sufficient supply of nitrite and nitrate for health and disease prevention. Understanding this pathway will provide the basis for new preventive or therapeutic strategies in diseases associated with NO insufficiency and new guidelines for optimal health. To date Dr. Bryan has published over 20 peer reviewed papers that have been cited over 1000 times. He has been invited to speak at a number of national and international meetings.

Dr. Bryan currently resides in Houston with his wife Kristen and their two sons Grant and Lincoln. The Bryans spend their weekends at their ranch near Caldwell where they raise cattle and horses and enjoy the great outdoors. Nathan enjoys playing golf and calf roping and team roping on his ranch and in competition.

Norman Hord, Ph.D., M.P.H., R.D.

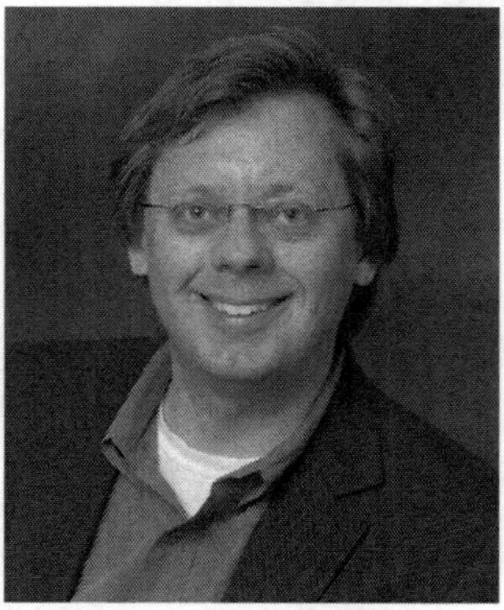

Norman Hord serves as an Associate Professor in Department of Food Science and Human Nutrition at Michigan State University (MSU), East Lansing, MI (USA). He received bachelor of science degree from Michigan State University, M.S. in nutrition from Clemson University, Ph.D. in nutrition from Purdue University, Master of Public Health degree from the Bloomberg School of Public Health from Johns Hopkins University and postdoctoral training as a Cancer Prevention Fellow at the National Cancer Institute. Dr. Hord is Chair of the Diet and Cancer Research Interest section of the American Society for Nutritional Sciences.

Dr. Hord supervises a research program that focuses on the role of dietary factors on phenotypes in colon epithelial cells related to colorectal cancer risk. His laboratory uses non-tumorigenic colon epithelial cell models to study dietary factor- and adipokine-induced cell behavior related to cancer risk. His laboratory is also characterizing the ability of probiotic bacteria to ameliorate the production of proinflammatory mediators caused by foodborne bacterial pathogens. Dr. Hord has received grant support from the USDA Higher Education Challenge Grant program, the National Cancer Institute (R03 grant program), the Kellogg Company, The J.F. Bell Institute for Health and Nutrition and various intramural funding sources. He has published research in nutrition, cancer research, cell biology and dietetics journals. He has served as a panel member of National Institutes of Health grant reviews, USDA NRI grant panel ad hoc reviewer and manuscript reviewer for cancer, cell biology, nutrition and dietetics journals.

Dr. Hord teaches courses in the undergraduate dietetics program and lectures in the Colleges of Human and Osteopathic Medicine as well as the Department of Epidemiology at MSU. He has served on the faculty of the Division of Cancer Prevention's Summer Curriculum in Cancer Prevention for the past ten years. He developed the MSU Dietetic Internship Program and currently serves as faculty coordinator for this program. This program recently received 10 year accreditation from The American Dietetic Association.

Dr. Hord advises forty undergraduate and two graduate students as well as two postdoctoral research associates. He serves on numerous theses and dissertation committees as well as on departmental, college and university committees.

REFERENCES

1. Liu, Q.; S.S., G. Binding sites of nitric oxide synthases. *Methods Enzymol* 268:311–324; 1996.
2. Feelisch, M.; Fernandez, B. O.; Bryan, N. S.; Garcia-Saura, M. F.; Bauer, S.; Whitlock, D. R.; Ford, P. C.; Janero, D. R.; Rodriguez, J.; Ashrafian, H. Tissue Processing of Nitrite in Hypoxia: An Intricate Interplay of Nitric Oxide-Generating and -Scavenging Systems. *J Biol Chem* 283:33927–33934; 2008.
3. Bjorne, H. H.; Govoni, M.; Tornberg, D. C.; Lundberg, J. O.; Weitzberg, E. Intragastric nitric oxide is abolished in intubated patients and restored by nitrite. *Crit Care Med* 33:1722–1727; 2005.
4. McKnight, G. M.; Smith, L. M.; Drummond, R. S.; Duncan, C. W.; Golden, M.; Benjamin, N. Chemical synthesis of nitric oxide in the stomach from dietary nitrate in humans. *Gut* 40:211–214; 1997.
5. Dejam, A.; Hunter, C. J.; Schechter, A. N.; Gladwin, M. T. Emerging role of nitrite in human biology. *Blood Cells Mol Dis* 32:423–429; 2004.
6. Gladwin, M. T.; Schechter, A. N.; Kim-Shapiro, D. B.; Patel, R. P.; Hogg, N.; Shiva, S.; Cannon III, R. O.; Kelm, M.; Wink, D. A.; Espey, M. G.; Oldfield, E. H.; Pluta, R. M.; Freeman, B. A.; Lancaster, J. R. J.; Feelisch, M.; Lundberg, J. O. The emerging biology of the nitrite anion. *Nature Chemical Biology* 1:308–314; 2005.
7. Bryan, N. S.; Fernandez, B. O.; Bauer, S. M.; Garcia-Saura, M. F.; Milsom, A. B.; Rassaf, T.; Maloney, R. E.; Bharti, A.; Rodriguez, J.; Feelisch, M. Nitrite is a signaling molecule and regulator of gene expression in mammalian tissues. *Nature Chemical Biology* 1:290–297; 2005.
8. Feelisch, M.; Martin, J. F. The early role of nitric oxide in evolution. *TREE* 10:496–499; 1995.
9. Gladwin, M. T.; Schechter, A. N.; Kim-Shapiro, D. B.; Patel, R. P.; Hogg, N.; Shiva, S.; Cannon, R. O., 3rd; Kelm, M.; Wink, D. A.; Espey, M. G.; Oldfield, E. H.; Pluta, R. M.; Freeman,

B. A.; Lancaster, J. R., Jr.; Feelisch, M.; Lundberg, J. O. The emerging biology of the nitrite anion. *Nature chemical biology* 1:308–314; 2005.

10. Lundberg, J. O.; Weitzberg, E.; Gladwin, M. T. The nitrate-nitrite-nitric oxide pathway in physiology and therapeutics. *Nat Rev Drug Discov* 7:156–167, 2008.
11. Bryan, N. S. Nitrite in nitric oxide biology: Cause or consequence? A systems-based review. *Free Radic Biol Med* 41:691–701; 2006.
12. Rassaf, T.; Kleinbongard, P.; Kelm, M. The L-arginine nitric oxide pathway: avenue for a multiple-level approach to assess vascular function. *Biological chemistry* 387:1347–1349; 2006.
13. Xia, Y.; Dawson, V. L.; Dawson, T. M.; Snyder, S. H.; Zweier, J. L. Nitric oxide synthase generates superoxide and nitric oxide in arginine-depleted cells leading to peroxynitrite-mediated cellular injury. *Proceedings of the National Academy of Sciences of the United States of America* 93:6770–6774; 1996.
14. Yoshida, K.; Kasama, K.; Kitabatake, M.; Imai, M. Biotransformation of nitric oxide, nitrite and nitrate. *Int Arch Occup Environ Health* 52:103–115; 1983.
15. Reutov, V. P.; Sorokina, E. G. NO-synthase and nitrite-reductase components of nitric oxide cycle. *Biochemistry (Mosc)* 63:874–884; 1998.
16. Vareille, M.; Rannou, F.; Thelier, N.; Glasser, A. L.; de Sablet, T.; Martin, C.; Gobert, A. P. Heme oxygenase-1 is a critical regulator of nitric oxide production in enterohemorrhagic Escherichia coli-infected human enterocytes. *J Immunol* 180:5720–5726; 2008.
17. Ambs, S.; Ogunfusika, M. O.; Merriam, W. G.; Bennett, W. P.; Billiar, T. R.; Harris, C. C. Up-regulation of inducible nitric oxide synthase expression in cancer-prone p53 knockout mice. *Proceedings of the National Academy of Sciences of the United States of America* 95:8823–8828; 1998.
18. Ambs, S.; Merriam, W. G.; Bennett, W. P.; Felley-Bosco, E.; Ogunfusika, M. O.; Oser, S. M.; Klein, S.; Shields, P. G.; Billiar, T. R.; Harris, C. C. Frequent nitric oxide synthase-2 expression in human colon adenomas: implication for tumor angiogenesis and colon cancer progression. *Cancer research* 58:334–341; 1998.
19. Hanahan, D.; Weinberg, R. A. The hallmarks of cancer. *Cell* 100:57–70; 2000.
20. Dalsgaard, T.; Simonsen, U.; Fago, A. Nitrite-dependent vasodilation is facilitated by hypoxia and is independent of known NO-generating nitrite reductase activities. *American journal of physiology* 292:H3072–3078; 2007.
21. Bryan, N. S.; Calvert, J. W.; Gundewar, S.; Lefer, D. J. Dietary nitrite restores NO homeostasis and is cardioprotective in endothelial nitric oxide synthase-deficient mice. *Free Radic Biol Med* 45:468–474; 2008.
22. Bryan, N. S.; Calvert, J. W.; Elrod, J. W.; Gundewar, S.; Ji, S. Y.; Lefer, D. J. Dietary nitrite supplementation protects against myocardial ischemia-reperfusion injury. *Proceedings of the National Academy of Sciences of the United States of America* 104:19144–19149; 2007.
23. Li, H.; Cui, H.; Kundu, T. K.; Alzawahra, W.; Zweier, J. L. Nitric oxide production from nitrite occurs primarily in tissues not in the blood: Critical role of xanthine oxidase and aldehyde oxidase. *The Journal of biological chemistry;* 2008.
24. Bryan, N. S.; Fernandez, B. O.; Bauer, S. M.; Garcia-Saura, M. F.; Milsom, A. B.; Rassaf, T.; Maloney, R. E.; Bharti, A.; Rodriguez, J.; Feelisch, M. Nitrite is a signaling molecule and regulator of gene expression in mammalian tissues. *Nature chemical biology* 1:290–297; 2005.
25. Spiegelhalder, B.; Eisenbrand, G.; Preussmann, R. Influence of dietary nitrate on nitrite content of human saliva: possible relevance to in vivo formation of N-nitroso compounds. *Food and cosmetics toxicology* 14:545–548; 1976.
26. Duncan, C.; Dougall, H.; Johnston, P.; Green, S.; Brogan, R.; Leifert, C.; Smith, L.; Golden,

M.; Benjamin, N. Chemical generation of nitric oxide in the mouth from the enterosalivary circulation of dietary nitrate. *Nat Med* 1:546–551; 1995.

27. Lundberg, J. O.; Weitzberg, E.; Lundberg, J. M.; Alving, K. Intragastric nitric oxide production in humans: measurements in expelled air. *Gut* 35:1543–1546; 1994.
28. McKnight, G. M.; Smith, L. M.; Drummond, R. S.; Duncan, C. W.; Golden, M.; Benjamin, N. Chemical synthesis of nitric oxide in the stomach from dietary nitrate in humans. *Gut* 40:211–214; 1997.
29. Bjorne, H. H.; Petersson, J.; Phillipson, M.; Weitzberg, E.; Holm, L.; Lundberg, J. O. Nitrite in saliva increases gastric mucosal blood flow and mucus thickness. *The Journal of clinical investigation* 113:106–114; 2004.
30. Bjorne, H.; Weitzberg, E.; Lundberg, J. O. Intragastric generation of antimicrobial nitrogen oxides from saliva—physiological and therapeutic considerations. *Free Radic Biol Med* 41:1404–1412; 2006.
31. Jansson, E. A.; Huang, L.; Malkey, R.; Govoni, M.; Nihlen, C.; Olsson, A.; Stensdotter, M.; Petersson, J.; Holm, L.; Weitzberg, E.; Lundberg, J. O. A mammalian functional nitrate reductase that regulates nitrite and nitric oxide homeostasis. *Nature chemical biology* 4:411–417; 2008.
32. Li, H.; Cui, H.; Kundu, T. K.; Alzawahra, W.; Zweier, J. L. Nitric oxide production from nitrite occurs primarily in tissues not in the blood: critical role of xanthine oxidase and aldehyde oxidase. *J Biol Chem* 283:17855–17863; 2008.
33. Alzawahra, W. F.; Talukder, M. A.; Liu, X.; Samouilov, A.; Zweier, J. L. Heme proteins mediate the conversion of nitrite to nitric oxide in the vascular wall. *American journal of physiology;* 2008.
34. Minneci, P. C.; Deans, K. J.; Shiva, S.; Zhi, H.; Banks, S. M.; Kearns, S.; Natanson, C.; Solomon, S. B.; Gladwin, M. T. Nitrite reductase activity of hemoglobin as a systemic nitric oxide generator mechanism to detoxify plasma hemoglobin produced during hemolysis. *Am J Physiol Heart Circ Physiol*; 2008.
35. Cosby, K.; Partovi, K. S.; Crawford, J. H.; Patel, R. K.; Reiter, C. D.; Martyr, S.; Yang, B. K.; Waclawiw, M. A.; Zalos, G.; Xu, X.; Huang, K. T.; Shields, H.; Kim-Shapiro, D. B.; Schechter, A. N.; Cannon III, R. O.; Gladwin, M. T. Nitrite reduction to nitric oxide by deoxyhemoglobin vasodilates the human circulation. *Nature Medicine* 9:1498–1505; 2003.
36. Rassaf, T.; Flogel, U.; Drexhage, C.; Hendgen-Cotta, U.; Kelm, M.; Schrader, J. Nitrite reductase function of deoxymyoglobin: oxygen sensor and regulator of cardiac energetics and function. *Circ Res* 100:1749–1754; 2007.
37. Li, H.; Samouilov, A.; Liu, X.; Zweier, J. L. Characterization of the effects of oxygen on xanthine oxidase-mediated nitric oxide formation. *J. Biol Chem* 279:16939–16946; 2004.
38. Carlsson, S.; Wiklund, N. P.; Engstrand, L.; Weitzberg, E.; Lundberg, J. O. Effects of pH, nitrite, and ascorbic acid on nonenzymatic nitric oxide generation and bacterial growth in urine. *Nitric Oxide* 5:580–586; 2001.
39. Takahama, U.; Yamamoto, A.; Hirota, S.; Oniki, T. Quercetin-dependent reduction of salivary nitrite to nitric oxide under acidic conditions and interaction between quercetin and ascorbic acid during the reduction. *Journal of agricultural and food chemistry* 51:6014–6020; 2003.
40. Lundberg, J. O.; Weitzberg, E. NO generation from nitrite and its role in vascular control. *Arteriosclerosis, thrombosis, and vascular biology* 25:915–922; 2005.
41. Dejam, A.; Hunter, C. J.; Tremonti, C.; Pluta, R. M.; Hon, Y. Y.; Grimes, G.; Partovi, K.; Pelletier, M. M.; Oldfield, E. H.; Cannon, R. O., 3rd; Schechter, A. N.; Gladwin, M. T. Nitrite infusion in humans and nonhuman primates: endocrine effects, pharmacokinetics, and tolerance formation. *Circulation* 116:1821–1831; 2007.

42. Nohl, H.; Staniek, K.; Sobhian, B.; Bahrami, S.; Redl, H.; Kozlov, A. V. Mitochondria recycle nitrite back to the bioregulator nitric monoxide. *Acta Biochim Pol* 47:913–921; 2000.

43. Veselik, D. J.; Divekar, S.; Dakshanamurthy, S.; Storchan, G. B.; Turner, J. M.; Graham, K. L.; Huang, L.; Stoica, A.; Martin, M. B. Activation of estrogen receptor-alpha by the anion nitrite. *Cancer research* 68:3950–3958; 2008.

44. Gonzalez, F. M.; Shiva, S.; Vincent, P. S.; Ringwood, L. A.; Hsu, L. Y.; Hon, Y. Y.; Aletras, A. H.; Cannon, R. O., 3rd; Gladwin, M. T.; Arai, A. E. Nitrite anion provides potent cytoprotective and antiapoptotic effects as adjunctive therapy to reperfusion for acute myocardial infarction. *Circulation* 117:2986–2994; 2008.

45. Kelm, M. Nitric oxide metabolism and breakdown. *Biochimica et Biophysica Acta* 1411:273–289; 1999.

46. Shiva, S.; Wang, X.; Ringwood, L. A.; Xu, X.; Yuditskaya, S.; Annavajjhala, V.; Miyajima, H.; Hogg, N.; Harris, Z. L.; Gladwin, M. T. Ceruloplasmin is a NO oxidase and nitrite synthase that determines endocrine NO homeostasis. *Nature chemical biology* 2:486–493; 2006.

47. Vanin, A. F.; Bevers, L. M.; Slama-Schwok, A.; van Faassen, E. E. Nitric oxide synthase reduces nitrite to NO under anoxia. *Cell Mol Life Sci* 64:96–103; 2007.

48. Larsen, F. J.; Weitzberg, E.; Lundberg, J. O.; Ekblom, B. Effects of dietary nitrate on oxygen cost during exercise. *Acta physiologica* (Oxford, England) 191:59–66; 2007.

49. Lundberg, J. O.; Govoni, M. Inorganic nitrate is a possible source for systemic generation of nitric oxide. *Free radical biology & medicine* 37:395–400; 2004.

50. Allen, J. D.; Cobb, F. R.; Gow, A. J. Regional and whole-body markers of nitric oxide production following hyperemic stimuli. *Free radical biology & medicine* 38:1164–1169; 2005.

51. Rassaf, T.; Lauer, T.; Heiss, C.; Balzer, J.; Mangold, S.; Leyendecker, T.; Rottler, J.; Drexhage, C.; Meyer, C.; Kelm, M. Nitric oxide synthase-derived plasma nitrite predicts exercise capacity. *British journal of sports medicine* 41:669–673; discussion 673; 2007.

52. Lauer, T.; Heiss, C.; Balzer, J.; Kehmeier, E.; Mangold, S.; Leyendecker, T.; Rottler, J.; Meyer, C.; Merx, M. W.; Kelm, M.; Rassaf, T. Age-dependent endothelial dysfunction is associated with failure to increase plasma nitrite in response to exercise. *Basic research in cardiology* 103:291–297; 2008.

53. Gago, B.; Lundberg, J. O.; Barbosa, R. M.; Laranjinha, J. Red wine-dependent reduction of nitrite to nitric oxide in the stomach. *Free Radic Biol Med* 43:1233–1242; 2007.

54. Peri, L.; Pietraforte, D.; Scorza, G.; Napolitano, A.; Fogliano, V.; Minetti, M. Apples increase nitric oxide production by human saliva at the acidic pH of the stomach: a new biological function for polyphenols with a catechol group? *Free Radic Biol Med* 39:668–681; 2005.

55. Ignarro, L. J.; Byrns, R. E.; Sumi, D.; de Nigris, F.; Napoli, C. Pomegranate juice protects nitric oxide against oxidative destruction and enhances the biological actions of nitric oxide. *Nitric Oxide* 15:93–102; 2006.

56. Sobko, T.; Reinders, C. I.; Jansson, E.; Norin, E.; Midtvedt, T.; Lundberg, J. O. Gastrointestinal bacteria generate nitric oxide from nitrate and nitrite. *Nitric Oxide* 13:272–278; 2005.

57. Sobko, T.; Huang, L.; Midtvedt, T.; Norin, E.; Gustafsson, L. E.; Norman, M.; Jansson, E. A.; Lundberg, J. O. Generation of NO by probiotic bacteria in the gastrointestinal tract. *Free Radic Biol Med* 41:985–991; 2006.

58. Zweier, J. L.; Wang, P.; Samouilov, A.; Kuppusamy, P. Enzyme-independent formation of nitric oxide in biological tissues. *Nat Med* 1:804–809; 1995.

CHAPTER 11

Nutrition and General Health

SAMUEL GRIEF and BRAZOS MINSHEW
University of Illinois at Chicago Medical School, Trivita, Inc

NUTRITION is a science in evolution. Historically, many different ancient and modern societies have established nutrition norms. The ancient Greeks, for example, ate a relatively modest and moderate diet, full of variety, including: seasonal vegetables and fruits, cereals, whole grains, dairy products such as yogurt and cheese, meat in small quantities, poultry and fish in abundance, olive oil as the main source of fat, many oily foods and modest consumption of wine during dinner. Today's so-called Mediterranean Diet can also be called "The ancient Greek diet" given their similarities. Hippocrates himself was quoted as stating "neither satiety nor hunger nor any other thing which exceeds the natural bounds can be good or healthful" [1].

Scientific discoveries of the last several hundred years have shed light on a myriad of nutrients found in food stuff. These discoveries have served as the foundation for medical and health practitioners to develop concrete and explicit nutrition guidelines for a wide variety of medical and health conditions. Twenty-first century medicine is now able to outline nutrition regimens that will help prevent and treat disease. The most recent discoveries discussed in this book are revolutionary in terms of identifying new molecules in foods that promote health and well-being. This knowledge is powerful. Yet, its application to our modern day society has been challenging.

Recent studies regarding cancer, heart disease and diabetes clearly point the arrow at high-quality nutrients in the diet as directly impacting one's overall risk for these top three diseases afflicting Americans. Eating more fruits and vegetables, eating heart-healthy fish and low-fat cuts of meat and poultry, consuming low-fat dairy products and choosing food products without partial hydrogenation and drinking alcohol and related beverages in moderation can all positively influence a population's health. The goal of this chapter is to review a broad array of currently available nutrition information to emphasize the importance of diet and how modest changes can drastically affect our health and well being. We will shift gears a bit to discuss the general context of nutrition and health irrespective of nitric oxide. There are well established guidelines for nutrition and we feel compelled to include these in a broad context to present the latest state of the art in terms of nutrition and general health. We will review contemporary guidelines for an optimal diet with the hope that the new concepts presented in this book can be integrated into accepted guidelines.

HEART HEALTH AND NUTRITION

The American Heart Association promotes a heart-healthy nutrition plan, emphasizing the following:

- Choose lean meats and poultry without skin and prepare them without added saturated and trans fat.
- Select fat-free, 1 percent fat, and low-fat dairy products.
- Cut back on foods containing partially hydrogenated vegetable oils to reduce *trans* fat in your diet.
- Cut back on foods high in dietary cholesterol. Aim to eat less than 300 milligrams of cholesterol each day.
- Cut back on beverages and foods with added sugars.
- Choose and prepare foods with little or no salt. Aim to eat less than 2,300 milligrams of sodium per day.
- If you drink alcohol, drink in moderation. That means one drink per day or less if you're a woman and two drinks per day or less if you're a man.
- Follow the American Heart Association recommendations when you eat out, and keep an eye on your portion sizes [http://www.americanheart.org/presenter.jhtml?identifier=851].

Notice that the emphasis is on moderation and cutting back or limiting foods that are more likely to induce obesity, high cholesterol or high blood pressure, all conditions known to be associated with NO insufficiency. Obesity will be dealt with in a later section.

Cholesterol, a waxy substance that is necessary for every almost every cell in our body, is also known as one of the main culprits in heart disease. The well-known Framingham study established cholesterol as one of the primary risk factors for heart disease [http://www.framinghamheartstudy.org/about/history.html]. Information from Chapter 2 revealed that a high cholesterol diet leads to a decline in nitric oxide production and a heightened state of oxidative stress that can inactive NO once produced. Following a low-saturated fat diet was, for many years, the cornerstone of treating high cholesterol. The late Robert Atkins challenged this dietary approach by introducing his diet book "The Atkins Diet Revolution" with its main principle of carbohydrate restriction. Posthumously, Atkins' dietary concept has been proven highly effective in lowering cholesterol and modulating the lipid parameters, including lowering total cholesterol, raising HDL cholesterol and reducing triglycerides [2]. Details presented in earlier chapters revealed that foods rich in nitrite and nitrate can combat the harmful vascular effects of a high cholesterol diet.

High blood pressure (hypertension) is a well-known risk factor for heart disease. The Dietary Approach to Stop Hypertension (DASH) diet has been promulgated as the leading dietary pattern to help lower blood pressure among the estimated 50 million Americans with hypertension. Nitric oxide is the most important molecule our body produces to regulate and maintain normal blood pressure. Eating unhealthy diets can lead to the rapid inactivation of NO and even lead to a decline in production. The DASH diet emphasizes moderate consumption of a variety of fruits and vegetables, whole grains, low-fat diary products, lean meats, poultry and fish, and nuts, seeds and legumes. Heart-healthy oils, such as olive and canola oil are encouraged, and the DASH diet typically confers approximately 25–30% of calories from these types of fat. [3]. We learned in chapter 4 that the DASH diet also provides additional nutrients in the form of nitrite and nitrate that can enhance and replete nitric oxide activity.

CANCER AND NUTRITION

Diet is a known risk factor for many cancers. Scientific evidence suggests that about 1/3 of the cancer deaths that occur in the US each year are due to nutrition and physical activity factors, including excess weight. (Reference: American Cancer Society. Cancer Facts & Figures 2008.) Obesity is implicated in numerous forms of cancer, including: colorectal, breast, uterine (endometrial), gallbladder, esophageal, pancreas, kidney (renal cell carcinoma), prostate, and thyroid. Experts aren't sure why extra fat can lead to malignancies, but changes in the circulating levels of various hormones (insulin, insulin-like growth factors and sex steroids) might explain the link [3]. In fact, it is estimated that overweight and obesity in the United States account for 14% of all cancer deaths in men and 20% in women [4].

Alcohol is an established cause of cancers of the following: mouth, pharynx, larynx, esophagus, liver, and breast. (Reference: American Cancer Society. Cancer Facts & Figures 2008.) Red meat and fiber have both been taken for granted as de facto players in the cancer and nutrition link. In fact, there still remains controversy surrounding both of these prominent elements in the western diet regarding their cancer effects [5,6].

Fat has been much maligned for its relation to obesity and cardiovascular disease. Not surprisingly, the results of animal experiments and various sorts of retrospective human epidemiologic studies indicate that high total fat intakes increase the risk for various cancers. As an example, there have been six cohort studies that specifically analyzed the association between fat intake and the risk of prostate cancer. In four of these, total fat intake was positively associated with risk of prostate cancer and the other two studies showed a trend toward significance [7]. The type of fat consumed directly impacts one's risk for cancer. It seems clear that high dietary intakes of omega-6 (n-6) polyunsaturated fatty acid (PUFA) increase the risk for developing breast cancer, whereas high intakes of omega-3 (n-3) polyunsaturated fatty acid (fish oils) reduce the risk. Similarly, a high ratio of n-6 to n-3 PUFA in the diet is a risk factor for colon cancer. A ratio of 1:1-2:1 (n-6:n-3) seems to be the most protective effect against the development and growth of mammary and colon tumors [8].

Enhanced whole grain intake has also been linked to a reduction in cancer risk. Jacobs *et. al.* [9] concluded, based on a meta-analysis of 40 case-control studies, that whole grain intake is associated with decreased risk for various cancers, particularly those of the colon/rectum and stomach. Several compounds present in whole grains, including phytate, phytoestrogens (such as lignan, plant stanols, and sterols), and several vitamins and minerals, may contribute to the observed lower risk of cancer. Additionally, high fiber content in whole grains may lead to satiation and lower overall energy consumption.

In 1997, the American Institute for Cancer Research and the World Cancer Research Fund summarized information arising from several hundred case-control and cohort studies involving fruits, vegetables and cancer risk as follows: *There exists an inverse association between fruit and vegetable intake and numerous cancers.* Most Americans do not eat enough fruits and veggies—in a recent study with NHLBI-screened subjects, Djousse *et. al.* found that the average daily servings of fruits/veggies were 3.2 and 3.5 for adult men and women, respectively [10].

It is not surprising that some types of vegetables surface more fre-

TABLE 11.1 Examples of Dietary Phytochemicals that May Be Protective Against Cancer.

Phytochemical	Dietary Sources
Allyl sulfur compounds	Onions, garlic
Catechins	Tea, berries
Ellagic acid	Grapes, strawberries, raspberries, walnuts
Indoles	Cruciferous vegetables
Isoflavones	Soybeans and other legumes
Isothiocyanates	Cruciferous vegetables
Lycopene	Tomatoes and tomato products
Quercetin	Onion, red grapes, citrus fruit, broccoli
Resveratrol	Grapes (skin), red wine
Terpenes	Citrus fruits
Thioethers	Garlic, onions

Reference: Nutritional Health: Strategies for Disease Prevention, 2nd Ed. Edited by Temple, *et.al.* Humana Press, 2006, pp. 154–155.

quently as protective against cancer, including carrots and green, cruciferous *(A member of the family of vegetables that includes kale, collard greens, broccoli, cauliflower, cabbage, Brussels sprouts, and turnips)*, and allium *(A genus of plants, including the onion, garlic, leek, chive, etc.)* vegetables. The explanation: *bioactive food components.*

ANTIOXIDANTS AND NUTRITION

Antioxidants are substances or compounds that have the ability to neutralize molecules known as 'free radicals'. Free radicals are by-products of the body's normal operations. These highly reactive and unstable by-products are also found in food, drink, smoke and other environmental toxins. Their instability often results in minor cellular damage, easily repaired by the body's own antioxidant defenses. On occasion, the cellular damage is serious and includes destruction of normal cellular architecture and functioning. It is these destructive changes that wreak havoc on the body's well being over time and cause disease.

Ingested antioxidants are mostly found in food substances. As a class of antioxidant-rich food, fruits and vegetables rank #1. Table 11.2 lists the top 20 antioxidant-containing food items.

There are several categories of antioxidants, including flavonoids, carotenoids, polyphenols, several vitamins, and other compounds. Many scientists have begun to look at the health benefits of antioxidants in general and flavonoids in particular.

Flavonoids are a group of antioxidants found in many different foods. As discussed in Chapter 7, the main sources of flavonoids are tea, onions, soy and wine. Foods such as cocoa, red wine and tea that have been culturally and historically thought to have healing or protective are actually rich in flavonoids. From cancer to heart disease, researchers have been investigating the role of flavonoids in preventive health care. While there is still much research to be done on this topic, current studies shed some light on the role these micronutrients may play in disease treatment and prevention.

Since cellular damage plays a role in cancer progression and antioxidants have a role in preventing cellular damage, deductive reasoning would say antioxidants have a role in preventing cancer. While this is a promising avenue for research, the results are mixed. The Zutphen Elderly Study done in 1994 [11] investigated the possible connection between dietary flavonoids and cancer risk. This study concluded, "Intake of flavonoids, mainly from tea, apples, and onions, does not predict a reduced risk of all-cause cancer or of cancer of the alimentary and respiratory tract in elderly men." A more recent study done at Northwestern University Feinberg School of Medicine [12] investigated the potential role for flavonoids in the treatment and prevention of pancreatic cancer. The researchers concluded "It is likely that flavonoids will move into the clinical arena as therapeutic or preventive tools for cancer." Perhaps as research continues on these powerful micronutrients, their role in cancer prevention will be better defined.

The role flavonoids may play in cardiovascular disease has been ex-

TABLE 11.2 List of Top 20 Antioxidant-Containing Foods.

1. Blueberry	11. Beetroot
2. Blackberry	12. Red Pepper
3. Garlic	13. Red Grape
4. Strawberry	14. Orange
5. Kale	15. Cherry
6. Spinach	16. Kiwi Fruit
7. Brussels Sprouts	17. Pink Grapefruit
8. Broccoli Floret	18. White Grape
9. Plum	19. Onion
10. Alfalfa Sprouts	20. Corn

amined by several prospective cohort studies. Results of these investigations have found that flavonoid intake is significantly inversely associated with coronary heart disease. In addition to the data regarding flavonoids and cancer, the Zutphen Elderly Study also reported that a flavonoid intake of 0 to 19.0 mg/day was found to be associated with a coronary heart disease mortality rate of 18.5 per 1000 person years whereas a mortality rate of 7.8 per 1000 person years was found among participants that consumed more than 29.9 mg/day (or approximately 5 to 6 cups of tea per day). Indications that flavonoids may play a beneficial role in cardiovascular disease stems from evidence that some flavonoids, such as phenolic substances in red wine, inhibit LDL oxidation [13]. Moreover, additional research has shown that flavonoids may inhibit platelet aggregation and adhesion, which may be an explanation for its effects on cardiovascular disease. Many of these effects may be due to the facilitated reduction of nitrite to NO. However, there is a necessity to conduct long-term, randomized trials of flavonoids to fully determine the contributions of these anti-oxidants to cardiovascular disease.

There remains much uncovered ground regarding the role of flavonoids in health maintenance and prevention. While research focusing on the health benefits of flavonoids found in natural products is significant, additional data is still needed to fully understand the safety and potential effects of flavonoids used as dietary supplements.

WHOLE GRAINS AND HEALTH EFFECTS

Grains are a staple food product of our daily lives. The whole grain, as it is known, contains three parts: the bran (outer husk), the endosperm (starchy part) and the germ (seed). Grains that are refined or processed lose both the bran and germ layers, thus stripping the grain of its main nutritional benefits. In fact, the bran layer is full of fiber, B-vitamins, up to 80% of the grain's minerals and a variety of *phytochemicals*—biological substances thought to be nutritionally important. The germ is also full of B-vitamins, vitamin E, other trace minerals, healthful unsaturated fats, phytochemicals and some antioxidants. The large endosperm portion is not without valuable nutrition and contains complex carbohydrates, protein and smaller amounts of B-vitamins.

Due to increased awareness of how nutrition directly contributes to overall health, medical and other health professionals have been promoting heightened attention among the lay public to eating more balanced meals, choosing heart-healthy food and increasing fiber (from sources such as whole grains) in the diet. It is this push towards improved public nutritional habits that has placed the limelight directly onto whole grains. The Food and Drug Administration (FDA) has approved the use by manufacturers of the following health claim: "Diets rich in whole grain foods and other plant foods, and low in total fat, saturated fat and cholesterol, may reduce the risk of heart disease and certain cancers." This health claim is affixed to all food products containing more than 50% whole grain by weight.

Fiber is a well-known food substance conferring many health benefits and is found in abundance in whole grain foods. In fact, one serving of a high-fiber, whole grain bread or cereal can provide more than half the daily dietary intake recommended by nutritional pundits. Whole grains are also rich in vitamin E, vitamin B-6 and the minerals calcium, magnesium, potassium, manganese, copper and zinc. Incorporating high-fiber, whole grain foods into the diet is very likely to not only improve health, but will almost certainly reduce the risk for suffering from one or more of the common diseases that affect millions of Americans.

OBESITY AND NUTRITION

Obesity has now become one of the leading health problems in the United States. Obesity is defined as body mass index (BMI) of more than 30 kg/m^2, while overweight is having a BMI of 25–29.9 kg/m^2. An estimated 97 million adults in the U.S. are obese or overweight. The magnitude of obesity all over the U.S. has continued to increase dramatically in recent years [14,15]. Approximately, two-thirds of the U.S. adult population is overweight or obese based on a recent survey in 2003–2004 compared to only one-half in 1988–1994 [14,15]. This increasing trend has been illustrated among states participating in the Behavioral Risk Factor Surveillance System. Based on this study in 1990, the prevalence

TABLE 11.3 The International Classification of Adult Underweight, Overweight and Obesity (BMI) Adapted from WHO 2004.

Classification	BMI (kg/m^2)
Underweight	< 18.50
Normal	18.50–24.99
Overweight	≥ 25.00
Obese	≥ 30.00

Data Source: Adapted from WHO, 1995, WHO, 2000 and WHO 2004.

TABLE 11.4 BMI for Age Among Children.

Classification	Percentile Range
Underweight	Less than the 5th percentile
Normal	5th percentile to less than the 85th percentile
At risk of Overweight	85th to less than the 95th percentile
Overweight	Equal to or greater than the 95th percentile

of obesity was less than or equal to 15% for all participating states. By 1998, there were 7 states with a prevalence of obesity between 20–24%. In 2006, there were 22 states, which had a prevalence of obesity equal or greater than 25%. [15]

Obesity is not only a problem among the adult population. Obesity is now the most common chronic illness in childhood [16]. One third of all children in the U.S. aged 2–19 year old are overweight (obese) or at risk for overweight. Among children aged 2–19 year old, the prevalence of at risk for overweight, defined as BMI of 85th to less than the 95th percentile was 19.5% [15,16]. The prevalence of overweight or obese, defined as BMI equal to or greater than the 95th percentile was 17.1 based on the 2003–2004 NHANES study. On June 8th, 2007, an Expert Committee, comprised of representatives from 15 professional organizations, was convened by the American Medical Association (AMA) and co-funded in collaboration with the Department of Health and Human Services' Health Resources and Services Administration (HRSA) and the Centers for Disease Control and Prevention (CDC). The Expert Committee recommended that for children and adolescents 2 to 18 years of age, new definitions for overweight and obesity be enacted as follows:

- Individuals with a BMI ≥ 95th percentile for age and gender, should be considered obese.
- Individuals with BMI ≥ 85th percentile, but < 95th percentile for age and gender, should be considered overweight, and this term replaces "at risk of overweight."

Unfortunately, pediatric overweight and obesity are increasing. The prevalence of overweight among children aged 6 to 11 more than doubled in the past 20 years, going from 7% in 1980 to 18.8% in 2004. The rate among adolescents aged 12 to 19 more than tripled, increasing from 5% to 17.1% [14,15].

Obesity is associated with multiple medical morbidities, psychological stress and social stigmatization in both adults and children [17,18]. Overall morbidity and mortality escalates with increase in BMI. In adults, disease and death risk are greater among individuals with BMI greater than 25 kg/m^2 [18,19]. Also, waist circumference measurement greater than 40 inches (102 cm) in men or 35 inches (89 cm) in women is associated with a higher risk of obesity-related co-morbidities such as cardiovascular diseases [19]. Medical co-morbidities include hypertension, dyslipidemia, DM type II, coronary artery disease (CAD), stroke, gallbladder disease, certain types of cancer, reduced fertility, osteoarthritis, orthopedic complications, sleep apnea, asthma, etc [18–21]. The risk for DM type II with a BMI above 35kg/m^2 increases by 93-fold in women and by 42-fold in men. The risk for CAD is increased 86% by a 20% rise in weight in males, while in women, there is a 3.6-fold increase in risk with BMI above 29 kg/m^2. Gallbladder disease is increased 2.7-fold [20].

The medical health problems associated with obesity in adults can also be seen in children [17,22]. In addition to the medical problems, pediatric obesity greatly influences the psychological and social aspects of childhood. The psychological stress may be a result of altered social interactions with peer group, poor self-concept, and depression. Obesity during childhood is a risk factor itself for much of adult morbidity and mortality. The probability of childhood obesity persisting into adulthood is estimated to increase from 20% at 4 years of age to 80% by adolescence [17].

Multiple factors come into play influencing the rise of obesity in the U.S. Among these factors, diet and reduced physical activity are the most commonly cited. However, issues such as policy governing the US food industry, primary education meal programs, and urban planning also play a role in the epidemic. Many of these factors do not discriminate in their impact on adults and children. Understanding the prevalence of obesity requires an understanding of the interactions between these factors.

Obesity can be attributed to the imbalance between energy intake and energy expenditure [19]. Intake of calories greater than the daily-recommended level for the average American results in weight gain. Individuals eating a diet replete with high-calorie, energy-dense, processed foods as well as, a diet depleted of fiber, micronutrients and antioxidants are predisposed to co-morbidities associated with obesity. The popularity of fast-food restaurants has only worsened the problem. Fast food consumption has been associated with excess total energy intake and increased bodyweight in adolescents and adults [23–25].

Aside from the increase in popularity of fast food, there has been a 300% increase in the consumption of soft drinks over the past 20 years [26]. The additional 120 calories of one serving of sugar-sweetened soft drink per day produces a 50 kg increase in body mass over 10 years.

Sugar-sweetened beverage consumption has been associated with obesity among adolescents [26]. Sugar-sweetened beverages have a high glycemic index, which increase the postprandial blood glucose and decrease insulin sensitivity. Also, a compounding effect has been shown wherein consumption of foods high in sugar result in a decreased satiety level, thus increasing the likelihood of greater food intake. An additional 835 calories are taken in by children who drink at least 8 oz. of sweetened beverage per day as compared to those who do not. Furthermore those who drink regular soft drinks eat more food than those who do not [27].

Loose regulations on the U.S. food industry have influenced unhealthy food choices by inattention to highly saturated fatty foods and sugar content available in the market. However, given recent media attention on the prevalence of obesity in the US, lawmakers are now pressured into paying closer attention to the issue [28]. Adolescents and children are not excluded when it comes to dietary behaviors. Studies suggest that both obese adolescents and their normal weight counterparts practice dieting [29]. In 2003, 73 percent of Americans said that they were trying to lose weight. This number decreased to 59% in 2007. Almost three quarters of the American population agree it's important to have a support network when trying to lose weight yet it appears those support networks do not exist. Despite efforts to lose weight by dieting, obesity is still pervasive.

In spite of the flood of diets currently on the market and increased public health initiatives to target unhealthy eating behaviors, the prevalence of obesity continues to increase. This can be largely attributed to the predominantly sedentary lifestyle that Americans are living [19]. Lack of physical activity and sedentary behavior has contributed to the increase in prevalence of obesity. Recent surveys on the American public's level of physical activity continue to show a low level of participation in physical fitness activities. Based on a CDC study, more than 50% of adults do not meet recommended level of physical activity and 24% do not engage in physical activity at all during their leisure time. Physical inactivity is not only seen in adults but in the young population as well. Among adolescents and children between grades 9–12, two thirds are not participating in physical activity at the recommended level.

Do physicians/providers counsel their patients on obesity management, good nutrition habits and regular physical activity? The United States Preventive Services Task Force (USPSTF) recommends that screening for obesity and counseling to promote regular physical activity as a routine part of health visits. Tailored counseling that incorporates shared decision-making, a written prescription, printed materials, and follow-up has been shown to increase the likelihood of success [30]. In one study, the number of patients who improved their physical activity level increased by 50 percent after receiving physician advice [31]. Nutritional counseling can be delegated to ancillary health care providers if time constraints exist.

Physical activity and good nutrition are considered essential elements to prevent chronic diseases and obesity, as outlined in the Centers for Disease Control and Prevention 2007 guide to promoting physical activity and good nutrition. Unfortunately, a majority of Americans do not participate in regular physical activity nor apply healthy dietary habits to every day meals. Despite the proven benefits of physical activity, more than 50% of U.S. adults do not get enough physical activity to provide health benefits; 24% are not active at all in their leisure time. About two thirds of young people in grades 9–12 are not engaged in recommended levels of physical activity. Based on the NHLBI guidelines, physical activity is a vital component of weight loss initially. Thirty to forty five minutes of moderate physical activity on 3 to 5 days per week initially is encouraged (Evidence category A). An accumulated 30 minutes or more of moderate physical activity on most days of the week should be set as a long-term goal among adults (Evidence category B). Daily exercise increases nitric oxide production and therefore provides additional benefits related to NO.

On the nutrition front, educating the public on the health benefits of healthy eating patterns and helping people implement these habits is an important undertaking. A large gap remains between healthy dietary patterns and what Americans actually eat. In 2005, only one-fourth of U.S. adults ate five or more servings of fruits and vegetables each day [32]. To help people improve their eating habits, the USDHHS and the U.S. Department of Agriculture publish Dietary Guidelines for Americans (available at http://www.healthierus.gov/dietaryguidelines). Some proposed calorie-lowering strategies from the Dietary Guidelines for Americans include eating foods that are low in calories (e.g., many kinds of vegetables and fruits and some soups). The healthiest way to reduce calorie intake is to reduce one's intake of added sugars, fats, and alcohol, which all provide calories but few or no essential nutrients. Special attention should be given to portion sizes, which have increased significantly over the past two decades. The Dietary Guidelines for Americans' key recommendations regarding weigh are:

1. To maintain body weight in a healthy range, balance calories from foods and beverages with calories expended.
2. To prevent gradual weight gain over time, make small decreases in food and beverage calories and increase physical activity.

In order to more assertively promote physical activity and good nutrition, the primary care provider should establish collaborative partnerships with nutrition specialists and physical education trainers. Results of these collaborations have been highly successful in promoting widespread behavior changes and achieving weight loss in different populations. The use of a coordinated multidisciplinary team effort is critical to the success of medically supervised weight loss. Physicians often have a referral network of nutrition specialists with which they collaborate. If no such network is available, the American Dietetic Association offers a tool for locating a nutrition specialist in your area at http://www.eatright.org/cps/rde/xchg/ada/hs.xsl/home_4874_ENU_HTML.htm. Most medical centers have specific departments dedicated to nutrition and physical education/therapy. A growing number of medical centers have an affiliation with nutrition and wellness centers, so-called for their emphasis on nutrition, weight management, diabetes education, physical activity education, psychological services, and in some cases bariatric surgical care. Since many third party insurers have recognized the value of these nutrition and wellness center services, many patients can benefit from the expert counseling provided at a modest cost.

Traditional, supervised weight loss center-sponsored dietary approaches to weight loss can work, but attrition rates over time are high [33]. Commercial weight loss diet plans, such as the Atkins diet, South Beach diet, Zone diet, and others are well known for their short term success in achieving modest weight loss of between 5–15% within the first 6–12 months [2,34]. Long-term success beyond one year in maintaining weight loss has been rarely reviewed; results for each diet plan are almost equivalent [35]. Individuals who attempt weight loss have identified specific components of a weight loss program that contribute to success and that make success difficult. Long-term support, having an exercise program or personal trainer, accountability/self-monitoring, and flexibility are key components to weight loss success. Difficulty making and maintaining lifestyle change, no time, lack of support, food is everywhere, and feelings of deprivation are common obstacles to success [35]. Studies are conflicting regarding overall success in achieving long-term weight loss through supervised weight loss programs. Research to date supports the conclusion that scientifically-supported diet regimens can produce weight loss of 9–13% of total body weight at 52–72 weeks, and that programs aided by pharmacotherapy can result, at most, in a 10–15% weight loss, even over the long-term.

In summary, obesity has become the predominant nutritional and medical condition afflicting the health and welfare of a majority of Americans. Addressing this condition is not optional.

AGING AND NUTRITION

It is no secret that living a long and healthy life is a universal goal shared by all. The 20th century was a boom for achieving this universal goal: there has been an explosion of the fraction of people who are now 65 years or older. Over 12% of Americans are now 65 years and older. Many scientists have endeavored to uncover the mysteries of aging. While we do know the cellular process by which aging occurs, not all of the reasons for aging are still clear. One thing that is clear is the combination of factors that accelerate the aging process: smoking, weak immunity, stress, insufficient rest, and most importantly—improper nutrition! It is this last factor that is the focus of the following discussion. Interestingly all these factors listed that accelerate the aging process are also associated with diminished NO production. It is known that as we age we lose our ability to produce NO from L-arginine [36–39].

What is the best way to eat in order to slow down, possibly reverse the aging process? Rat models provide the answer. Early in the 20th century, research conducted on these mammalian cousins confirmed that dietary restriction (DR) led to a longer mean, average and overall lifespan. DR meant providing only 60% of the body's caloric needs during the adult life span. While DR seems a bit stringent for the average American, there is certainly some wiggle room among many Americans to lower their caloric intake to effect a change for the better. Researchers are still unsure why DR retards the aging process and results in a longer life for rats. Is it simply less fat in the diet? Less weight leading to less disease? Or is it related to the body's enhanced ability to neutralize oxidative stress related to food and oxygen by-products? The current consensus is that multiple factors are likely to lead to a longer, more healthful life among humans by extrapolating the rat longevity data. First, eating less will translate into lower weight. Americans between the ages of 40–59 are the heaviest group on record. Not surprisingly, it is also this age group that becomes afflicted with most of the common chronic diseases facing Americans, including hypertension, diabetes, cancer and heart disease. Second, many diseases may be prevented or eliminated by certain food products. Examples include calcium-rich foods and osteoporosis, broccoli and lung cancer, tomato-based products and prostate enlargement, lutein-laden foods and age-related macular degeneration (ARMD), and more. This last condition, ARMD, affects about 2 million Americans yearly and is the leading cause of blindness. Eating foods rich in lutein, including eggs, as well as other antioxidants (mentioned earlier in this chapter) will help prevent this life-altering disease and may also lower your risk for other disease-shortening medical conditions. The mantra "eat three colors of foods with every meal" is another way of saying that variety is truly likely to contribute to a longer, healthier life.

Third, although fat has been much maligned in the 20th century as the leading cause of disease in the western world, 21st century science has confirmed that good fats do exist and are necessary for better health. Cold water fish, nuts, avocadoes and other heart-healthy, fat-containing foods are absolutely recommended for their ability to provide excellent nutrition, enhance absorption of fat-soluble vitamins, lessen the consumption of pro-inflammatory fats, and lower the risk for the most common chronic diseases facing Americans.

Chronic diseases, such as cancer, heart disease, diabetes, asthma, arthritis and others are typically due to a combination of genetic and environmental influences. All of these chronic diseases listed above are directly impacted by the amount and type of foods consumed in one's diet. For example, recent research has shown that lowering the glycemic index (GI) of one's diet may be a better treatment approach for people with adult onset diabetes than other dietary approaches [40]. Diabetes typically results in volatile and inconsistent blood sugars, sometimes with a precipitous fall in blood sugar and more often with excessive rise in blood sugar. This rise usually occurs following meals and is termed "post-prandial hyperglycemia" (PPH) among scientists and medical professionals. It is PPH that has generated more focus of late in regards to complications related to diabetes and its oxidative stress on the human body [41,42]. Dietary control of PPH can be accomplished by eating portion-controlled meals, carefully counting and/or restricting carbohydrates, and consuming a variety of hues of foods which provide various antioxidants and other vitamins and minerals with disease-altering effects.

CONCLUSION

Nutrition is at the foundation of good health. Learning how and what to eat in order to fend off disease is an evolving science. With the above information, and with future innovations in nutritional science, medical professionals and the lay public will be well-prepared to have meaningful and fruitful discussions about one of the most basic human needs: eating and nutrition. It is hoped that the future of nutrition will be an open book, allowing all who wish to learn to be able to access the information systematically and seamlessly. The new concepts of restoring nitric oxide homeostasis through diet will certainly help us to devise new strategies for disease prevention through nutrition.

ABOUT THE AUTHORS

Dr. Samuel N. Grief, MD, FCFP

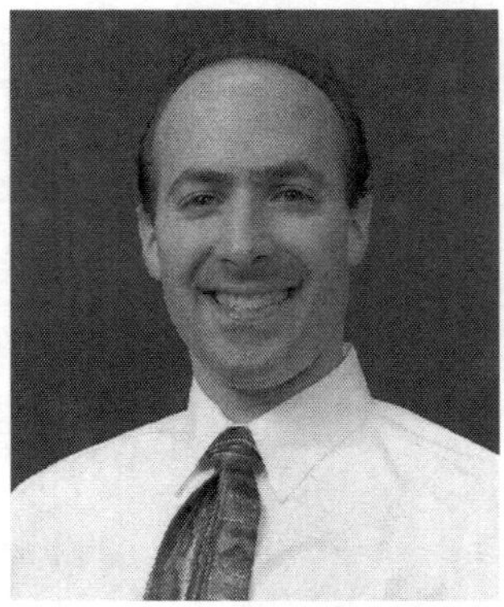

Dr. Samuel N. Grief, MD, FCFP is a Family Physician since 1991. He has worked in a variety of clinical settings, including community health centers, private practice and in academia. Currently, he is associate professor in clinical family medicine at the University of Illinois at Chicago (UIC) and the medical director for the UIC Campus Care health insurance. His field of expertise is obesity and nutrition.

Dr. Grief is a former radio show host of "The New England Health Hour" and "UIC Health Chat". He has been an invited guest speaker for many radio, television, and multimedia interviews and presentations.

Dr. Grief is also an accomplished writer. He is the co-author of "The End of Obesity", published in 1998. He is the editor of the award-winning nutrition newsletter "Nutri-Talk". He is a freelance author for several health and medical publications.

Dr. Brazos Minshew

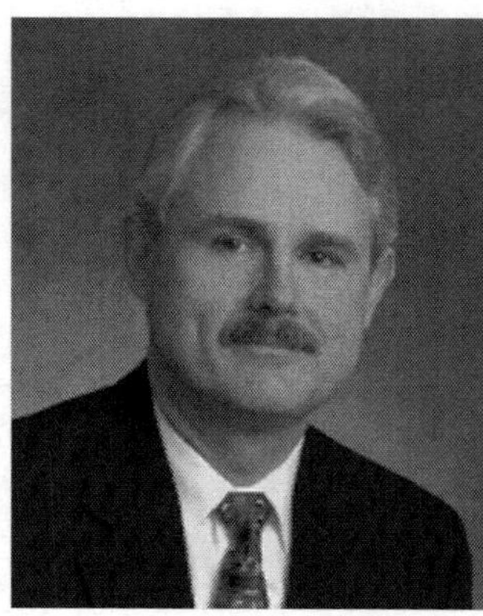

Dr. Minshew is the Chief Science Officer at TriVita. He has been in Practice since 1982. He served as a research associate in cancer research at Occidental Institute for six years, as a stress management counselor with Baylor Hospital and as director of Complimentary and Alternative Medicine at TienaHealth in Dallas, Texas. Dr. Minshew is an author, inventor and teacher.

REFERENCES

1. Merikas, G., Hippocratic Aspects of Dietetics. *Nutrtion-Dietetics,* 1992. 4(2): p. 65–70.
2. Gardner, C.D., et al., Comparison of the Atkins, Zone, Ornish, and LEARN diets for change in weight and related risk factors among overweight premenopausal women: the A TO Z Weight Loss Study: a randomized trial. *Jama*, 2007. 297(9): p. 969–77.
3. Temple, ed. *Nutritional Health: Strategies for Disease Prevention.* 2nd ed. 2006, Humana Press.
4. Calle, E.E., et al., Overweight, obesity, and mortality from cancer in a prospectively studied cohort of U.S. adults. *N Engl J Med,* 2003. 348(17): p. 1625–38.
5. Chao, A., et al., Meat consumption and risk of colorectal cancer. *Jama*, 2005. 293(2): p. 172–82.
6. Fuchs, C.S., et al., Dietary fiber and the risk of colorectal cancer and adenoma in women. *N Engl J Med,* 1999. 340(3): p. 169–76.
7. Fleshner, N., et al., Dietary fat and prostate cancer. *J Urol,* 2004. 171(2 Pt 2): p. S19–24.
8. Chajes, V. and P. Bougnoux, Omega-6/omega-3 polyunsaturated fatty acid ratio and cancer. *World Rev Nutr Diet,* 2003. 92: p. 133–51.
9. Jacobs, D.R., Jr., et al., Whole-grain intake and cancer: an expanded review and meta-analysis. *Nutr Cancer,* 1998. 30(2): p. 85–96.
10. Djousse, L., et al., Fruit and vegetable consumption and LDL cholesterol: the National Heart, Lung, and Blood Institute Family Heart Study. *Am J Clin Nutr,* 2004. 79(2): p. 213–7.
11. Hertog, M.G., et al., Dietary flavonoids and cancer risk in the Zutphen Elderly Study. *Nutr Cancer,* 1994. 22(2): p. 175–84.
12. Roginsky, A.B., et al., On the potential use of flavonoids in the treatment and prevention of pancreatic cancer. *In Vivo,* 2005. 19(1): p. 61–7.
13. Maron, D.J., Flavonoids for reduction of atherosclerotic risk. *Curr Atheroscler Rep,* 2004. 6(1): p. 73–8.
14. Flegal, K.M., et al., Prevalence and trends in obesity among US adults, 1999–2000. *Jama,* 2002. 288(14): p. 1723–7.
15. Ogden, C.L., et al., Prevalence of overweight and obesity in the United States, 1999-2004. *Jama*, 2006. 295(13): p. 1549–55.
16. O'Brien, S.H., R. Holubkov, and E.C. Reis, Identification, evaluation, and management of obesity in an academic primary care center. *Pediatrics,* 2004. 114(2): p. e154–9.
17. Committe on Nutrition. Prevention of pediatric overweight and obesity. *Pediatrics,* 2003. 112(2): p. 424–430.
18. Campbell, I., The obesity epidemic: can we turn the tide? *Heart,* 2003. 89 Suppl 2: p. ii22–4; discussion ii35–7.
19. McInnis, K.J., B.A. Franklin, and J.M. Rippe, Counseling for physical activity in overweight and obese patients. *Am Fam Physician,* 2003. 67(6): p. 1249–56.
20. Jung, R.T., Obesity as a disease. *Br Med Bull,* 1997. 53(2): p. 307–21.
21. Stein, C.J. and G.A. Colditz, The epidemic of obesity. *J Clin Endocrinol Metab,* 2004. 89(6): p. 2522–5.
22. Nichols, M.R. and D. Livingston, Preventing pediatric obesity: assessment and management in the primary care setting. *J Am Acad Nurse Pract,* 2002. 14(2): p. 55–62; quiz 63–5.
23. French, S.A., L. Harnack, and R.W. Jeffery, Fast food restaurant use among women in the Pound of Prevention study: dietary, behavioral and demographic correlates. *Int J Obes Relat Metab Disord*, 2000. 24(10): p. 1353–9.

24. French, S.A., et al., Fast food restaurant use among adolescents: associations with nutrient intake, food choices and behavioral and psychosocial variables. *Int J Obes Relat Metab Disord,* 2001. 25(12): p. 1823–33.
25. Binkley, J.K., J. Eales, and M. Jekanowski, The relation between dietary change and rising US obesity. *Int J Obes Relat Metab Disord,* 2000. 24(8): p. 1032–9.
26. Harrington, S., The role of sugar-sweetened beverage consumption in adolescent obesity: a review of the literature. *J Sch Nurs,* 2008. 24(1): p. 3–12.
27. Ludwig, D.S., K.E. Peterson, and S.L. Gortmaker, Relation between consumption of sugar-sweetened drinks and childhood obesity: a prospective, observational analysis. *Lancet,* 2001. 357(9255): p. 505–8.
28. Nestle, M. and M.F. Jacobson, Halting the obesity epidemic: a public health policy approach. *Public Health Rep,* 2000. 115(1): p. 12–24.
29. Talamayan, K.S., et al., Prevalence of overweight misperception and weight control behaviors among normal weight adolescents in the United States. *ScientificWorldJournal,* 2006. 6: p. 365–73.
30. Kreuter, M.W., S.G. Chheda, and F.C. Bull, How does physician advice influence patient behavior? Evidence for a priming effect. *Arch Fam Med,* 2000. 9(5): p. 426–33.
31. Meriwether, R.A., et al., Physical activity counseling. *Am Fam Physician,* 2008. 77(8): p. 1129–36.
32. Nebeling, L., et al., Still not enough: can we achieve our goals for Americans to eat more fruits and vegetables in the future? *Am J Prev Med,* 2007. 32(4): p. 354–5.
33. Bacon, L., et al., Evaluating a 'non-diet' wellness intervention for improvement of metabolic fitness, psychological well-being and eating and activity behaviors. *Int J Obes Relat Metab Disord,* 2002. 26(6): p. 854–65.
34. Dansinger, M.L., et al., Comparison of the Atkins, Ornish, Weight Watchers, and Zone diets for weight loss and heart disease risk reduction: a randomized trial. *Jama,* 2005. 293(1): p. 43–53.
35. Burke, L.E., et al., A descriptive study of past experiences with weight-loss treatment. *J Am Diet Assoc,* 2008. 108(4): p. 640–7.
36. Reckelhoff, J.F., et al., Changes in nitric oxide precursor, L-arginine, and metabolites, nitrate and nitrite, with aging. *Life Sci,* 1994. 55(24): p. 1895–902.
37. Tominaga, M., et al., Hypertension and ageing impair acetylcholine-induced vasodilation in rats. *J Hypertens,* 1994. 12(3): p. 259–68.
38. Chauhan, A., et al., Aging-associated endothelial dysfunction in humans is reversed by L-arginine. *J Am Coll Cardiol,* 1996. 28(7): p. 1796–804.
39. Andrawis, N., D.S. Jones, and D.R. Abernethy, Aging is associated with endothelial dysfunction in the human forearm vasculature. *J Am Geriatr Soc,* 2000. 48(2): p. 193–8.
40. Jenkins, D.J., et al., Effect of a low-glycemic index or a high-cereal fiber diet on type 2 diabetes: a randomized trial. *Jama,* 2008. 300(23): p. 2742–53.
41. Ceriello, A., Postprandial hyperglycemia and diabetes complications: is it time to treat? *Diabetes,* 2005. 54(1): p. 1–7.
42. McNulty, P.H., et al., Effect of simulated postprandial hyperglycemia on coronary blood flow in cardiac transplant recipients. *Am J Physiol Heart Circ Physiol,* 2007. 293(1): p. H103–8.

CHAPTER 12

Paradigm Shift: From Toxic Food Additive to Indispensable Nutrient

NATHAN S. BRYAN

Brown Foundation Institute of Molecular Medicine, The University of Texas Health Science Center, Houston, TX 77030

NITRIC OXIDE is one of the most studied molecules in modern times. Since its discovery in the 1980s, clear evidence has emerged demonstrating that it is one of the most important signaling molecules in the human body. There are a number of diseases associated or caused by an insufficiency of NO [1]. NO status is routinely assessed by steady state nitrite and/or nitrate concentrations, therefore these diseases also suggest a deficiency in both anions which have recently shown biological activity; nitrite by itself [2] and nitrate through its ability to be reduced to nitrite and NO [3]. The demonstration of NO formation by an enzyme in vascular endothelial cells in 1987 [4,5] has since had profound implications in research and medicine. The revelation that EDRF is NO and is synthesized by mammalian cells from L-arginine through a complex oxidation reaction catalyzed by the flavo-hemoprotein NO synthase (NOS) was revolutionary. However, if any of the co-factors or prosthetics groups are not accessible or functional, NOS produces superoxide instead of NO and this is the basis for the onset of many diseases. The complex regulation and production of NO provides many opportunities for malfunction from high levels of asymmetric dimethyl arginine (ADMA), a competitive inhibitor of NOS, inefficient or lack of L-arginine transport and uptake, cofactor oxidation and enzyme uncoupling to name a few. Therefore, the notion that there may be an alternate source of NO from that produced by NOS which can compensate for NO insufficiency and rescue individuals with endothelial dysfunction is exciting and revolutionary. We now know that there are a number of diseases associated or characterized by a deficiency in NO production. Due to the very complex and complicated reaction to make NO from L-arginine and its quick reactivity and extremely short half life, developing strategies to enhance NO production in humans to combat or treat disease has had mixed results. Today the dogma still exists to supplement L-arginine to enhance NO output. While this may work in healthy individuals with functional NOS, it cannot and will not work in individuals with endothelial dysfunction. In fact it is this dysfunction that puts them at risk for disease. The population of people who may be NO insufficient due to endothelial dysfunction and vascular disease are exactly the population that can benefit from an alternative source of NO. Simple changes in dietary habits to include foods rich in nitrite and nitrate will likely provide benefit. Perhaps an awareness of this dietary NO pathway will stimulate better strategies to restore NO homeostasis and combat cardiovascular disease. I wish to briefly summarize the main concepts presented here.

Nitrite is now known to be an intrinsic signaling molecule [2,6] capable of producing NO under appropriate conditions as well as form nitrosothiols [2,7]. Nitrite is shown to increase regional blood flow [8] that can increase oxygen delivery to hypoxic tissues. Enhancing nitrite availability through therapeutic intervention by administering bolus nitrite prior to cardiovascular insult has shown remarkable effects in reducing the injury from myocardial infarction, ischemic liver and kidney injury, stroke and cerebral vasospasm [9–14] in animal models. These first reports on the efficacy of nitrite in cytoprotection have lead to nine current clinical trials for the use of nitrite and/or nitrate in both healthy volunteers and patients with specific cardiovascular complications (www.clinicaltrials.gov). Most recently nitrite has been shown to precondition the myocardium when given 24 hours prior to ischemic insult due to the modulation of mitochondrial electron transfer [15] as well as augment ischemia induced angiogenesis and arteriogenesis [16]. Nitrite is also showing remarkable efficacy at promoting regional blood flow in sickle cell patients [17]. Plasma nitrite levels increase in response to exercise in healthy individuals whereby in aged patients with endothelial dysfunction there is no increase in nitrite from exercise [18]. Nitrite has also been shown to predict exercise capacity in humans [19]. Physical activity can even prevent age-related impairment in nitric oxide availability in elderly athletes [20]. We now know that nitrite is just as efficacious when given orally at restoring NO biochemistry [21], reversing hypertension from NOS inhibition [22] and protecting from myocardial ischemia-reperfusion injury [23]. This provides proof of concept that dietary sources of nitrite have physiological function.

Nitrite is used as a preservative in meat products to inhibit the growth of pathogens, most notably *Clostridium botulinum,* and these antibacterial effects have been attributed to NO formation [24]. The discovery of endogenous nitrite reduction to NO in the acidic stomach triggered researchers to explore therapeutic uses for acidified nitrite as an antimicrobial agent. Indeed, acidified nitrite results in the generation of NO and other nitrogen oxides, which have potent antibacterial activity against a range of pathogens, including *Salmonella, Yersinia* and *Shigella* species, *H. pylori,* and *Pseudomonas aerguinosa* [25–28]. These antibacterial effects of nitrite have recently been investigated in the airways. In an animal model resembling cystic fibrosis, acidified nitrite successfully cleared the airways of mucoid *P. aeruginosa,* a pathogen commonly infecting the airways of patients with cystic fibrosis [29]. Infected urine typically contains considerable amounts of nitrite, owing to bacterial reduction of urinary nitrate. Although nitrite is stable at neutral or alkaline conditions, it is reduced to NO and has potent antibacterial effects if the urine is mildly acidified (to pH 5–6); these effects are potentiated in the presence of the reducing agent vitamin C [28]. In fact, the *in vitro* antibacterial potency of nitrite and ascorbic acid is fully comparable to that of traditional antibiotics such as nitrofurantoin and trimetoprim. Acidification of urine—for example, by vitamin C intake—has been used in traditional medicine for the prevention and treatment of urinary tract infections. This effect may be related to the formation of antibacterial nitrogen oxides from the acidified nitrite [3,30].

Nitrite can also be derived from reduction of salivary nitrate by commensal bacteria in the mouth and gastrointestinal tract [27,31,32]. About 25% of orally ingested available nitrate is actively secreted into the saliva. This nitrate is partially converted to nitrite by oral bacteria and then disproportionates with formation of NO after entering the acidic environment of the stomach, helping to reduce gastrointestinal tract infection, increase mucous barrier thickness and increase gastric blood flow [33]. Proton pump inhibitors or chronic administration of antacids can adversely affect NO formation from nitrite in the stomach [31]. Commensal bacteria that reside within and on the human body can reduce nitrate thereby supplying a large and alternative source of nitrite. Therefore dietary and enzymatic sources of nitrate are a potentially large source of nitrite in the human body. Dietary nitrate supplementation has been shown to reduce diastolic blood pressure in healthy volunteers [34] protect from ischemia-reperfusion injury and inhibit platelet aggregation [35]. Dietary nitrate supplementation, in an amount achievable through a diet rich in vegetables, results in a lower oxygen demand during submaximal work [36], protect from non-steroidal anti-inflammatory drug (NSAID)-induce gastric ulcers [37] and enhance gastric mucosal blood flow and mucosal defense [38]. Most of the effects of nitrate are ablated by spitting and not swallowing demonstrating the essential nature of the enterosalivary circulation of nitrate [39]. The acute increase in plasma nitrite seen after a nitrate load is critically dependent on nitrate reduction in the oral cavity by commensal bacteria. Therefore the removal of these bacteria with an antibacterial mouthwash or antibiotics will very likely attenuate the NO-dependent biological effects of dietary nitrate [40]. This presents an interesting paradox to modern hygienic practices to prevent infection or illness from bacteria which may be adversely affecting our cardiovascular health. Our society today is compulsive about anti-bacterials. There are anti-bacterial soaps, mouthwashes, detergents and lotions. It is unknown what long term effects eradicating the commensal bacteria on or in our body will cause.

Perhaps the most compelling argument for implication for nitrite and nitrate requirements in the diet comes from breast milk of nursing mothers and the nutritional and immunological benefits to the infant. Breast milk is nature's most perfect food. Ongoing studies in our lab reveal the presence of high concentrations of nitrite and nitrate in human breast milk consistent with previous reports [41]. Breast milk from certain mothers contained the highest nitrite concentration of any food or beverage product tested (near 50 μM—Hord and Bryan unpublished observations). Human breast milk contains high concentrations of nitrate and nitrite in the early postpartum period and the relative concentrations of the two anions change from colostrum to transition milk to mature milk. In fact nitrite and nitrate in breast milk is found at concentrations much higher than that found in commercial baby formulas. The nitrite consumed by the infant enters the acidic environment of the stomach leading to the generation of nitric oxide in the gastric lumen. We know of the effects of NO in adult stomachs in terms of gastric mucosal integrity and blood flow from the reduction of nitrate to nitrite to NO. At birth, the gastrointestinal tract of the infant is sterile, and it is rapidly colonized by bacteria originating from the mother and the environment [42,43]. The first colonizing bacteria are aerobic bacteria, such as staphylococci, enteroccoci, and enterobacteria [44]. Then, anaerobic bacteria, such as *Bacteroides, Bifidobacterium,* and *Clostridium* species, gradually colonize the gastrointestinal tract [44]. We now appreciate that reduction of nitrate to nitrite requires the commensal bacteria that normally reside in our body. However in newborn infants this pathway has not developed. Therefore breast milk high in nitrite relative to nitrate overcomes the nature's deficiency early in life. At later stages of development nitrate becomes the predominant anion when a symbiosis exists with the colonized bacteria. This becomes extremely interesting in terms of levels of exposure based of nitrite ingestion based and body weight of an infant (near 1 mg/kg). The Joint Food and Agricultural Organization/World Health Organization has set the Acceptable Daily Intake (ADI) for the nitrate ion is set at 3.7 mg/kg body weight and for the nitrite ion at 0.06 mg/kg body weight [45]. You begin to see the humor and ignorance in terms of regulation of nitrite and nitrate exposure. If there were merits to any of the claims of nitrite and nitrate in promoting carcinogenesis, we would expect a higher incidence of cancer of breast fed infants compared to formula fed. In fact there is a recognized and huge disparity in the health of breast fed vs formula fed babies. Current dogma is that it is due to immunoglobulins transferred from mother to baby are responsible for the benefits of breast milk. A strong case can be made for nitrite as an essential molecule in the development and immune function of infants. Nature has devised a perfect system to nourish and foster the growth and development of nursing babies. Nitrite appears to be one of those indispensable nutrients.

Traditional Chinese medicine (also known as TCM) includes a range of traditional medical practices originating in China. It is considered a Complementary or Alternative Medical system in much of the western world while remaining as a form of primary care throughout most of Asia. TCM practices include treatments such as herbal medicine, acupuncture, dietary therapy, Tui na and Shiatsu massage. TCM theory is extremely complex and originated thousands of years ago through meticulous observation of nature, the cosmos, and the human body. In China, herbal medicine is considered as the primary therapeutic modality of internal medicine. Of the approximately 500 Chinese herbs that are in use today, 250 or so are very commonly used. Rather than being prescribed individually, single herbs are combined into formulas that are designed to adapt to the specific needs of individual patients. An herbal formula can contain anywhere from 3 to 25 herbs. As with diet therapy, each herb has one or more of the four flavors/functions and one of five "temperatures" ("Qi") (hot, warm, neutral, cool, cold). Ongoing studies in our lab at the Institute of Molecular Medicine in Houston reveal that many of these traditional Chinese medicine extracts contain very large amounts of nitrite and nitrate in the extracts given to patients. There are a number of published reports on the association of TCM and nitric oxide related effects [46,47]. I am confident that many of the described benefits of these ancient medications are due to their inherent nitrite and/or nitrate content. Treatments that have been used for centuries are now found to be rich in nitrite and nitrate.

The need to include fresh plant food or raw animal flesh in the diet to prevent disease was known from ancient times. Native peoples living in marginal areas incorporated this into their medicinal lore. For example, spruce needles were used in temperate zones in infusions, or the leaves from species of drought-resistant trees in desert areas. In 1536, the French explorer Jacques Cartier, exploring the St. Lawrence River, used the local natives' knowledge to save his men who were dying of scurvy. He boiled the needles of the arbor vitae tree to make a tea that was later shown to contain 50 mg of vitamin C per 100 grams [48]. It is known that plants are generally a good source of vitamin C, the amount in foods of plant origin depends on: the precise variety of the plant, the soil condition, the climate in which it grew, the length of time since it was picked, the storage conditions, and the method of preparation. The exact same conditions hold true for the amount of nitrite and nitrate in plants. One can not help but notice the emerging physiological data on nitrite are strikingly analogous to a vitamin. "Vitamine" or vital amine was the term coined by Casimir Funk (1884–1967) for the unidentified substances present in food which could prevent the diseases scurvy, beriberi, and pellagra. A vitamin is by definition any of a group of organic substance essential in small quantities to normal metabolism, found in minute amounts in natural foods or sometimes produced synthetically: deficiencies of vitamins produce specific disorders. We know that nitrite is produced in relatively small quantities in normal metabolism of L-arginine and reduction of nitrate and is found in minute amounts in natural foods. This is becoming remarkably similar to the ascorbic acid story years ago. It became apparent that vitamin C deficiency caused scurvy. This was prevented by eating certain foods known to contain ascorbic acid. Certain foods contain ascorbic acid such as citrus fruits whereas other foods do not. Therefore benefit is only gained from eating those foods rich in ascorbic acid. Throughout history, the benefit of plant food to survive long sea voyages has been occasionally recommended by authorities. While the earliest documented case of scurvy was described by Hippocrates around the year 400 BC, the first attempt to give scientific basis for the cause of this disease was by a ship's surgeon in the British Royal Navy, James Lind. Scurvy was common among those with poor access to fresh fruit and vegetables, such as remote, isolated sailors and soldiers. John Woodall, the first appointed surgeon to the British East India Company, recommended the preventive and curative use of lemon juice in his book "The Surgeon's Mate", in 1617. The Dutch writer, Johann Bachstrom, in 1734, gave the firm opinion that *"scurvy is solely owing to a total abstinence from fresh vegetable food, and greens; which is alone the primary cause of the disease."* Could it be then that if one does not eat sufficient foods rich in nitrite and nitrate specific disorders such as cardiovascular disease occur? Chapter 4 was devoted to identifying food sources rich in nitrite and nitrate. Not surprisingly there are some foods enriched with both nitrite and nitrate and others that contain undetectable levels. Therefore depending on which foods you eat will determine if you are getting sufficient nutrient in the form of nitrite and nitrate. Our animal studies reveal that nitrite insufficiency exacerbates I/R injury and increases mortality from I/R [23]. There are a host of diseases which are associated with decreased NO availability as measured by nitrite. Becoming more evident is the enormous benefit of exogenous dietary nitrite and nitrate in a number of disease models in animals and even in humans. A simple ubiquitous molecule we have been advised to avoid may be an indispensable nutrient that many are lacking.

In fact this type of thinking and rationale is not new. Orthomolecular medicine is a form of complementary and alternative medicine which aims to prevent and treat disease with substances which are natural to the body. Prescriptions typically focus on providing nutrients, either through dietary supplements or modified diets which provide proper nutrition and eliminate deleterious substances such as allergens, refined foods, sugar and transfats. The term "orthomolecular" was first coined in a 1967 letter by Nobel Prize winner Linus Pauling and later elaborated on in a 1968 paper [49] on micronutrients and psychiatry to express the idea of "the right molecules in the right amounts" (ortho is Greek for right). In this paper, Pauling indicated that the right molecules are "substances that are normally present in the human body." Proponents state that orthomolecular treatments are based on patients' personal biomolecules, particularly nutrients such as vitamins. That same premise can be applied to the NO biochemistry of patients. Preclinical and clinical studies now reveal that nitrite can replete NO metabolites and correct conditions associated with NO insufficiency.

According to the World Health Organization, cardiovascular disease (CVD) is the number one killer of both men and women in the United States. These deaths represent a staggering 40% of all deaths. Close to 1 million people die each year and more than 6 million are hospitalized. The cost of CVD, in terms of health care and lost productivity, is over $270 billion and increasing as the baby boom population ages. Ischemic heart disease, as the underlying cause of most cases of acute myocardial infarction, congestive heart failure, arrhythmias, and sudden cardiac death, is the leading cause of morbidity and mortality in all industrialized nations. In the United States, ischemic heart disease causes nearly 20% of all deaths (≈600 000 deaths each year), with many of these deaths occurring before the patient arrives at the hospital. Heart disease is very likely the result of a dysfunctional endothelium. One of the most important substances released by our body is nitric oxide (NO). The discovery that the human body makes nitric oxide from L-arginine revolutionized science and medicine. Continuous generation of NO is essential for the integrity of the cardiovascular system and a decreased production and/or bioavailability of NO is central to the development of cardiovascular disorders. It is also important for communication in our nervous system and a critical molecule which our immune system using to kill invading pathogens, including bacteria and cancer cell. Reduced nitric oxide (NO) availability is a hallmark of a number of disorders, including cardiovascular disease. Understanding strategies to enhance and restore NO homeostasis is critical to developing treatments to cardiovascular disease and more importantly strategies to prevent disease from developing. Nothing affects our health more than what we choose to eat. It has long been recognized that a poor diet contributes to disease or at least makes us more susceptible. To the contrary a healthy diet rich in fruits and vegetables and low in fats and calories protects us from many diseases. The exact mechanism of the beneficial effects of certain foods in largely unknown although the general dogma is that it is due to their high antioxidant capacity. The notion that there may be certain foods that can enrich nitric oxide within our body is revolutionary.

Several chapters have reviewed the latest reports of the potential benefits of nitrites and nitrates in physiology. Although these agents have been used for hundreds of years as meat and food preservatives to minimize bacterial contamination, it has been feared that these substances could be carcinogenic. This misbelief has hopefully been corrected with current and ongoing studies. These are naturally occurring molecules in our diet as well as our body, and can function as reservoirs or prodrugs to be converted to nitric oxide. Nitric oxide is probably one of the most important signaling molecules in our body to regulate numerous physiological functions including blood flow to tissues and organs. The conversion of nitrite and nitrate to nitric oxide in our tissues is obviously an important finding. Interestingly formulations of topical nitrite preparations are effective in wound and burn healing. Clinical trials for such uses as well as diabetic skin ulcers are also underway. It appears that dietary manipulations of nitrites and their topical uses will be effective and inexpensive therapies to restore nitric oxide.

The early Roman physician Galen based his description of the vascular system on the concept of "pneuma" or spirits, a vital principle consisting of matter in a finely divided or ethereal state that flowed through the vascular and nervous systems and animate the entire organism. Many diseases were thought to owe their origin to some disturbances of these ethereal spirits. Although these ideas were fanciful, this paradigm actually prevented the advancement of medical science for centuries. Today evidence on the production and effects of such an ethereal substance, NO, exists. Nitric oxide is indeed formed in many organs and as previously mentioned has important roles in physiology and pathophysiology.

An optimal diet may then consist of a sufficient supply of nitrite and nitrate for health and well being. Regular intake of nitrite-containing and rich anti-oxidant food such as green leafy vegetables may ensure that blood and tissue levels of nitrite and NO pools are maintained at a level sufficient to compensate for any disturbances in endogenous NO synthesis. Since low levels of supplemental nitrite have been shown to enhance blood flow, dietary sources of NO metabolites could therefore improve circulation and oxygen delivery. This dietary pathway may not only provide essential nutrients for NO production but also provide a rescue or protective pathway for people at risk for cardiovascular disease.

I have invited the world's experts (from both academia and industry) in their particular discipline to contribute individual chapters. I hope this approach has provided a fair and balance view of nitric oxide biochemistry, nitrite and nitrate chemistry in physiology and in the food sciences. Therapeutics is the branch of medicine concerned with the remedial treatment of disease. It is prudent at this juncture to take a step back and look at nitrite and nitrate as a means of prevention of a number of diseases associated with NO insufficiency. Early intervention to restore NO/nitroso homeostasis through natural dietary means may prove to be a cost effective and natural means to prevent disease. There is, by design, enormous redundancy in physiology where there are multiple pathways and regulatory processes for critical biological functions. This redundancy ensures that if one pathway is absent or dysfunctional, then there is a backup plan to produce and regulate critical signaling molecules and pathways. It is becoming increasingly clear that a deficiency in nitric oxide is a hallmark of a number of disease conditions. It is highly unlikely that Nature devised a singular pathway which requires a complex five-electron oxidation of a semi-essential amino acid requiring multiple co-factors and prosthetic groups. Maintenance of NO homeostasis by nitrite may be that redundant backup system in NO biology. A simple one-electron reduction of nitrite to form NO or bimolecular reaction with thiols to form nitrosothiols is a viable and effective system for recapitulating NO biochemistry. Since at least half of our body's pool of nitrite is derived from what we eat, we can, at will, affect NO biochemistry through dietary means. Discovery and recognition of this pathway is likely to affect public health and strategies to prevent and/or treat disease. We are currently faced with an enormous public health crisis as our aging baby boomers succumb to disease, particularly cardiovascular disease. Treatment and care of our greatest generation is a tremendous economic burden. Developing strategies to prevent disease or reduce injury from a cardiovascular accident will improve patient outcome and enhance their quality of life. Recognizing a natural and inexpensive regimen of foods rich in nitrite and nitrate to restore NO homeostasis can have profound effects on public health. It is my hope that this book will stimulate dialogue between health care professionals, clinical nutritionists, dieticians, food scientists and epidemiologists as a means to better understand and appreciate contemporary views of nitrite and nitrate in the context of indispensable nutrients. As with anything remedy or treatment a risk benefit assessment should be considered. I predict the benefits will strongly outweigh any potential risks, particularly for patients with conditions of NO insufficiency.

ABOUT THE AUTHOR

Nathan S. Bryan, Ph.D.

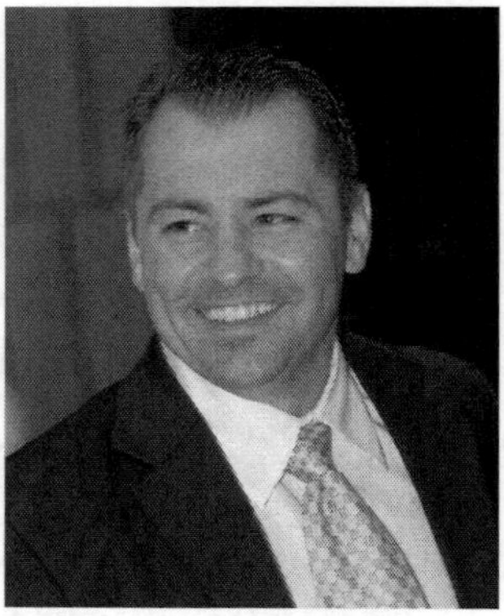

Dr. Bryan was born in Bryan Texas in November 1973. Nathan grew up in small town Texas. He spent his grade school years in Lexington (population 1000) and attended High School in Caldwell (population 3000). He earned his undergraduate Bachelor of Science degree in Biochemistry from the University of Texas at Austin and his doctoral degree from Louisiana State University School of Medicine in Shreveport where he was the recipient of the Dean's Award for Excellence in Research. He pursued his post-doctoral training as a Kirschstein Fellow at Boston University School of Medicine in the Whitaker Cardiovascular Institute. Dr. Bryan joined the Institute of Molecular Medicine, University of Texas Health Science Center in Houston, in June 2006 in the Center for Cell Signaling. He is also a faculty member of the Department of Integrative Biology and Pharmacology and Graduate School of Biomedical Sciences at the UT Houston Medical School. He is an active member of the Nitric Oxide Society, Society for Free Radical Biology and Medicine and the American Heart Association.

Dr. Bryan's research is dedicated to providing a better understanding of the interactions of nitric oxide (NO) and related metabolites with their different biological targets at the molecular and cellular level and the significance of these reactions for physiology and pathophysiology. Attempts are made to identify what particular changes in NO-related signaling pathways and reaction products occur in disease states such as endothelial dysfunction, ischemia/reperfusion, tissue/cardiac protection, diabetes, atherosclerosis and inflammation with the aim of testing their amenability as biomarkers for diagnosis and/or treatment of specific disease.

Current research is directed to understand the interactions of exogenous dietary nitrite/nitrate (NOx) on the endogenous NO/cGMP pathway and how perturbations in each system affect cardiovascular health. This involves mechanisms of nitrite transport and cellular uptake as well as mechanism of nitrite reduction back to NO and via direct NO-independent signaling actions of nitrite. Work in Dr. Bryan's lab involves molecular biology and analytical biochemistry utilizing gas phase chemiluminescence and HPLC in multiple organ systems and blood. Much of the work involves *in vivo* characterization of NO/nitrite metabolism using a number of transgenic and knockout animal models of disease. Dr. Bryan and colleagues recently discovered that nitrite is a biologically active molecule which was previously thought to be an inert breakdown product of NO production. These findings have unveiled many beneficial effects of nitrite in the treatment and prevention of human disease. These discoveries may provide the basis for new preventive or therapeutic strategies in diseases associated with NO insufficiency and new guidelines for optimal health. Since nitrite and nitrate are common constituents of many fruits and vegetables, changes in dietary habits may have profound effects on many diseases associated with NO insufficiency. NO insufficiency is a hallmark of a number of diseases including cardiovascular disease. The notion that nitrite can recapitulate NO biochemistry and serve as an alternative and compensatory mechanism of NO production is revolutionary. It may also serve as the endocrine mediator of NO signaling. Moreover, the direct signaling actions of nitrite may represent a novel NO independent pathway for nitrite. If our current understanding is true, then an optimal diet may then consist of a sufficient supply of nitrite and nitrate for health and disease prevention. Understanding this pathway will provide the basis for new preventive or therapeutic strategies in diseases associated with NO insufficiency and new guidelines for optimal health. To date Dr. Bryan has published over 20 peer reviewed papers that have been cited over 1000 times. He has been invited to speak at a number of national and international meetings.

Dr. Bryan currently resides in Houston with his wife Kristen and their two sons Grant and Lincoln. The Bryans spend their weekends at their ranch near Caldwell where they raise cattle and horses and enjoy the great outdoors. Nathan enjoys playing golf and calf roping and team roping on his ranch and in competition.

REFERENCES

1. Voetsch, B.; Jin, R. C.; Loscalzo, J. Nitric oxide insufficiency and atherothrombosis. *Histochemistry and cell biology* 122:353–367; 2004.
2. Bryan, N. S.; Fernandez, B. O.; Bauer, S. M.; Garcia-Saura, M. F.; Milsom, A. B.; Rassaf, T.; Maloney, R. E.; Bharti, A.; Rodriguez, J.; Feelisch, M. Nitrite is a signaling molecule and regulator of gene expression in mammalian tissues. *Nature chemical biology* 1:290–297; 2005.
3. Lundberg, J. O.; Weitzberg, E.; Cole, J. A.; Benjamin, N. Nitrate, bacteria and human health. *Nat Rev Microbiol* 2:593–602; 2004.
4. Palmer, R. M. J.; Ferrige, A. G.; Moncada, S. Nitric oxide release accounts for the biological activity of endothelium-derived relaxing factor. *Nature* 327:524–526; 1987.
5. Ignarro, L. J.; Buga, G. M.; Wood, K. S.; Byrns, R. E.; Chaudhuri, G. Endothelium-derived relaxing factor produced and released from artery and vein is nitric oxide. *Proc. Natl. Acad Sci. USA* 84:9265–9269; 1987.
6. Gladwin, M. T.; Schechter, A. N.; Kim-Shapiro, D. B.; Patel, R. P.; Hogg, N.; Shiva, S.; Cannon III, R. O.; Kelm, M.; Wink, D. A.; Espey, M. G.; Oldfield, E. H.; Pluta, R. M.; Freeman, B. A.; Lancaster, J. R. J.; Feelisch, M.; Lundberg, J. O. The emerging biology of the nitrite anion. *Nature Chemical Biology* 1:308–314; 2005.
7. Angelo, M.; Singel, D. J.; Stamler, J. S. An S-nitrosothiol (SNO) synthase function of hemoglobin that utilizes nitrite as a substrate. *Proceedings of the National Academy of Sciences of the United States of America* 103:8366–8371; 2006.
8. Cosby, K.; Partovi, K. S.; Crawford, J. H.; Patel, R. K.; Reiter, C. D.; Martyr, S.; Yang, B. K.; Waclawiw, M. A.; Zalos, G.; Xu, X.; Huang, K. T.; Shields, H.; Kim-Shapiro, D. B.; Schechter, A. N.; Cannon III, R. O.; Gladwin, M. T. Nitrite reduction to nitric oxide by deoxyhemoglobin vasodilates the human circulation. *Nature Medicine* 9:1498–1505; 2003.
9. Lu, P.; Liu, F.; Yao, Z.; Wang, C. Y.; Chen, D. D.; Tian, Y.; Zhang, J. H.; Wu, Y. H. Nitrite-derived nitric oxide by xanthine oxidoreductase protects the liver against ischemia-reperfusion injury. *Hepatobiliary Pancreat Dis Int* 4:350–355; 2005.
10. Duranski, M. R.; Greer, J. J.; Dejam, A.; Jaganmohan, S.; Hogg, N.; Langston, W.; Patel, R. P.; Yet, S. F.; Wang, X.; Kevil, C. G.; Gladwin, M. T.; Lefer, D. J. Cytoprotective effects of nitrite during in vivo ischemia-reperfusion of the heart and liver. *The Journal of clinical investigation* 115:1232–1240; 2005.
11. Webb, A.; Bond, R.; McLean, P.; Uppal, R.; Benjamin, N.; Ahluwalia, A. Reduction of nitrite to nitric oxide during ischemia protects against myocardial ischemia-reperfusion damage. *Proc Natl Acad Sci USA* 101; 2004.
12. Pluta, R. M.; Dejam, A.; Grimes, G.; Gladwin, M. T.; Oldfield, E. H. Nitrite infusions to prevent delayed cerebral vasospasm in a primate model of subarachnoid hemorrhage. *Jama* 293:1477–1484; 2005.
13. Jung, K. H.; Chu, K.; Ko, S. Y.; Lee, S. T.; Sinn, D. I.; Park, D. K.; Kim, J. M.; Song, E. C.; Kim, M.; Roh, J. K. Early intravenous infusion of sodium nitrite protects brain against in vivo ischemia-reperfusion injury. *Stroke*; a journal of cerebral circulation 37:2744–2750; 2006.

14. Tripatara, P.; Patel, N. S.; Webb, A.; Rathod, K.; Lecomte, F. M.; Mazzon, E.; Cuzzocrea, S.; Yaqoob, M. M.; Ahluwalia, A.; Thiemermann, C. Nitrite-derived nitric oxide protects the rat kidney against ischemia/reperfusion injury in vivo: role for xanthine oxidoreductase. *J Am Soc Nephrol* 18:570–580; 2007.
15. Shiva, S.; Sack, M. N.; Greer, J. J.; Duranski, M. R.; Ringwood, L. A.; Burwell, L.; Wang, X.; MacArthur, P. H.; Shoja, A.; Raghavachari, N.; Calvert, J. W.; Brookes, P. S.; Lefer, D. J.; Gladwin, M. T. Nitrite augments tolerance to ischemia/reperfusion injury via the modulation of mitochondrial electron transfer. *Journal of Experimental Medicine* 204:2089–2102; 2007.
16. Kumar, D.; Branch, B. G.; Pattillo, C. B.; Hood, J.; Thoma, S.; Simpson, S.; Illum, S.; Arora, N.; Chidlow, J. H., Jr.; Langston, W.; Teng, X.; Lefer, D. J.; Patel, R. P.; Kevil, C. G. Chronic sodium nitrite therapy augments ischemia-induced angiogenesis and arteriogenesis. *Proceedings of the National Academy of Sciences of the United States of America* 105:7540–7545; 2008.
17. Mack, A. K.; McGowan Ii, V. R.; Tremonti, C. K.; Ackah, D.; Barnett, C.; Machado, R. F.; Gladwin, M. T.; Kato, G. J. Sodium nitrite promotes regional blood flow in patients with sickle cell disease: a phase I/II study. *British journal of haematology* 142:971–978; 2008.
18. Lauer, T.; Heiss, C.; Balzer, J.; Kehmeier, E.; Mangold, S.; Leyendecker, T.; Rottler, J.; Meyer, C.; Merx, M. W.; Kelm, M.; Rassaf, T. Age-dependent endothelial dysfunction is associated with failure to increase plasma nitrite in response to exercise. *Basic research in cardiology* 103:291–297; 2008.
19. Rassaf, T.; Lauer, T.; Heiss, C.; Balzer, J.; Mangold, S.; Leyendecker, T.; Rottler, J.; Drexhage, C.; Meyer, C.; Kelm, M. Nitric oxide synthase-derived plasma nitrite predicts exercise capacity. *British journal of sports medicine* 41:669–673; discussion 673; 2007.
20. Taddei, S.; Galetta, F.; Virdis, A.; Ghiadoni, L.; Salvetti, G.; Franzoni, F.; Giusti, C.; Salvetti, A. Physical activity prevents age-related impairment in nitric oxide availability in elderly athletes. *Circulation* 101:2896–2901; 2000.
21. Bryan, N. S.; Calvert, J. W.; Gundewar, S.; Lefer, D. J. Dietary nitrite restores NO homeostasis and is cardioprotective in endothelial nitric oxide synthase-deficient mice. *Free Radic Biol Med* 45:468–474; 2008.
22. Tsuchiya, K.; Kanematsu, Y.; Yoshizumi, M.; Ohnishi, H.; Kirima, K.; Izawa, Y.; Shikishima, M.; Ishida, T.; Kondo, S.; Kagami, S.; Takiguchi, Y.; Tamaki, T. Nitrite is an alternative source of NO in vivo. *American journal of physiology* 288:H2163–2170; 2005.
23. Bryan, N. S.; Calvert, J. W.; Elrod, J. W.; Gundewar, S.; Ji, S. Y.; Lefer, D. J. Dietary nitrite supplementation protects against myocardial ischemia-reperfusion injury. *Proceedings of the National Academy of Sciences of the United States of America* 104:19144–19149; 2007.
24. Reddy, D.; Lancaster, J. R., Jr.; Cornforth, D. P. Nitrite inhibition of Clostridium botulinum: electron spin resonance detection of iron-nitric oxide complexes. *Science* 221:769–770; 1983.
25. Dykhuizen, R. S.; Frazer, R.; Duncan, C.; Smith, C. C.; Golden, M.; Benjamin, N.; Leifert, C. Antimicrobial effect of acidified nitrite on gut pathogens: importance of dietary nitrate in host defense. *Antimicrobial agents and chemotherapy* 40:1422–1425; 1996.
26. Dykhuizen, R. S.; Fraser, A.; McKenzie, H.; Golden, M.; Leifert, C.; Benjamin, N. Helicobacter pylori is killed by nitrite under acidic conditions. *Gut* 42:334–337; 1998.
27. Benjamin, N.; O'Driscoll, F.; Dougall, H.; Duncan, C.; Smith, L.; Golden, M.; McKenzie, H. Stomach NO synthesis. *Nature* 368:502; 1994.
28. Carlsson, S.; Wiklund, N. P.; Engstrand, L.; Weitzberg, E.; Lundberg, J. O. Effects of pH, nitrite, and ascorbic acid on nonenzymatic nitric oxide generation and bacterial growth in urine. *Nitric Oxide* 5:580–586; 2001.

29. Yoon, S. S.; Coakley, R.; Lau, G. W.; Lymar, S. V.; Gaston, B.; Karabulut, A. C.; Hennigan, R. F.; Hwang, S. H.; Buettner, G.; Schurr, M. J.; Mortensen, J. E.; Burns, J. L.; Speert, D.; Boucher, R. C.; Hassett, D. J. Anaerobic killing of mucoid Pseudomonas aeruginosa by acidified nitrite derivatives under cystic fibrosis airway conditions. *The Journal of clinical investigation* 116:436–446; 2006.

30. Carlsson, S.; Govoni, M.; Wiklund, N. P.; Weitzberg, E.; Lundberg, J. O. *In vitro* evaluation of a new treatment for urinary tract infections caused by nitrate-reducing bacteria. *Antimicrobial agents and chemotherapy* 47:3713–3718; 2003.

31. Lundberg, J. O.; Weitzberg, E.; Lundberg, J. M.; Alving, K. Intragastric nitric oxide production in humans: measurements in expelled air. *Gut* 35:1543–1546; 1994.

32. Spiegelhalder, B.; Eisenbrand, G.; Preussmann, R. Influence of dietary nitrate on nitrite content of human saliva: possible relevance to in vivo formation of N-nitroso compounds. *Food Cosmet Toxicol* 14:545–548; 1976.

33. Bjorne, H. H.; Petersson, J.; Phillipson, M.; Weitzberg, E.; Holm, L.; Lundberg, J. O. Nitrite in saliva increases gastric mucosal blood flow and mucus thickness. *The Journal of clinical investigation* 113:106–114; 2004.

34. Larsen, F. J.; Ekblom, B.; Sahlin, K.; Lundberg, J. O.; Weitzberg, E. Effects of dietary nitrate on blood pressure in healthy volunteers. *The New England journal of medicine* 355:2792–2793; 2006.

35. Webb, A. J.; Patel, N.; Loukogeorgakis, S.; Okorie, M.; Aboud, Z.; Misra, S.; Rashid, R.; Miall, P.; Deanfield, J.; Benjamin, N.; MacAllister, R.; Hobbs, A. J.; Ahluwalia, A. Acute blood pressure lowering, vasoprotective, and antiplatelet properties of dietary nitrate via bioconversion to nitrite. *Hypertension* 51:784–790; 2008.

36. Larsen, F. J.; Weitzberg, E.; Lundberg, J. O.; Ekblom, B. Effects of dietary nitrate on oxygen cost during exercise. *Acta physiologica* (Oxford, England) 191:59–66; 2007.

37. Jansson, E. A.; Petersson, J.; Reinders, C.; Sobko, T.; Bjorne, H.; Phillipson, M.; Weitzberg, E.; Holm, L.; Lundberg, J. O. Protection from nonsteroidal anti-inflammatory drug (NSAID)-induced gastric ulcers by dietary nitrate. *Free Radic Biol Med* 42:510–518; 2007.

38. Petersson, J.; Phillipson, M.; Jansson, E. A.; Patzak, A.; Lundberg, J. O.; Holm, L. Dietary nitrate increases gastric mucosal blood flow and mucosal defense. *Am J Physiol Gastrointest Liver Physiol* 292:G718–724; 2007.

39. Lundberg, J. O.; Govoni, M. Inorganic nitrate is a possible source for systemic generation of nitric oxide. *Free Radic Biol Med* 37:395–400; 2004.

40. Govoni, M.; Jansson, E. A.; Weitzberg, E.; Lundberg, J. O. The increase in plasma nitrite after a dietary nitrate load is markedly attenuated by an antibacterial mouthwash. *Nitric Oxide* 19:333–337; 2008.

41. Iizuka, T.; Sasaki, M.; Oishi, K.; Uemura, S.; Koike, M.; Shinozaki, M. Non-enzymatic nitric oxide generation in the stomachs of breastfed neonates. *Acta Paediatr* 88:1053–1055; 1999.

42. Fujita, K.; Murono, K. Nosocomial acquisition of Escherichia coli by infants delivered in hospitals. *The Journal of hospital infection* 32:277–281; 1996.

43. Mandar, R.; Mikelsaar, M. Transmission of mother's microflora to the newborn at birth. *Biology of the neonate* 69:30–35; 1996.

44. Orrhage, K.; Nord, C. E. Factors controlling the bacterial colonization of the intestine in breastfed infants. *Acta Paediatr Suppl* 88:47–57; 1999.

45. Authority, E. F. S. Nitrate in vegetables: scientific opinion of the panel on contaminants in the food chain. *The EFSA Journal* 689:1–79; 2008.

46. Gillis, C. N. Panax ginseng pharmacology: a nitric oxide link? *Biochemical pharmacology* 54:1–8; 1997.
47. Chen, X. Cardiovascular protection by ginsenosides and their nitric oxide releasing action. *Clinical and experimental pharmacology & physiology* 23:728–732; 1996.
48. Martini, E. Jacques Cartier witnesses a treatment for scurvy. *Vesalius* 8:2–6; 2002.
49. Pauling, L. Orthomolecular psychiatry. Varying the concentrations of substances normally present in the human body may control mental disease. *Science* 160:265–271; 1968.

Index